Preventing Bullying
AND School Violence

Preventing Bullying
AND School Violence

BY

Stuart W. Twemlow, M.D.

Frank C. Sacco, Ph.D.

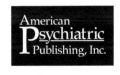

American Psychiatric Publishing, Inc.

Washington, DC
London, England

Copyright © 2012 American Psychiatric Association
ALL RIGHTS RESERVED

Manufactured in the United States of America on acid-free paper
15   14   13   12   11   5   4   3   2   1
First Edition

Typeset in Adobe's Minion and Bell Gothic

American Psychiatric Publishing, Inc.
1000 Wilson Boulevard
Arlington, VA 22209-3901
www.appi.org

Library of Congress Cataloging-in-Publication Data
Twemlow, Stuart W.
    Preventing bullying and school violence / by Stuart W. Twemlow, Frank C. Sacco
— 1st ed.
        p. ; cm.
    Includes bibliographical references and index.
    ISBN 978-1-58562-384-6 (pbk. : alk. paper) 1. Bullying—Psychology. 2. Bullying—Prevention. 3. School children—Conduct of life. 4. School violence. I. Sacco, Frank C., 1949–   II. Title.
    [DNLM: 1. Bullying—psychology. 2. Adolescent. 3. Child. 4. Community–Institutional Relations. 5. Schools. 6. Violence—prevention & control.   WS 350.8.A4]
    BF637.B85T94 2012
    371.5′8—dc22

                                                                                                2011004932

British Library Cataloguing in Publication Data
A CIP record is available from the British Library.

To Karl A. Menninger, M.D., whose inspiration is the seed of all of our work, and to all of the children he loved, sick and well, in whose hands the future of the planet earth rests.

Contents

About the Authors

Stuart W. Twemlow, M.D., is Professor of Psychiatry in the Menninger Department of Psychiatry and Behavioral Sciences, Baylor College of Medicine, and Senior Psychiatrist, The Menninger Clinic, Houston, Texas; Faculty Member, Houston-Galveston Psychoanalytic Institute, Houston, Texas; and Honorary Professor of Psychoanalytic Studies, Deakin University, Melbourne, Australia.

Frank C. Sacco, Ph.D., is President of Community Services Institute in Boston and Springfield, Massachusetts; and Adjunct Professor at Western New England College in Springfield, Massachusetts.

Foreword

Peter Fonagy, Ph.D., F.B.A.

MENTAL health interventions for children increasingly are being integrated into their daily lives (Durlak et al. 2011; Kavanagh et al. 2009). The model of mental health care delivery based uniquely around the consulting room has come to be outmoded. As clinicians have come to recognize that the child's environment impacts so powerfully on the uptake, and ultimately the value, of clinical consultation, it makes sense for interventions to take place closer to where these environmental influences are most intensely felt—in the child's family and also his or her school. Children are simply more affected by what happens around them than are adults, which is not surprising, given the biological task of childhood preparation for a lifetime of adaptation. The two quintessentially formative environmental influences, home and school, have increasingly become the preferred contexts for effective intervention. Multisystemic therapy, for example, has been able to address behavioral challenges that eluded clinic-based interventions by moving into the family home.

As an essential communitywide resource for children and young people, schools have enormous potential to optimize the extent to which mental health interventions are socially inclusive and do not perpetuate inequalities in health care accessibility, which we know to be toxic for the well-being of society as a whole (Marmot 2010). School-based interventions for emotional disorders have successfully reached groups of children who might normally elude clinical attention. Young people are as much as 10 times more likely to access a school-based mental health service than a non-school-based one (Catron et al. 1998; Kaplan et al. 1998). In one study, almost 75% of students indicated that their preference would be to see a mental health worker in a school context rather than outside of school (Quinn and Chan 2009). The reason for this may be obvious: first, there is ease of access; second, there is familiarity; and finally, there is an economic argument, perhaps more important for policy makers, that a school location may make mental health services less expensive (American Academy of Pediatrics 2004).

In recent years, we have witnessed dramatic developments in the creation and delivery of a wide range of school-based mental health interventions (Durlak et al. 2011). Many of these have been oriented toward schoolwide, universal-level programs, which have been shown to generate a very wide range of social, emotional, cognitive, and academic improvements. It seems that these universal interventions are less valuable in preventing or treating serious forms of psychological distress—as shown, for example, by the limited effectiveness of depression prevention programs at the schoolwide level (Stice et al. 2009). There is good evidence, however, that programs targeted toward individuals at high risk of or showing symptoms of mental distress can be effectively treated in the school context (Baskin et al. 2010). The key requirement appears to be the presence of a conceptual framework that guides the work of the mental health professional.

There is an evident gap in the literature for models for mental health professionals to adopt when working within schools. Understandably, mental health professionals have a bias and follow the path of least resistance. We use the clinical models finally honed in the clinic or the consulting room in another room, albeit one perhaps more sparsely furnished, but one which, in our minds, serves as a replacement consulting room and provides a "secure base." We tend to import our training, practice, techniques, and habits from our natural habitat—be that a hospital, a community mental health center, or a private consulting room—to the school environment, and with these also our thinking. But do the clinical models derived from the consulting room work in the context of these alternative environments? Do we have the model to address generic childhood problems in these alternative contexts?

Systemic therapies have arguably evolved highly efficacious strategies alongside a comprehensive theoretical framework for addressing childhood mental disorder in the context of a child's family life. These technical modifications came with a new psychology of families that has been a source of inspiration to clinicians throughout the world (e.g., Minuchin 1974; Selvini Palazzoli et al. 1978, 1980). Do we have a similar psychology of schools that enables us to look at behavioral problems generated in, and to some degree by, the school environment in the educational context? We do now.

This book is about empowering mental health professionals to work confidently in educational settings, to advise in relation to educational structure, knowing how and where systemwide intervention might generate an amelioration of behavioral problems. It also offers what is effectively a psychology of schools, an opportunity to step into the virtual mind of social systems that we normally entrust with the education of our young ones. Constructing a psychology of schools is an ambitious agenda. The authors identify a specific target and go a considerable way toward achieving their declared goal of providing a model for tackling violent behavior in the school context. They have taken a necessarily broad and dynamic approach to the problem. They see schools as representative of the communities in which they exist, but also as organizations that make a major contribution to the character of the communities housing them.

Bullying and violence in schools is a problem not just of the individual, but also of the social context in which the person must exist in collaboration and in dependent relationships with others. School bullying is a characteristic of the social system, not of the bully and the victim. It is the social tensions from which violence emerges and that violence can then create in a school which this book aims to provide a successful model addressing. At the heart of the book is the notion of relationships and their significance in generating social problems. We all know the individual factors that increase the risk of violent behavior; poverty, low maternal education, and single parenting are sociodemographic risk factors that are mostly strongly correlated with parental behavioral factors, such as less sensitive and involved parenting, withdrawal, inconsistency, and absence of positive interactions. This book does not engage with these risk factors, but rather with those that enable individuals with such backgrounds to become a problem. The book, perhaps for the first time, gives a robust and informative guiding framework for mental health professionals to work as agents of effective change in schools and colleges. The learning in these contexts can be extended to other environments. We are indebted to these authors for offering a creative, original, yet highly practical vision for working effectively in schools. They also help to provide a conceptual bridge, which most of us have been missing, to take full advantage of the opportunities that school environments offer for reducing the distress and enhancing the psychological well-being of the children under our stewardship.

References

American Academy of Pediatrics: Policy statement: school-based mental health services. Pediatrics 113:1839–1845, 2004

Baskin TW, Slaten CD, Crosby NR, et al: Efficacy of counseling and psychotherapy in schools: a meta-analytic review of treatment outcome studies. The Counseling Psychologist 38:878–903, 2010

Catron T, Harris VS, Weiss B: Posttreatment results after 2 years of services in the Vanderbilt School-Based Counseling Project, in Outcomes for Children and Youths With Emotional and Behavioral Disorders and Their Families: Programs for Evaluating Best Practice. Edited by Epstein MH, Kutash K, Duchnowski A. Austin, TX, Pro-Ed, 1998, pp 633–656

Durlak JA, Weissberg RP, Dymnicki AB, et al: The impact of enhancing students' social and emotional learning: a meta-analysis of school-based universal interventions. Child Dev 82:405–432, 2011

Kaplan DW, Calonge BN, Guernsey BP, et al: Managed care and school-based health centers: use of health services. Arch Pediatr Adolesc Med 152:25–33, 1998

Kavanagh J, Oliver S, Caird J, et al: Inequalities and the Mental Health of Young People: A Systematic Review of Secondary School-Based Cognitive Behavioural Interventions. London, EPPI-Centre, Social Science Research Unit, Institute of Education, University of London, 2009

Marmot M: Fair Society, Healthy Lives—The Marmot Review: Strategic Review of Health Inequalities in England Post 2010. London, Marmot Review, 2010

Minuchin S: Families and Family Therapy. Cambridge, MA, Harvard University Press, 1974

Quinn P, Chan S: Scottish secondary school students' preferences for location, format of counselling and gender of counsellor: a replication study based in Northern Ireland. Counselling and Psychotherapy Research 9:204–209, 2009

Selvini Palazzoli M, Boscolo L, Cecchin G, et al: Paradox and Counter-Paradox. New York, Jason Aronson, 1978

Selvini Palazzoli M, Boscolo L, Cecchin G, et al: Hypothesizing-circularity-neutrality: three guidelines for the conductor of the session. Fam Process 19:3–12, 1980

Stice E, Shaw H, Bohon C, et al: A meta-analytic review of depression prevention programs for children and adolescents: factors that predict magnitude of intervention effects. J Consult Clin Psychol 77:486–503, 2009

Preface and Introduction

STUART W. TWEMLOW, M.D.
FRANK C. SACCO, PH.D.

ALL mental health professionals have unique skill sets: for psychologists, it is psychological testing; for psychiatrists, knowledge of the body and physical methods of treatment; for social workers, marshaling of community resources; for nurses and physician assistants, practicing independently and extending physicians' skills; and the list goes on. The shared connections between these mental health professionals need to be developed and understood—rather than assumed—in order to render the most effective health care possible and reduce the burgeoning problem of school violence.

There are currently few guidelines and precious little data to support how to accomplish our goals across a variety of types of schools. Amid today's social chaos, inadequate attention is paid to the crucial role of mental health professionals in shaping and managing community involvement when problem solving in schools. Mental health professionals can be vital in preventing illness by promoting various wellness programs in schools (as we describe in Chapter 11, "Effortless Wellness and Other Afterthoughts"). Furthermore, our experiences in schools throughout the United States, from the poorest schools to the wealthiest ones, have taught us that most schools have highly competent teachers who have taken it upon themselves to acquire the necessary psychological education, develop their own nonpunitive disciplinary techniques, and become knowledgeable about things that they know are necessary, beside the teaching of academics. Dedicated teachers are like all dedicated professionals in this regard: they are working for the good of the cause, not for a hefty paycheck.

What use will this book be to the busy mental health professional? It is full of hands-on practical knowledge, with clear "how to" approaches. It encourages the clinician to brainstorm and invent new strategies and approaches when traditional ones do not work, and the references are practical.

Chapter 1 describes the myriad factors that make school violence such a complex problem and discusses the tendency of clinicians to oversimplify the problem. We focus especially on how the roles of various individuals are often defined in the social system, creating a parallel between these roles and those played by the actors in a play, so to speak.

Chapter 2 hones in on one of the most important factors in creating a healthy academic environment: the connection between the family, the school, and the community. It is true that these entities operate separately; however, in our opinion, school violence can be effectively addressed only if the connection between the family, the school, and the community is so intimate that one *cannot* operate without the other. The mental health professional reading this book needs to see this connection and be involved with every element of it, beginning with knowledge and leadership and moving forward.

Chapters 3 and 4 directly address ways in which mental health professionals can work with service agencies that intervene in cases involving violent children. Although psychoanalytically trained professionals have a long history of development of group skills, especially small groups such as those led by Wilfred Bion, Fritz Redl, and Fred Pine, the management of large groups (more than 10 or 12 people) is very different, as Vamik Volkan has noted. We also include explanations of the mental health profiles and attitudes mental health professionals are likely to encounter when working within complex social bureaucracies, such as large schools. Chapter 4 presents case studies in a staging paradigm, to help clarify this complex situation.

Chapter 5 deals with bullying as a process, not a problem simply stemming from one person. In looking at the bullying process as a social rather than an individual problem, the scope of the mental health professional's intervention becomes more complicated, but also more effective. Our studies have proved that attempts to intervene with school bullying that focus on bullies and victims as disturbed children in need of either treatment or punishment (or both) lead to very poor general results. The Centers for Disease Control and Prevention (2007) considers that climate approaches are more important now than ever in approaching school violence. We have found that the bullying process is largely controlled by the bystanding audience, composed of all the other individuals in the school. In fact, we have gone as far as to say that the bully will only do what the bystander allows. In other words, bullying is a social phenomenon and a process within the school, not solely the independent actions of a disturbed individual. The overall health and welfare of children is much benefited by a more global climate approach, which in turn seems to improve academic standards. In our work, we have found that a major increase in academic performance occurs in young people who have internalized this idea of bullying as a process.

Chapter 6 deals with the fact that children must feel safe in order to learn. Many children with differences due to sexual orientation or physical and emotional difficulties do not feel safe in school, and thus there are significant problems for such students to learn. We believe that it is the responsibility of mental health professionals and school personnel to work together to create a secure environment in which students feel safe and are able to focus their attention on learning.

Chapter 7 is aimed at helping the mental health professional recognize and assess vulnerable children who need special attention because of mental illness and/or learning disabilities.

Chapters 8, 9, and 10 describe, respectively, therapeutic mentoring as a way of activating community resources, federal and state programs central to the medical leadership process, and the specialized but highly media-attractive threat assessment of homicidal children.

The final chapter in this book highlights the notion of wellness, summarizing how children can be kept well, preferably effortlessly. They will want to come to school, since they realize that school is an essential part of their intellectual, social, and emotional learning process. We focus not just on physical health, which is the focus of many wellness programs, but also on helping children adopt certain mental attitudes, like mentalization and altruism, that will enable them to cope with the complexities of life they will one day face. This extension of the idea of wellness to the mental realm provides a clear and essential role for the mental health professional.

While the scope of this overview might seem daunting to the busy practitioner, we have found that these principles, once grasped, can be gainfully incorporated into therapeutic practice, enhancing an effective and deeply rewarding clinical life.

Please read on!

Reference

Centers for Disease Control and Prevention: The effectiveness of universal school-based programs for the prevention of violent and aggressive behavior: a report on recommendations of the Task Force on Community Preventive Services. MMWR Recomm Rep 56(RR-7):1–12, 2007

Acknowledgments

WE would like to take this opportunity to express our thanks to those who have contributed to and supported our work.

Professor Peter Fonagy was intimately involved with the experimental phases of the Peaceful Schools Project and all our work ever since. Professor Fonagy wrote the section on developmental pathways for conduct disorder in Chapter 7 ("Assessment of At-Risk Children"), as well as the Foreword. For us he has been an invaluable guide and mentor in his usual gentle and helpfully critical fashion.

Dr. Glen Gabbard, a longtime friend, has provided us with an outstanding example of clinical excellence and scholarship, reminding us of the importance of being clear and straightforward in our writing.

Hundreds of teachers and thousands of students in nine elementary schools in the Midwest participated in the cluster randomized trial phase (1999–2001) of CAPSLE (Creating a Peaceful School Learning Environment), our systems- and mentalization-focused whole-school intervention to reduce school aggression. Professor Eric Vernberg and his master's and Ph.D. students at Kansas University also were central to this effort.

We have been fortunate to be involved in projects all over the world. Anne Kantor, Dr. Eugen Koh, and Carolyn Aston in Victoria, Australia, helped create a large-scale process establishing mentalization and well-being for Australian elementary schoolchildren. Jennifer Malcolm and Dave Konovitch organized Positive Vibrations for Peace in Negril, Jamaica, which has created a turnaround in the school system of this beautiful but immensely violent country. Renee Prillaman in North Carolina, with Sarah Stiegler of the North Carolina Psychoanalytic Foundation, started Peaceful Schools–North Carolina, a project that is flourishing by keeping buy-in high and devising individualized solutions for school problems that use a framework incorporating mentalization, power dynamics, natural leaders, and altruism in a climate where bullying is seen as a process, not a person, and part of the leader's task is to manage the group dynamics of the school as a whole. Sarah Fisher and Trish Morille in Houston,

Texas, created "+Works" (Positive Works), a "Momstinct"/"Dadstinct" grass-roots program focused on getting ahead of America's bullying epidemic through positive talk and action at school and in the home. Sarah and Trish have melded the basic elements of this approach into one that focuses on positive re-framing of negative thoughts and on education of parents. We also have active projects in Hungary and Finland.

Dr. Mary Ellen O'Toole, retired Special Supervisory Agent and profiler with the FBI, has been a friend and guide to the complexities of media exaggeration and fear of lethal violence from school shooters, and we greatly value our on-going relationship with her.

Dr. Robert Hales and John McDuffie and the editorial and publications staff at American Psychiatric Publishing guided us through a training process that we much appreciate. Iris Murdoch efficiently and pleasantly helped with typing. Finally, we offer our deepest gratitude to Dr. Erica Bernheim, a poet, who took the sharp edges off the manuscript, adding her gentle and crystal-clear touch to its roughness.

Source Credits

Portions of this book were previously published elsewhere. We gratefully acknowledge use of textual and graphical material from the following sources:

Twemlow S, Cohen J: Stopping school violence (guest editorial). Journal of Applied Psychoanalytic Studies 5:117–124, 2003

Twemlow S, Fonagy P, Sacco F: An innovative psychodynamically influenced approach to school violence. J Am Acad Child Adolesc Psychiatry 40:377–379, 2001

Twemlow S, Fonagy P, Sacco F: Feeling safe in school. Smith Coll Stud Soc Work 72:303–326, 2002

Twemlow S, Fonagy P, Sacco F, et al: Assessing adolescents who threaten homicide in schools. Am J Psychoanal 62:213–235, 2002

Twemlow S, Sacco F: Why School Antibullying Programs Don't Work. New York, Jason Aronson/Rowman & Littlefield, 2008

Permission has been obtained from the Copyright Clearance Center to reprint excerpts from the following sources:

Twemlow SW, Bennett T: Psychic plasticity, resilience, and reactions to media violence: what is the right question? American Behavioral Scientist 51:1155–1183, 2008

Twemlow S, Fonagy P, Sacco F: The role of the bystander in the social architecture of bullying and violence in schools and communities. Ann N Y Acad Sci 1036:215–232, 2004

1

School Violence

Range and Complexity of the Problem

The School Culture

School violence prevention programs have become a distinct form of behavioral health intervention performed by many levels of mental health professionals (MHPs) in the field. In recent years, increasing numbers of MHPs have been tapped to fill various roles within the community in the interest of intervening closest to the people experiencing problems. MHPs began as academics and were marshaled into action during the First and Second World Wars. Propelled by the War on Poverty of the 1960s, community mental health shaped how psychiatrists and other MHPs practiced. Psychiatry itself evolved from an insulated service for the privileged into a field that today offers a wide spectrum of services for any community.

Psychology also became integrated into the world of the schools, and this integration led to opportunities for MHPs to play active roles in schools, homes, and neighborhood clinics. Nurse practitioners, for example, are no longer shackled to

1

physicians or considered simply doctors' helpers, but have evolved into independent medical practitioners with increasing medical responsibilities in community settings. Social workers began close to the community, helping people cope with their basic needs; Jane Addams and the settlement houses were early examples of this (Knight 2005). Today, social workers are integral parts of multidisciplinary teams in school and community settings, doing a great deal more than case work. Many have made valuable direct and indirect contributions toward an improved understanding of the problem of school violence: Petti and Salguero (2005) have described the emerging roles of MHPs in community agencies.

School violence has likewise been addressed (Simon and Tardiff 2008) from a psychiatric perspective targeting a variety of violent behaviors that span the life cycle and involve a wide range of adult issues with aggression. Goldstein and Conoley (1997) provided an educational perspective that blends larger social systems theory with practical, everyday educational programming. They offered ideas that target the school climate and involve larger system changes designed to reduce violence at school.

Devine et al. (2004) took a wider perspective on school violence, using prevention as a unifying theme for exploring how violence evolves in a number of different contexts. Miller et al. (2003) approached school violence from a community vantage point, offering a social work perspective on interventions and prevention of violence at school.

From this brief review, it is clear that the development of approaches to counteract school violence has a rich history. In this book we focus on the MHP's role(s) in creating effective interventions, helping children, and contributing to prevention during that process. We realize that we are proposing expansion of the role of the MHP beyond consultation, supervision, and advice and thereby increasing the workload. Our clinical practice has clearly indicated that this work is needed and that even if the MHP occasionally donates the time, the referrals that will result easily compensate for the pro bono work.

The traditional or expected role of an MHP in responding to school violence has clearly changed dramatically over the past few decades. Unfortunately, there simply are not enough MHPs available to sit down with and treat every disturbed child that acts out at school. Instead, textbooks and manuals for school consultations in every profession from psychiatry to social work have had to adjust to evolving times. Violence can be tricky and is constantly changing. For instance, while the Internet offers the opportunity to create positive social networks for training and education, it is also a haven for pedophiles. Bullying through compulsive texting, which was not part of the zeitgeist even 5 years ago, has now become part of any conversation about creating safe academic environments. In other words, violence is a universal way in which children express a number of problems, from child abuse to parental neglect and beyond. All of these conflicts are then acted out on the "stage" provided by the school. The climate of the school can actually be the causal agent or the trigger for this compressed, con-flicted, and often traumatic energy in children.

School violence has become a way of expressing unmet behavioral health needs in children at both ends of the socioeconomic continuum. On one end, eco-nomic hardship and family dysfunction have ripped apart populations living in poverty, forming a high-risk subpopulation of multiple-problem families (Sacco et al. 2007) who are educated primarily in urban and rural-industrial public school systems. On the other end, we find suburban schools where parents are be-leaguered by a different set of stressors that make it difficult for them to act as full partners in educating their children. Attendance at high-achievement schools in affluent communities carries a still different set of pressures for students, parents, and teachers. When children feel valued, they think, use intention, open their minds, and learn; for that to occur, schools need to become safe and creative en-vironments that actively intervene and prevent pathological social aggression.

Our modern digital era has created a new climate, changing many of the rules for everybody involved. Young people today have far more computer skills than do most of their parents. Parents and school personnel may not even be aware of the extent of their lack of knowledge about students' online activities, as suggested by the school homicides planned on school-owned and "pro-tected" computers. When one thinks about how instant messaging, texting, and the Internet have collapsed the boundaries between home and school, one real-izes that the gap between school and home has virtually been eliminated. Chil-dren cannot escape problems at school simply by going home. This fact places a distinct pressure on behavioral health specialists to respond to the reality of how young people are now living day by day. A majority of the interventions sug-gested in this book will require a keen awareness of how the digital era has shaped the way children experience their home and school worlds. Many of the strategies contained here are guided by the principle of creating more consistent and positive signals for children from both home and school environments. When a child receives inconsistent signals from the home and school, violence is around the corner and disruption is its herald.

To counteract the new realities in school violence, we propose a shift in be-havioral health interventions, requiring at least a two-pronged attack for each school: 1) approaches targeting emerging mental health, learning, and behav-ioral problems; and 2) approaches targeting school climate and power dynam-ics. The first prong remains sophisticated behavioral health oversight for emerging psychiatric difficulties such as posttraumatic stress disorder (PTSD), attention-deficit/hyperactivity disorder (ADHD), oppositional defiant disorder (ODD), pervasive development disorders (PDDs), and a number of other dis-ruptive disorders. This part of the intervention will need to be accompanied by an deeper understanding of educational psychology, primarily focusing on nor-mal and abnormal development and how learning deficiencies early in a student's life can become primary sources of frustration and humiliation, leading to aggression in later years.

There clearly is a link between learning disabilities and delinquency. Aggression expressed at school often stems from a child's compensatory mechanisms to manage humiliation and frustration. In this way, a child learns to disrupt as a way to distract from his or her weaknesses in learning. This might be a matter of an information-processing weakness, or it might be a full-blown learning disorder, but regardless, the child cannot keep up with his or her "regular" classmates' educational pace and will become deeply frustrated at a young age. By the time children with undiagnosed or undiscovered learning disabilities reach third grade, they will be falling behind their classmates at a rapid rate. The teacher's maxim "you learn to read K–3; thereafter, you read to learn" may put some children in an untenable position, leaving them with a choice to become seen as bad or disruptive rather than to reveal their intellectual difficulties and risk being seen as "stupid." Thus, the behavioral health specialist needs to be aware of school disruption and violence as a strategy adopted to mask learning disorders. How and why does the MHP work within this complex of problems? There are four principles:

1. Become comfortable working with other disciplines and agencies (i.e., reach out beyond your defined discipline or comfort zone).
2. Realize that research and clinical practice strongly indicate that school violence cannot be approached, let alone resolved, without interdisciplinary collaboration.
3. Practical interventions (not simply theories) are what schools need.
4. The umbrella for all this work is *prevention,* not exclusively treatment:
    *   *Primary or universal prevention* (see Chapters 4, "Case Studies in School Violence," and 11, "Effortless Wellness and Other Afterthoughts"), in which you are promoting wellness and helping create disease-free climates.
    *   *Secondary or selected prevention* (see Chapters 6, "Children Need to Feel Safe to Learn," and 7, "Assessment of At-Risk Children"), in which you are identifying and helping at-risk children *before* problems become major or disruptive.
    *   *Tertiary or indicated prevention* (see Chapter 10, "Risk and Threat Assessment of Violent Children"), in which you are providing formal treatment opportunities for disturbed children and families and working with agencies and schools to prevent widespread disruption.

Regardless of the general nature of a particular school, parents and schools must send the same positive message to children about achievement, home and school preparation, and social behavior. This is especially true in the early grades, but it is important to continue spreading that message throughout the child's educational life cycle. Parents and schools need to be on the same page, with the child's best interests driving all decisions. This harmonious message must remain at the forefront in school violence interventions, regardless of type of school, level of resources, or country. The most effective clinical interventions in school settings begin with unifying the home–parent signal and ensuring that children receive consistent and clear communication about how to behave in school, during transitions or breaks between classes, after school, and at home in the community, with the help of the appropriate MHP.

In order to effectively prevent and intervene in school violence, the MHP must be attuned to the differences between urban and suburban school violence (described in more detail in Chapter 10, "Risk and Threat Assessment of Violent Children"). Many of the pressures felt in urban schools result from the skyrocketing incidence of child abuse and child removal due to caregiver aggression and neglect, as well as the decrease in available positive male role models within all communities. Unfortunately, a growing number of families are heroically maintained by single heads of households but lack the proper social support to ensure that children have healthy environments in which to grow. Disruptive behavior disorders are both environmentally induced and biologically based. Regardless of the etiology of the problem causing violence and disruption within schools, one ugly reality remains painfully clear: resources are shrinking while need is increasing exponentially. We can see proof of this in the increased medical expenditures in Medicaid, child abuse reporting, and independent reviews of poverty rates in children conducted by recognized agencies such as the Southern Poverty Law Center.

The public education system has no ability to screen or select students. Thus, public education is forced to deal with an overwhelming percentage of highly dysfunctional, often-mobile families and children living in unstable environments and exposed to the traumatic influences of parental addiction, removal from family, crime, poor housing, and the lack of consistent parental role models. Schools are now increasingly being expected to function as both parent and school. There is also a contradictory mandate for schools to increase academic achievement. We found in two experiments, one in the midwestern United States (Fonagy et al. 2005) and one in Jamaica (Twemlow et al., in press), that when children—especially at-risk older children—feel valued and bullying is discouraged, academic achievement increases. The MHP must learn to be sensitive to these inherent dual pressures on schools and to strategize accordingly.

The stressors potentially leading to violence in suburban schools are more related to social or interpersonal aggression than to any other factors. Families of low to middle socioeconomic status (SES) living in suburban environments often have two parents working. Many of these families are reblended, with the integration of siblings and mates at various stages of resolution of their personal difficulties. There is also an enormous amount of social aggression that exists in technologically advanced and equipped populations composed of increasingly younger individuals. It is not unusual to see 10-year-olds who are addicted to texting one another and who prematurely engage in coercive and negative behaviors. Suburban schools can be vicious fishbowls that become unavoidable breeding grounds for psychological pain, containing children trying desperately to fit into peer groups while competing with each other for attention.

Parental pressure on children to achieve and to succeed can also be a stressor, unintentionally fueling dangerous conditions for vulnerable youth. Parents in this difficult situation often feel overwhelmed and exhausted. They clearly have the best interests of their children at heart, yet the demands of everyday life have depleted their available energy. This can lead to a variety of responses from parents, ranging from dismissive attitudes to open hostility and litigiousness. These types of problems involve the potential for sudden deterioration in achievement, lethal school violence (as we have seen in school shooters), substance abuse, truancy, and even teenage suicide.

Regardless of the urban or suburban nature of the school, the role that the school plays in the social development of children is the same. Children move from their families into a school of peers supervised by another group of adults. When children first begin to venture out into the world, the school is their first real social stage. It is on this performing platform that adults can begin to recognize every child's needs and strengths. Anna Freud was a strong proponent of teachers' roles in understanding the psychological makeup and development of children. Her idea is more important today than ever. The most efficient way to reach children is to impact them where they have the highest percentage of contact from the earliest ages—that is, at school. There is little doubt that the earlier a child's needs can be identified, the simpler the intervention will be, increasing the likelihood of a successful outcome.

School is a prominent place in which children's identities are formed, and violence-related problems will first be recognized and responded to by someone other than the immediate family. Children who are already involved with state agencies may be highly mobile, changing from school to school frequently as caregivers change. These children may be prematurely included with other children who have not been exposed to such high levels of trauma and early childhood violence. Public schools have no choice but to cope with these mixings of different levels of disruptive behavior disorders. Even well-motivated children from involved families can become targets in environments where highly mobile and often predatory children are allowed to create victims before interventions are possible. This is where the second prong of our approach to school violence comes in, which targets the school climate, rather than the child. We further explore the power dynamics inherent in the bully–victim–bystander triangle to assist MHPs in designing climate interventions that will work. While Chapter 5, "Bullying Is a Process, Not a Person," elaborates on this concept, it remains a theme and concern in every chapter of this book.

Our current era presents MHPs with a unique set of challenges. They must think outside of the box, collect information from different types of places, and learn to identify the new roles they must play within specific disciplines. Traditional models focused simply on assisting problem children are clearly of little use in today's urban, suburban, and rural schools. At-risk children are a subclass needing special consideration from the community of MHPs working in close collaboration with local schools. There is also a pressing need for MHPs and the community at large to recognize that school violence often represents an entire community's way of responding to a variety of toxic environmental conditions, such as poor housing, low support for education, insufficient support services, and overall social deviance. Many types of aggression are easily recognized very early in the developmental cycle and have been shown to be resistant to change over the child's life cycle; school violence, for example, is easily recognized by Head Start teachers. The primary goal is to allow children to experience school without having their problems interfere with other children's rights (or their own rights) to get a good education.

Our approach also stresses the value of identifying what we describe as *natural leaders* (discussed in more detail in Chapters 5, "Bullying Is a Process, Not a Person," and 11, "Effortless Wellness and Other Afterthoughts"). There are people in every school across the world that children quickly identify as sources of protection and comfort, who perform their tasks away from the limelight and without the need to be publicly acknowledged as leaders. Natural leaders can assist schools by impacting the overall climate in a positive fashion. Behavioral interventions targeting climate require supervision by MHPs to assist school personnel in developing strategies that will prevent the evolution of coercion within the school environment. Understanding how unconscious power dynamics operate equips the MHP with the tools necessary to create interventions that prevent a school environment from becoming dismissive and encouraging school violence. Natural leaders can evolve at any age and can be children or adults. Clinicians need to keep their eyes open when working with schools to help teachers identify natural leaders and provide the opportunity to utilize their positive, often behind-the-scenes activity. A clinician's supervision of this process will enhance the consistency of its impact and allow flexible dialogue within the school. This step will strengthen the school's response to early signs of violence as has become necessary with the changing nature of school climate issues that affect children's learning every day.

Complex Problems Require Multidimensional Solutions

School violence is a complex and many-layered phenomenon, yet many antiviolence interventions may approach the problem from an oversimplified perspective or attempt to address only certain components of the problem in isolation. We have noticed an ongoing thread in literature on school violence, one that searches for specific programmatic solutions to behavioral problems, usually through add-ons to what is often an already overloaded curriculum. Besides discouraging staff, such solutions overburden teachers, who will often ignore the new curricula or approach them in a half-hearted way, which is then modeled by students. Biggs et al. (2008), among others, have shown clear differences in classroom adherence to interventions, even when a school-as-a-whole approach was used. Teachers tend to be very independent and need to fully buy into the idea. When we step back and examine the big picture, we realize that teaching is an enormously complex task. In addition to possessing intellectual skills, teachers must understand how children vary throughout the fastest growing phase of their lives (from age 4 or 5 years through young adulthood). Teachers must also be knowledgeable about psychopathology, parental health, the economics of funding schools, and a number of other issues.

Although individual psychopathology, genetic endowment, and stage of development impact how children interact with others, the expression of violence and difficult-to-handle behavior in schools is always heavily influenced by the social context. With rare exceptions, these individual factors can be modified if the child is attending a school that can manage social aggression. In other words, there are very few psychiatric conditions in which a child will become violent, irrespective of environmental influences. To achieve this objective, we believe that MHPs should target at least five specific dimensions of the individual child's social and emotional life when creating school violence interventions:

1. The capacity for self-reflection and mentalizing; that is, the ability of individuals to think about themselves, how they come across to others, and how others see them
2. The capacity to make, maintain, and deepen friendships
3. The ability to control, modulate, and sublimate impulses, including a deep understanding of the role of power dynamics in negotiating peaceful solutions to problems
4. The desire and ability to work in teams cooperatively and collaboratively
5. The capacity to behave altruistically toward others: peers, adults, others in need, and the environment, including a broader sense of social responsibility and respect for the quality of the social context within which they live

These capacities, when enhanced, ensure a solid foundation for academic progress and will reduce eruptions of school violence. In addition, the MHP needs to be aware of the macrosystem surrounding the child. There must be a multidimensional approach with good medical leadership and child-focused strategies. Finally, the MHP needs to assess the school's climate and evaluate the

---

TABLE 1–1.   Preliminary assessment of the school climate: some important questions

---

Preschool/elementary school

1. What makes boys and girls popular at your school?
2. What do you feel when you see a fight? Do you like it or does it scare you?
3. Do you see certain children frequently picked on or left out? What happens to them? What can a student do about it? Have you ever done something like that? Do you know what a bully is?
4. What individuals or groups bully kids?
5. Who is the scariest kid at your school? Why?
6. How does your school tell you how to handle bullies? What do you do?
7. If a kid looks strange or is quiet, do other students reach out to him/her, or is the student teased and excluded?
8. Do you ever not want to go to school because you might get picked on?

Middle/high school

1. Which groups or cliques can you clearly identify in your school? Is one group dominant?
2. Are there racial/ethnic groups who control the school?
3. Are there any gangs in your school? (see Scott 1994)
4. Do young people plan fights during the day and talk about when or where they will fight and who will win?
5. Do teachers appear intimidated at your school?
6. Are there teachers or counselors you can talk to about these problems?
7. What is security like at your school?
8. Have you ever reported a student being bullied? What happened?
9. What does your school tell you about how to handle bullying or what to do if you overhear someone threatening to hurt somebody?

---

power dynamics (bully–victim–bystander) within it. The MHP can anticipate problems for a child by knowing in advance the general nature of the school climate. A quick blueprint can be made by interviewing selected students from different grades with a trusted school counselor or social worker present, as illustrated in Table 1–1.

From a psychodynamic perspective, these capacities assume that the school provides the following elements for children: a background of safety and a feeling of well-being, a holding environment of adults who can respond appropriately to the children's developmental needs, and a setting that provides containment and helps children process negativity in relationships without being overwhelmed. Children must also have people to help them regulate affect, value relationships, and learn to mentalize in a secure attachment experience. Finally, children need support systems that encourage them to function as responsible members of the open social system of the community.

How Communities Respond to Violence

School violence is a community issue, and MHPs are advised to see the community as an active part of the solution as well as the social context for the development of the problems. The community is responsible for its younger citizens and thus bears the responsibility of embracing its schools and of offering them the maximum support possible. School violence will rattle the community. When a tragic suicide after "sexting" or a dramatic school shooting occurs, the community is shaken up and will act in ways to gain stability. Violence prevention is not a reaction, but a community state of mind. This is the essence of the theory underpinning all school violence interventions for either individual at-risk children or for school systems as a whole.

The events of 9/11 exposed many children to terrifying personal violence as well as to frightening community chaos. Poor children are likely to be exposed to violence on a regular basis, whether on the streets or between caregivers. It is the meanings that children attribute to these experiences as well as the attunement (or lack thereof) adults show that has the most profound impact on what the effects of violence will ultimately be in the lives of our children. The anxiety adults have about their own safety is contagious. Teachers are often parental surrogates, especially for very young children, who may know their teachers better than their often-absent and busy parents. After 9/11 we studied several schools in Massachusetts and found that the more stable teachers had fewer upset children, especially in K–4 grades. Chemtob et al. (2010) conducted a study of children's responses to 9/11 stress. In this study, 18- to 54-month-old children showed increased aggression and emotional liability only when their mothers had both depression and PTSD, but not with either alone. A great deal of reality testing for children happens through the efforts and examples presented by trusted adults.

School violence is, of course, also perpetrated by outsiders with varying grudges against schools. Their reasons for attacking and killing schoolchildren are often ones that are never discovered, and thus, complete prevention is impossible (see Chapter 10, "Risk and Threat Assessment of Violent Children"). When violence strikes a community, especially in the form of an attack on a school (either from within or outside), the community and its members—not only the direct family and the school officials and teachers, but also the surrounding community—react with disbelief and shock. There are some idiosyncratic reactions to acute trauma. For some, it is very difficult to remove the

TABLE 1–2. Four stages of community response to school violence

Stage		Reactive response	Proactive response
I	Denial/projection	Finger pointing/blaming others	Mobilization of the community behind the school during crisis
II	Anger	Quick-fix crisis response Legal responses Zero tolerance of perpetrator	Think through with an analytical team that is multidisciplinary
III	Depression/apathy	Return to stage I with a hopeless, helpless, or "It can't happen again at my school" response or brief, useless antiviolence programs	Long-term (5+ year) program that is fully integrated into the school culture with enthusiasm and patience
IV	Acceptance	Time heals and old patterns re-form without a new attitude	School and community buy-in continues; a visionary approach is maintained

Source. Patterned after Elisabeth Kubler-Ross: *On Death and Dying.* New York, Macmillan, 1969.

traumatic event from their minds. They may continue dreaming about it, suffering from insomnia and depression, and may ultimately need psychiatric care. Individuals also may become indecisive, may look to others to make decisions, and may even deny the reality of danger, holding onto a fantasy of rescue that is not possible or real. Some individuals act as if the person or situations are still a threat, even when they clearly are not. They may avoid strangers as well as friends; they may become suspicious of everybody. *Paranoia* may not be too extreme a term for such a reaction within a community, as Kai Erikson (1994) showed in his sociological study of disaster. This study focused on people who had lived side by side as close friends for many years, but attacked each other as the community disintegrated.

Communities are no different from individuals in many crucial ways. Table 1–2 lists reactive and proactive responses to serious school violence; unfortunately, even today, reactive responses tend to dominate the ways schools and communities respond. All too often, schools and communities do not work together, nor do they have much in the way of guidance or financial support for long-term palliation. The death of ideals provokes a pattern of responses as the community tries to adapt to an unthinkable event.

In the first stage, there is an attempt to project blame onto somebody, a form of omnipotent denial. This form of denial comes from the powerful infantile image of the grandiose infant screaming and finger pointing. The reactive response considers blaming the school, blaming law enforcement personnel, blaming teachers, as well as blaming the bully, or almost *anybody*. Since the acuteness of the trauma is overwhelming, the mind's capacity to reflect collapses; the mind functions poorly and in a narrowly focused, tunnel-vision fashion. Only the fear remains central to the community and to the individual. With prior planning, the proactive response would include preparation for the mobilization of the community behind the school during the crisis.

The second stage features anger unaccompanied by reflective, intelligent, or empathic responses to the trauma. Individuals begin looking to others for solutions because they feel helpless themselves, but their real desire is to run from solutions or to entertain fantasies that everything will return to normal soon. Anger dominates the community as well as the school. Often, quick-fix solutions, such as crisis intervention teams, are brought in, but their effects on students are often not helpful. In fact, these efforts can even prove harmful, since reliving a trauma by talking about it, especially close to the time of the trauma, is sometimes retraumatizing. Legal responses can also be remarkable. In the recent case of Phoebe Prince in South Hadley, Massachusetts, a young girl hanged herself in response to peer bullying. We saw that the entire state and community's response was anger, accompanied by all sorts of legal suggestions, such as mandatory reporting of bullying, massive lawsuits against the bullies and their parents, and criminal charges against the bullying girls. Such schools often institute zero tolerance of perpetrators—that is, they "bully bullies"—and thus are not modeling good examples to children. A productive response would instead create a team and "press the pause button," creating a well-thought-through response, one much more productive than a reactive angry one. A multidisciplinary team from the community and school can assist in planning what the school and community needs to do to prevent such violence and also how to respond to it.

The third stage is characterized by feelings of depression and apathy, often continuing months to years after the initial violence, defined by hopeless, helpless feelings or denial that "it can't happen *again* at my school." All too often, brief and useless antiviolence programs are introduced into schools in a perfunctory manner without much genuine hope of long-term success or belief that the program will actually help. By contrast, a proactive response would involve a long-term 5-year (or longer) program that is fully integrated into the school culture and becomes as routine for all members of the school as brushing their teeth. This type of response involves the whole school culture: children, parents, janitors, administrators, volunteers, and teachers.

The final stage, acceptance, stresses a proactive visionary approach. School administrators are very well aware that violence is with us and has been since the beginning of human history, and it is very unlikely to go away. Nonetheless, schools, working together with their local communities, can vastly reduce the impact of violence by building and maintaining collaborative, nonblaming working relationships. Buy-in is very, very important to sustain in schools. This means that everybody has to keep in mind constantly the potential dangers of violence and the necessity for children and adults to learn how to manage the types of conflict that could lead to more serious outcomes.

Ingredients of Effective Antiviolence Interventions in Schools

In the melting-pot culture of the United States, it seems only common sense that school interventions should take into account the culture, especially its understanding of interpersonal violence. Zoucha (2006) defined *culture* as the learned, shared, and transmitted beliefs, norms, and lifestyles of a particular population that guides its thinking, decisions, and actions in patterned ways and often intergenerationally. As an example of shared cultural beliefs, Zoucha (2006) mentioned the finding that among Potawatomi Native Americans, those who had experienced family violence believed that oppression by the dominant race was an important cause of such violence. The same attitude regarding the dominance of the white American was linked to patterns of alcohol and drug use, low self-esteem, and shame in the Potawatomis' lives (Zoucha 2006). Whatever the truth of these beliefs may be, any proposed intervention must take them into account.

There is a growing consensus that effective violence prevention in schools necessarily involves three overlapping processes: 1) identifying and intervening with "at-risk" students; 2) teaching students—largely through peer and teacher modeling—the skills and knowledge that promote the social and emotional competencies that provide the foundation for reflective learning and nonviolent problem solving; 3) developing systemic interventions that enhance safer, more caring, and more responsive schools and, optimally, communities (see Catalano et al. 2002 for a review). However, this work is all too rarely implemented in an effective manner.

Our studies have shown that at least six overlapping factors may inadvertently undermine effective violence prevention efforts in schools:

1. Lack of vision and multiyear commitment and funding
2. Failure to comprehensively understand the child as a thinking human being
3. Lack of an integrated approach to systemic factors in the school environment

4. Failure to distinguish social/emotional safety and physical security (i.e., a physically secure school might be socially and emotionally unsafe)
5. Insufficient training in recognizing at-risk students and understanding normal and abnormal child development
6. Lack of attention to adult role models of bullying and nonbullying behavior.

The U.S. government has made strides in improving these factors in the very recent past (see www.stopbullying.gov).

Effective violence prevention efforts need to rely on the school and its community vision and must be accompanied by a multiyear commitment to create a safe, caring, and responsive place where students will learn not only academically but also socially, emotionally, and ethically.

There must also be a comprehensive and integrative effort between educators, parents, and members of the community, both individually and systemically. Cognitive, social, emotional, physical, and moral development are integrally interrelated, and all potentially affect a child's ability to learn. Effective violence prevention efforts depend, in part, on understanding the relationships that people have in schools. When people are related in healthy ways, they recognize when others are in distress. They care and naturally "reach out." They ask, "What's going on?" They listen. When they become concerned ("This doesn't feel right"), they act.

Ultimately, all violence prevention programs come down to relationships—we must focus on our ability to listen to ourselves, to recognize other people's experience, and to use this information to solve problems, learn, and be creative together. Good teachers have always known this, and experienced teachers often comment that we were closer to the goal of peaceful schools 20 years ago than we are today, often rightly considering the cyber complications of having a world with no privacy and no time to self-reflect and self-regulate anxiety for our children. These teachers automatically reach out to connect with students. Gifted teachers appreciate that how students feel about themselves and others and how they (mis)manage relationships shapes their ability to learn, but for the most part, American education tends to view emotional life and the promotion of positive relationships with suspicion—as neither necessary nor part of the basic work of teaching.

It is only in recent years that there has been a burgeoning of research in how healthy relationships foster a student's ability to learn and to solve problems in nonviolent ways (Cohen 1999, 2001; Fonagy et al. 2009; Pianta 1999). Since families, peer groups, schools, and neighborhoods are interconnected systems, all of these sectors of life influence one another and influence children's development. For example, we know that aggression at home relates to aggression in school, and certain risk factors in the home predict aggression in schools (Loeber and Stouthamer-Loeber 1998). Research has provided mounting support for the notion that better violence prevention results will be achieved if school-based interventions are coordinated, collaborative endeavors that involve a vital school–home–community partnership (Cohen 1999, 2001; Swearer et. al 2010; Twemlow and Sacco 2008).

Learning to be part of a collaborative problem-solving team in schools is a complex and difficult task requiring mutual trust and understanding, and yet is vital for effective violence prevention, as well as for the promotion of health efforts. Many schools have developed these processes idiosyncratically, while others utilize data-driven models that delineate a series of steps and ways of evaluating the efficiency of given interventions (e.g., Carr et al. 2002). Both research-based and individually motivated efforts are all important to some extent in the prevention of youth violence (Pasi 2001).

There are a number of additional processes that impair collaborative problem-solving efforts: teachers and school administrators simply do not communicate with one another, and potentially helpful violence prevention efforts are fragmented. For example, many schools do not include cooperative learning, conflict resolution teaching, anger management, health education, antibullying efforts, sex education, and service learning in their health education efforts. All of these skills may directly and/or indirectly foster recognition of at-risk students and prevention of youth violence without much in the way of curriculum add-ons (Twemlow and Sacco 2008).

In recent years, the culture and climate of schools have become dominant concerns for many educational administrators as well as teachers. These considerations have been spotlighted not only because of lethal violence but also because educators appreciate that when students feel safe, academic achievement increases (Cohen 1999; Fonagy et al. 2005; Zins et al. 2004). However, administrators do not consistently take steps to effectively create safer, more caring, and more responsive schools. Too often, climate-focused approaches are passed over in favor of character, social, emotional, and educational efforts or inadequate and inappropriate "anger management" programs like those used at Columbine High School; predictably, such programs give administrators the (dangerous) illusion that they are doing something useful. At the tenth anniversary of the Columbine shootings, several scholarly tomes emerged (Cullen 2009; Langman 2009) that focus heavily on the inherent mental illness in the two boys involved. The contribution of the school climate (which made it hard for the boys to discuss their inner distress) is not dealt with in a sophisticated fashion in these writings, which by implication regard mental illness as a primary defect (i.e., existing independently of the environment).

Very few schools have personnel who are trained to recognize the signs that a student may be at risk of acting violently. Even fewer have sensitized school personnel to the range of subtle and dramatic ways that students (and sometimes teachers) are emotionally and socially abusive and violent to others. It is critical that school personnel understand the range of signs of physical, social, and emotional violence, because these signs provide the information needed to "stand up" and address the problem and/or to seek help from others. All too often we overfocus on the issue of physical safety without appreciating the critical importance of basic safety and well-being.

Research Perspectives on Bullying and Violence in Schools

There is a gargantuan amount of research literature on bullying and school violence. The United States alone has more than 300 programs proposed to ameliorate school violence. You may wonder what new information may still be available and what this book can tell you. When American Psychiatric Publishing wanted another book on school violence after the successful volume edited by Mohammad and Sharon Lee Shafii in 2001, we already knew that in spite of the good research work done (particularly in England, Norway, Finland, and the United States) since 2001, there had been disappointing results in the many and vigorous attempts to ameliorate violence in schools and communities.

In the meantime, there have been a number of authoritative references from the prestigious Institute of Criminology at Cambridge University (Farrington and Ttofi 2009), which was contracted to review the literature for the government of Sweden. The parameters of this comprehensive meta-analysis of the effectiveness of programs designed to reduce school bullying excluded many American studies, which were considered too focused on violence and aggression in schools rather than on bullying. Farrington's painstaking work, and a lot of his contact with us (our studies were excluded for these reasons), suggests that there is an internal "war" within the bullying/school violence literature. The typical Farrington bully, modeled after Olweus (Olweus and Limber 1999), is a disturbed individual who most likely would have strong antisocial traits, and also would be quite uncommon in most schools. The type of bully that Olweus followed and commented upon would often end up with criminal convictions in adult life. The Olweus approach pays close attention to the bully through careful watching, privilege restrictions, and "serious talks." Our research suggests, however, that these antisocial bullies comprise a very small part of the bullying and school violence population, although a single determined bully can bring a school to its knees on rare occasions. A stronger objection is that such pathologizing definitions of bullying aid in the denial of problems in schools where administrators do not want to acknowledge the problem, but instead scapegoat a single individual, and do little, if anything, to prevent further instances of school violence. (Chapter 4, "Case Studies in School Violence," provides several examples.)

In contrast, many children occasionally exhibit victimizing behavior and would not see themselves as bullies or be perceived that way by teachers or parents. The summative effect of multiple victimizing is often much more important than the social impact of single antisocial bullies. Some schools prefer the term "target" instead of "victim," and "victimizer" instead of "bully." We agree with this preference. International differences in how democracies evolve also affect the extent to which schools perform what authorities demand. While in Australia giving workshops and lectures on community and school violence, we had an epiphany, realizing that it wasn't so much the program that changes the school or communities, but how the context is prepared for change and how much it wants to change.

We wrote a book in 2008 for school staff and parents and school administrators and policy makers, *Why School Antibullying Programs Don't Work* (Twemlow and Sacco 2008), in which we listed ways to prepare the school context with much less emphasis on the specific program chosen. In our book, we concluded that school antibullying programs don't work very well, certainly in relation to the amount of research time and energy put into them. The teacher, student, and parent do not usually see much change in the school experience when these programs are implemented. When we decided to write this book, we wanted to focus on the essential leadership role of the MHP in changing that context so that a school would be more prepared and receptive to antiviolence interventions. MHPs (as with professionals in all fields) have, by social assignation, adopted a leadership role. A recurring question we heard was "What should and could clinicians do when called into schools, in addition to seeing mentally disturbed children, observing classrooms, and making referrals?" This school consultation model has been used for many decades and has been clinically useful. We concluded that for this new role, the clinician must understand the whole process, not just the clinical component of it, making connections between the various elements of the community, the school, and the MHP's role in it.

The Problem of Excellence: Achievement Pressure in Affluent Families and Schools

There are a number of fallacies about how lower-SES and higher-SES families differ. It is not just wealthy parents who are interested in having their children attend good schools. There are many lower-income parents who sacrifice to send their children to school, wanting them to have a better chance than they did. We saw this often in developing countries like Jamaica, where tragically impoverished parents would pay for taxis to take their children to school and would insist on giving them money for lunch, even if they themselves were unable to eat much. We see this in the United States, where one affluent community we were assisting had to make special arrangements for the influx of poor families who wanted their children to go to academically better schools. Wealthy families, despite their material possessions, may bring up their children very poorly, not necessarily due to malicious intent, but through the unconscious actions of their mental illness and limited attachment experiences on their caring and nurturing capacities. In other words, poverty needs to be distinguished from dysfunction.

We have worked in a number of countries, including Australia, New Zealand, Hungary, the United States, and Finland. In countries where affluence dominates, children are often afflicted with the "problem of excellence." They are driven by their parents toward high achievement in ways that can be quite depressing and anger-producing. We saw that this problem of excellence was often complicated by wealthy parents who were professionals—doctors, attorneys, and CEOs—who had been brought up in a success-focused ethic and who themselves often suffered from insecurely attached parenting—that is, the effects of growing up without secure, loving parents available to help their children develop a feeling of safety and self-knowledge. For example, a suicidal twelfth grader was berated by her father, a physician, after a suicide attempt, when she tearfully mentioned that she had received a 95% on a school test. The father replied, "If you'd done what I told you, you would have got 98%." This man was not being deliberately malicious or sadistic to his child; he was merely ignorant of a set of values that required the recognition of something other than material attainment and success. In another example, a CEO impulsively took his family to New Orleans just after Hurricane Katrina to do good works and help the poor and dispossessed. They were met in the streets by gunfire, warring, and distressed people and out-of-control police. They narrowly escaped with their lives. This CEO father lacked the humility to perceive how risky to his family his actions were; instead, he assumed that his success in business would translate into success in a completely foreign setting. We have spent some time discussing affluent schools because they are often used as examples within which to configure the rehabilitation of the ghetto environment.

From our work in many academically outstanding private, charter, and well-endowed public schools in affluent residential areas, we have observed that social aggression in these settings is often more cruel and less understandable than in much poorer settings. We conceptualize the power dynamic in affluent schools as being vertical rather than horizontal. In the nonaffluent schools, gangs and cliques create a way to survive. Protection, money, and status are a given with gangs. Attacks in less affluent settings usually involve violent actions, like maiming and homicide, but are often in the service of self-protection or occur as a result of other desperate situations in which mentalization for the individual and community is virtually impossible.

By contrast, in the vertical power dynamic observed in more affluent school settings, the more powerful children and parents in the school directly influence the less powerful, often through cruel, sadistic forms of bullying. In our opinion, some of these forms of social aggression are actually worse in content and tone, even if less physically coarse, than what we have seen in poorer school settings. In more affluent schools, the social pecking order creates the formation of cliques within the school, and these are also likely to reflect parental behavior. Most children will have two financially stable or affluent parents who are determined to have their children well educated and are willing to pay for it. "Well educated," then, is defined largely in terms of gaining the intellectual skills that will enable a child to enter an excellent university and one day have a job that provides stability, growth, and social status. We are not criticizing these values or attitudes. Most parents, across class lines, begin with these attitudes and will go to extraordinary lengths and will work menial jobs just to educate their children. President Obama's background provides one such example of a mother who sacrificed a great deal so that her son could have an excellent education.

So what is at the core of the "problem of excellence"? In our work with affluent schools, we have often found that a dynamic exists in which the children will tend to hate each other, but will want to gain status with the teacher and other authority figures. This creates a no-holds-barred competition. The intensity of this competition is often reflected in the dynamics around cheerleading, which today is often a form of competition between mothers acting out their repressed wishes for prominence through their teenage girls. Even in academically oriented schools, athletic success tends to be overemphasized, and the hatred and lethal violence that can result from that is graphically illustrated in the details of the 1999 massacre at Columbine High School, which was regarded as one of the best high schools in the country.

Affluent children can be extremely frightened of their own parents. One very intelligent young girl took 3 weeks to write a letter to her parents, particularly her father, with a simple statement that she was depressed and felt that she needed to visit a therapist. Her father's view was that this was "mental health bunk," and that all his daughter needed was a "swift kick in the butt." In one middle school, a father said to a teacher, in front of his child and the class, "My child has embarrassed the family by not achieving perfect grades." This family was from an Asian country where academic success can be highly competitive, but the victim of all this was the child himself, who was miserably depressed and feeling victimized by both family as well as "friends." At another affluent school, a group of advanced and highly gifted schoolchildren who had achieved entrance into Ivy League schools spoke openly of the pressures of having to achieve very high grade point averages. One child said that anything less, including admission to a very high-quality state school, would be seen as a serious failure to her parents and would lead to mockery at school and punishment at home.

In some families, we have treated parents who have become seriously mentally ill as a result of their children's failure to achieve as highly as their parents feel that they should. A highly driven professional parent with a spouse who similarly pushes academic performance to the extreme will create a problem of excellence, which is a bad model and can result in problems for the child that may well be transgenerational. The child then becomes a victim of the parents' problems, which can lead to a lifetime of psychiatric illness and a continuation of the vicious cycle. Clearly, this represents a poor attachment model and a poor parenting model, in spite of the good intentions, intelligence, and academic and material success of the parents.

In one school we intervened in, the parents were resistant to even anonymous assessment of school environment, let alone open discussion of school violence and bullying. As one parent said, "We may create a problem just by identifying bullying as a problem, and then all children will start being bullies." These more affluent schools also tend to choose school climate assessment of a general type that truly reveals nothing about specific behavioral issues and problems within the school. Questions such as, "How do you like being in school?" are not unlike the patient satisfaction questionnaires one sees in a hospital setting. Perhaps you do find that 95% of the schoolchildren are very satisfied with the school and you may be proud of that, except that it only took two who were unhappy at Columbine to engineer a massacre. Asking questions about specific pathological behaviors, while more painful, is a much more realistic and ultimately rewarding approach.

Secure Attachment in the Home, School, and Community

Those who have worked in severely disturbed and violent schools have seen how positive changes in children can inspire parents to change. Children who are insecurely attached to a dysfunctional home base can be transformed in a securely attached school—that is, a school that provides a safe, peaceful working environment in which children are encouraged to function well socially as well as intellectually and emotionally. Often, schools will take over certain significant parenting functions, and the quality of life of the child improves. When parents notice improvement in their children's functioning, it gives them hope and can lead them to make positive changes in their own lives. In one example of this effect, a highly disturbed child who had set his mother's car on fire and was considered psychotic and mentally retarded was placed in an "educable mentally retarded" classroom. After 2 years in a school with a good climate focus, he settled down and was eventually placed in a gifted classroom. He is now a highly successful college graduate. His mother, who had 14 children with no in-home father figure, became quite interested in why the boy wanted to go to school so regularly. She is now running a Walmart store and has also changed her life for the better. This mother was flexible enough to be curious about her child's "unusual" interest in going to school. It is this parent–school connection that forms the backbone of the structure that changes the school–community connection.

Fundamentally, then, securely attached parents may be rich or poor, white or black, and may live in the city, rural areas, or in any country. The security of attachment of parents makes children feel fundamentally safe and at home within themselves and where they are, and provides them a feeling of being contained and held, with a feeling of safety and well-being (Twemlow et al. 2002). Hartman et al. 2003 have shown that overly negative, critical, bullying parental behavior contributes to conduct problems in children, and that interventions that therapeutically challenge such parental behavior can do much to reverse the conduct problems.

Although this book addresses what the MHP needs to know about school, family, and community attachment issues,[1] some MHPs may still say, "I'm just going to focus on examining at-risk and disturbed children and refer them on for treatment." An important issue for such MHPs to realize is that not only does such treatment often not help the individual child, there are many problem children who will take the place of the one in treatment unless the school changes.

What is still seriously lacking in research approaches is interventions that are low-cost, nonpathologizing, and practical and do not interfere with the educational process. An impossible task? Probably not, but given the almost infinite variations in everyday reality, each school will likely need to create its own approach. Randomized trials can point out appropriate directions but cannot answer how an intervention works or help distinguish which type of intervention is best for which school. "Clinical"—that is, individualized—experience will always be needed to answer such questions and, we feel, is more likely to help the unique school situation, just as personalized medicine is the preference for patients in the twenty-first century.

---

[1]*Attachment issues* in this context refers to the earlier life experiences of parents that shape their knowledge and comfort in raising their own children.

KEY CLINICAL CONCEPTS

- School violence is a complex phenomenon that is often oversimplified and dealt with in isolation.

- MHPs have expanded roles—whether as physicians and nurse practitioners or psychologists, counselors, and social workers—in responding to school violence.

- School violence can be approached from a variety of different perspectives, ranging from the purely medical to the community-based orientation of social work.

- School violence reflects the major discomforts of children living in multiple settings of the home, school, and community.

- The digital era has changed school violence dramatically, providing a compressor for shame that can infect a school and lead to lethal consequences for students.

- School violence intervention blends the traditional behavioral health intervention models with prevention models that work to impact and prevent bullying or coercion in a school environment.

- Urban and suburban schools suffer from different but still very powerful forces that drive violence outward or inward toward students and adults.

- Changing schools needs natural leaders who work behind the scenes and build healthy communities.

- MHPs need to include a child's macrosystems in school violence interventions and not try to isolate problems.

- School violence is a community issue. Communities react to violent events in their schools like individuals do to bereavement, proceeding through several stages of response not dissimilar to the process of grieving.

- Effective violence prevention involves three elements:
  1. Identifying at-risk children
  2. Using peers to build programs
  3. Developing systemic solutions that involve the community

- Research on bullying and school violence offers many (often conflicting) ideas about school violence and bullying.

- Secure attachment of parents to their children, and vice versa, is found in all ethnic groups and at all SES levels and plays a key role in preventing school violence.

References

Biggs BK, Vernberg EM, Twemlow SW, et al: Teacher adherence and its relation to teacher attitudes and student outcomes in an elementary school-based violence prevention program. School Psych Rev 37:533–549, 2008

Carr E, Dunlap G, Horner R, et al: Positive behavioral support evolution of an applied science. Journal of Positive Behavioral Interventions 4:4–16, 2002

Catalano R, Berglund L, Ryan J, et al: Positive youth development in the United States: research findings on evaluations of positive youth development programs. Prevention and Treatment, 2002. Available at: www.journals.apa.org/prevention/volume5/pre005001a.html. Accessed December 2, 2010.

Chemtob CM, Nomura Y, Rajendran K, et al: Impact of maternal posttraumatic stress disorder and depression following exposure to the September 11 attacks on preschool children's behavior. Child Dev 81:1129–114, 2010

Cohen J (ed): Educating Minds and Hearts: Social and Emotional Learning and the Passage Into Adolescence. New York, Teachers College Press, 1999

Cohen J (ed): Caring Classrooms/Intelligent Schools: The Social Emotional Education of Young Children. New York, Teachers College Press, 2001

Cullen D: Columbine. New York, Twelve, 2009

Devine J, Gilligan J, Micrek KA, et al: Youth violence: scientific approaches to prevention. Ann NY Acad Sci 1036, 2004

Erikson K: A New Species of Trouble: Explorations in Disaster, Trauma, and Community. New York, WW Norton, 1994

Farrington D, Ttofi M: School based programs to reduce bullying and victimization. Campbell Systematic Reviews 6, 2009. 10.4073/csr.2009.6.

Fonagy P, Twemlow SW, Vernberg E, et al: Creating a peaceful school learning environment: impact of an antibullying program on educational attainment in elementary schools. Med Sci Monit 11:317–325, 2005

Fonagy P, Twemlow S, Vernberg E, et al: A cluster randomized controlled trial of a child-focused psychiatric consultation and a school systems-focused intervention to reduce aggression. J Child Psychol Psychiatry 50:607–616, 2009

Goldstein AP, Conoley JC: School Violence Intervention: A Practical Handbook. New York, Guilford, 1997

Hartman RR, Stage SA, Webster-Stratton C: A growth curve analysis of parent training outcomes: examining the influence of child risk factors (inattention, impulsivity, and hyperactivity problems), parental and family risk factors. J Child Psychol Psychiatry 44:388–398, 2003

Knight L: Citizen: Jane Addams and the Struggle for Democracy. Chicago, IL, University of Chicago Press, 2005

Langman P: Why Kids Kill: Inside the Minds of School Shooters. New York, Palgrave Macmillan, 2009

Loeber R, Stouthamer-Loeber M: Juvenile aggression at home and school, in Violence in American Schools. Edited by Elliott D, Hamburg B, Williams K. New York, Cambridge University Press, 1998, pp 94–126

Miller J, Martin IR, Schamess G: School Violence and Children in Crisis: Community and Social Interventions for Social Workers and Counselors. Denver, CO, Love Publishing, 2003

Olweus D, Limber S: Blueprints for Violence Prevention: Bullying Prevention Programs: Book Nine. Boulder, CO, University of Colorado at Boulder Institute of Behavioral Sciences, Center for the Study and Prevention of Violence, 1999

Pasi R: Challenging and Caring Schools: A Guide for Bringing Social Emotional Learning Into the Building, New York, Teachers College Press, 2001

Petti TA, Salguero C: Community Child and Adolescent Psychiatry: A Manual of Clinical Practice and Consultation. Washington, DC, American Psychiatric Publishing, 2005

Pianta R: Enhancing Relationships Between Children and Teachers. Washington, DC, American Psychological Association, 1999

Sacco FC, Twemlow SW, Fonagy P: Secure attachment to family and community: a proposal for cost containment within higher user populations of multiple problem families. Smith College Studies in Social Work 77(4):31–51, 2007

Scott C: Juvenile violence. Psychiatr Clin North Am 22:71–83, 1994

Shafii M, Shafii SL: School Violence: Assessment, Management, Prevention. Washington, DC, American Psychiatric Publishing 2001

Simon RI, Tardiff K: Textbook of Violence Assessment and Management. Washington, DC, American Psychiatric Publishing, 2008

Swearer S, Espelage D, Vaillancourt T, et al: What can be done about school bullying? Linking research to educational practice. Educational Researcher 39:38–47, 2010

Twemlow SW, Sacco F: Why School Antibullying Programs Don't Work. New York, Jason Aronson, 2008

Twemlow SW, Fonagy P, Sacco FC: Feeling safe in school. Smith Coll Stud Soc Work 72:303–326, 2002

Twemlow SW, Fonagy P, Sacco FC, et al: Reducing violence and prejudice in a Jamaican all-age school using attachment and mentalization approaches. Psychoanal Psychol (in press)

Zins J, Weissberg R, Wang M, et al: Building Academic Success on Social and Emotional Learning: What Does the Research Say? New York, Teachers College Press, 2004

Zoucha R: Considering culture in understanding interpersonal violence. J Forensic Nurs 2:195–196, 2006

2

The Family–School–
Community Connection

THIS chapter presents our approach to constructing interventions that incorporate the school, the family, and the community in concrete care plans that target specific problems that present themselves in schools. This approach presents a "geography" of the subsystems that must be coordinated in order to achieve a sustained therapeutic response to the types of underlying problems that often lead to school violence. This approach is a specific treatment strategy that begins with the problems exhibited by children, following the many connections that sustain those problems or are protective factors that mitigate the unhealthy effects of the problems.

Targeting Interlocking Systems

Figure 2–1 illustrates the relationships between many of the complex problems and solutions facing today's mental health professional (MHP): power dynamics that affect the resolution of family, school, and community problems; altru-

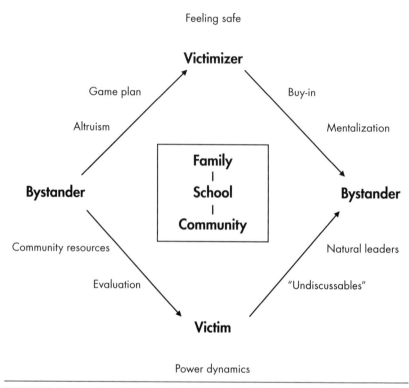

Feeling safe

FIGURE 2–1.   The family–school–community connection.

istic actions, natural leaders, and other factors that mobilize people (creating what we call "buy in"); and feelings of safety in community and school. There are always hidden agendas and problems that also have a vast influence on schools' abilities to function healthily, including teachers who bully students and parents who bully teachers, to name only two.

Let us further explore this approach by viewing an example of how this style of intervention connecting family, school, and community might be put into practice.

Case Example: Nick, "the Bully"

Nick was a 9½-year-old African American boy whose school reported him as having a bullying problem that had erupted into regular conflicts with both peers and teachers. He was referred to an outpatient mental health clinic that provided home-based family therapy. Nick was referred for a psychological evaluation to determine whether the problems experienced at school were a re-sult of attention-deficit/hyperactivity disorder (ADHD) or some other type of impairment that could be helped by the involvement of a psychiatrist or other services. The home-based therapist was an African American woman who worked closely with Nick's mother in weekly sessions that often revolved around trying to understand why he was having such trouble in school. Nick's mother reported to the therapist that she did not have the same type of problems with him at home, that he was respectful and responded to her boundaries, requests, and limits.

The therapist reported that she had been working with Nick's mother for approximately 4 months and had noticed a significant conflict between how his mother experienced this child's difficulties and how the school presented the problems to the therapist. The therapist had consulted with the vice principal at Nick's school and was informed that Nick was often disrespectful of other children's space, he displayed impulsive responses, had difficulty in attending and staying on task, exhibited irritability and hyperactivity, and was generally hard to manage in a regular classroom setting.

Nick's mother had reported to the therapist that her child was frequently bullied at school. This child did not present a genuinely strong male image and was, in fact, more effeminate in his presentation. This frequently would elicit an aggressive response from the other children at school. His mother reported to the therapist that Nick would frequently tell her that when he went to school he was teased about being a sissy, and that often children would surround him and taunt him. She also reported that Nick spent most of his time after school at home playing on his computer, as well as being very interested in fashion. This was quite unpleasant for his mother, as she was trying to encourage him to be more of a boy, rather than exhibiting the play preferences and behaviors more common in a young girl.

The therapist worked during weekly sessions to assist Nick's mother in adjusting her ideas about the value of the child being in "a real man" and shifted more toward his academic success and his ability to live at home in a peaceful fashion. The therapist was struck by how differently the school and the parent viewed Nick's problem. The therapist also noted the mounting conflict between the mother and the school about how Nick was perceived when he was at school. His mother was becoming increasingly frustrated with the school, because she would receive at least one or two calls a week from the school, informing her that her son had been asked to leave a classroom or was assigned yet another in-school suspension. Nick's mother and his therapist agreed that Nick needed to be assessed, and that the school needed to create a special education plan to assist him in having a better education and a safer, healthier social experience at school. His mother did not trust that the school would do an accurate assessment and asked the therapist's assistance in obtaining a psychoeducational assessment that could answer some of the questions about what the etiology of her son's difficulties at school might be.

The therapist was a master's-level social worker and had initially diagnosed this child as having ADHD, based on reports from school indicating that he met DSM-IV-TR (American Psychiatric Association 2000) criteria for ADHD. Nick was impulsive, had difficulty paying attention, was often inattentive, and had random bursts of excess energy that were not easily contained in a regular education classroom. The therapist had originally suggested that the mother consider a psychiatric consultation to review the possibility that medication might be useful. Nick's mother was very strongly against medication and urged the therapist to try to help him using psychotherapy and consultations with the school.

A referral was made to the psychologist working as part of the multidisciplinary team at the therapist's clinic, and psychological testing was initiated as a way to formulate a treatment plan and to assist in making a differential diagnosis. There was a real question as to whether or not Nick's symptoms constituted ADHD and whether or not a referral to a psychiatrist would be indicated. His mother agreed to follow through with recommended treatment if the assessment demonstrated that her son was indeed suffering from an attentional impairment that could be helped through medication.

When Nick reported for psychological testing, the first step of the assessment was a clinical interview with the therapist. During this interview, the therapist informed the psychologist of the background information and the problems that both the mother and the child were experiencing at school. The therapist offered the psychologist the background information and provided the referral question that targeted a differential diagnosis and educational assessment to determine whether the child needed special services at school or not. The psychologist's first interview was significant in picking up on the gender identity issues. Nick began the initial clinical interview by playing with a dollhouse in the room. He took an immediate interest in combing a doll's hair and arranging the dollhouse in a fashionable way. There were no indications that this was causing Nick conflict; however, the psychologist noted that this gender identity issue was still a significant factor in understanding Nick's difficulties at school. The therapist reported to the psychologist that the mother was not open to discussing the child's gender confusion and instead took a more hard-line stance, constantly encouraging her child to engage in more traditionally masculine activities.

The intelligence testing was helpful in determining that Nick had the ability to attend to incoming stimuli. His Wechsler Intelligence Scale for Children—Fourth Edition (WISC-IV; Wechsler 2004) IQ was 89, with a significant difference between subtest scores. The test indicated an impoverishment of working memory and processing speed. While these are common findings for children with ADHD, there was a clear pattern of this child being able to attend and concentrate throughout the intelligence testing. The IQ estimates, in other words, were not providing a true reflection of his abilities. On the human figure-drawing portion, it became quite obvious that Nick had an unusual perception of himself in the world. When asked to draw a picture of a person, he drew an abstract artistic representation of just a head. When asked to explain the picture, he said, "I only do portraits." The psychologist began to realize that this was a child who was brighter than his measured IQ. The use of the word "portrait" was inconsistent with the low IQ scores and suggested that his somewhat humorous approach of insisting that he only does portraits reinforced the idea that he had an idiosyncratic way of experiencing the world. This was a further reflection of some of his gender identify confusion; he assumed a somewhat elitist approach to any and all of his work.

The Rorschach test was quite revealing in that Nick offered over 60 responses. This is quite unusual in children, and the psychologist noted that these responses were not very elaborate, instead consisting of rapid-fire, single-word images that the child had difficulty integrating into a whole response. His responses were accurately perceptions but it seemed as though the images were "shotgunned out" in an unintegrated fashion. This way of approaching the Rorschach suggested that Nick was having difficulty with sensory integration. In other words, his projective responses displayed signs of an inability to order and integrate his perceptions. The Rorschach also showed an absence of any movement or other indications of fantasy production, and instead had a combination of quick images followed by pure color responses. This suggested that the impulsivity and difficulty were related to Nick's difficulty in integrating his sensory simulation.

Nick's Thematic Apperception Test (TAT) stories confirmed that he always identified with the female figure, and all of his stories were indicative of his wish to be female. All of the figures, whether male or female, were responded to as if they were female, and there was a consistent message of frustration and sadness.

The psychological evaluation suggested that this was a child who might be struggling with a mild case of Asperger's disorder, in addition to grappling with clear gender identity issues. The psychologist ruled out ADHD, despite the fact that several criteria could be understood as symptoms of ADHD. Nick's acting out at school was diagnosed by the psychologist as part of an Asperger's social inhibition. His difficulty in maintaining his focus and controlling his behaviors in a regular classroom were also connected to Nick's difficulty with visuospatial integration and sensory integration. He was interested in fashion and other feminine interests, but not to the level of a ritual preoccupation that is more common with Asperger's or children on the autism spectrum. Nevertheless, the psychologist was convinced that Nick needed special education services and that many of his difficulties stemmed from an inability to integrate and/or screen out sensation and stimulation from his environment. Nick's aggression was seen as a response to frustration. The psychologist recommended that Nick be considered a special education child and that a plan be developed to reduce the amount of stimulation that he would experience on any given day. The psychologist also recommended that the school consider creating social skills classes and that the teachers be made aware of Nick's difficulties with sensory integration and of the possibility that he may be a mild Asperger's child.

The therapist was then faced with creating a solution that would be helpful not only to the mother but also to the school and surrounding community. The intervention would be too narrow if it simply identified the diagnostic classification of Asperger's disorder and gender identity disorder without in some way addressing how these diagnoses were handled at home, in school, and by the community. Nick spent virtually all of his after-school and weekend time at home engaged in solitary and somewhat ritualistic activities involving dolls and fashion. There was little doubt that he was not an aggressive child and was unlikely to be the initiator of bullying in a school setting. The therapist and psychologist both agreed that Nick's most likely risk would be as a victim because of his effeminate presentation in an urban public school dominated by children who were much more aggressive and intolerant of children with unresolved sexual identities.

To approach this situation, the diagnostic picture would be similar of that of a DSM-IV-TR biopsychosocial approach. It would take four levels of functioning—psychiatric diagnosis, school climate, home, and community—and assign a diagnostic component to each that could be used in structuring an intervention that could target the interlocking systems of home, family, and community.

TABLE 2–1. Sample diagnostic formulation for Nick

Psychiatric diagnosis

Asperger's disorder, gender identity confusion

School climate

Bullying is at a dangerous level, with dismissive school personnel blaming
victims or targets. The most likely role for this child at school would be that
of a victim, despite the fact that the school sees him as a bully interfering with
the rights of others. Psychologist is clear in cautioning/advising that risks for
Nick are more likely to be self-focused and over time could result in suicidal
or other self-defeating or self-destructive behaviors.

Home

Mother is unwilling to acknowledge issues with gender identity confusion and
is in conflict with the school concerning the responses to and diagnoses of
her child's misbehavior at school.

Community

Lack of resources for nonathletic children with cross-gender interests. Child
spends considerable time at home, disconnected from more gender-specific
community activities. No resources available in community to engage with
child for the purpose of building a sense of self-esteem and value. Child is not
interested in sports, and there are no other after-school activities that meet
his interests.

A therapist may not be in a place to deliver all of the services but must be aware
of the child's needs. This will provide an opportunity to prevent violence by reducing the victim pool. Table 2–1 presents a sample diagnostic formulation for
Nick.

This sample diagnostic formulation was designed to develop a coordination
plan of interventions targeting not only Nick's psychiatric symptoms but also
the way he is treated at school and how the school understood his problems, as
well as how his mother interacts with the school and deals with her son's gender
confusion, and finally targeting the community, which seemed to be barren of
resources that could offer him a full life. This multilayered diagnostic formulation offers the opportunity to develop interventions that decrease the pressure
on at-risk children and increase their support so they are not caught in situations where they will feel that people do not like them and that they must fight
everybody who does not understand them, and so they do not remain isolated at
home engaging in solitary activities around their own special interests. There is
no question that it was critical to understand the psychiatric and psychological
issues that were impacting Nick.

This approach views the child as a reflection of larger social system forces and begins by understanding the child's psychiatric and psychological problems. This is the beginning of developing a geography that traces how the child moves through his or daily life from home to school and through the community. This is a modern version of what Anna Freud understood at the turn of the century: children come first and everything should revolve around the "best interests of the child" (Goldstein et al. 1996). This legal standard was the result of collaboration between Anna Freud and Yale University that continues today between the Anna Freud Centre in London and the Yale Child Study Center in New Haven, CT. The concept of the "best interests of the child" drives most ethics in psychological evaluation for family law. In fact, this "best interests" principle drives judicial thinking when evaluating the rights of parents in custody struggles. Children develop the same way as humans now as then, but culture has accelerated at an unimaginable pace. What remains constant is that children are sentient beings that need to be understood. Our approach is designed to be active in all fronts that impact the well-being of children.

Hierarchy of Treatment Needs: A Multidisciplinary Assessment

Assessment of school violence problems demands a clear and comprehensive hierarchy-of-needs assessment. Well-designed tools are available that can help guide such evaluations; for example, in 2009, Massachusetts implemented a statewide domain-specific assessment instrument called Child and Adolescent Needs and Strengths (CANS) Comprehensive Multisystem Assessment (Praed Foundation 1999). This instrument offers a three-point rating scale of strengths and weaknesses for children and adolescents. The CANS provides a comprehensive overview of key areas of a child's functioning in areas of school, family, and community life. It is a free instrument that is in the public domain and it also has excellent psychometric properties.

Step One: Home Safety and Stability

The first step in approaching a school violence problem is an assessment of the safety and basic survival needs of the children. School violence often stems from the fact that aggressive children or their victims are living in homes that have child abuse, domestic violence, addiction, overpressured parents, and other forces that may lead to aggressive actions at school. Often, referrals to mental health clinics consist of children attending urban public schools who have already experienced a protective services intervention or are in state custody and may be receiving services from various child welfare agencies.

Many of these families have already been identified because of instances of child abuse and neglect, reported by either a primary care physician or a member of the school community. State agencies may already be intervening in the family, and a service plan may be in place to determine whether or not a child is living in a safe home or experiencing stressors at school. It is critical to establish the child's basic safety prior to moving on to the medical or psychiatric diagnosis. The MHP must be certain that the child is living in a safe home. It is key to remember that child abuse and neglect are not just related to urban schools or disadvantaged areas but may be present at all levels of income and in every type of family. The exact correlation between child abuse and socioeconomic status (SES) is not a fixed one and varies considerably with a wide range of other risk factors (Trickett et al. 1991). For example, in a study of more than 350,000 children in South Australia (Hirte 2010), there was a strong relationship between income as measured by SES index and rates of reported child abuse. The indigenous population was most "at risk" and had the highest rates of reported child abuse. Even in this study, 5%–9% of the child abuse occurred in higher-SES families. There was an even distribution of substantiated emotional abuse among lower- and higher-SES families.

The first step in this assessment process involves knowing who the child's custodian is and whether or not that custodian is capable of maintaining a safe and stable household. If the custodian is not the parent and the child lives in a foster home or lives at home under the custodial arrangements of child protective services, the assessment must begin with an understanding of the risks and protective factors active at home that impact on the child's daily life at school.

Safety at home can also present as a juvenile court issue. In many cases, adolescents will be connected to a juvenile court through either a Child in Need of Services (CHINS) or a Person in Need of Supervision (PINS) designation,[1] or by virtue of a criminal charge that is being monitored by a juvenile probation office. In these cases, the question of safety at home or within the community is being managed by a court-appointed probation officer. The assessment begins with the responsible custodial officer, who provides information that can assure the clinician that the child or adolescent in question is living in a safe home and

---

[1]CHINS and PINS are discussed in more detail in Chapter 9, "Role of Medical Leadership in Unlocking Resources to Address School Violence." These terms refer to a family law procedure where parents and schools can make a filing in juvenile court because of school truancy, running away, or other status offenses typically seen in oppositional defiant disorder (ODD).

that measures have been taken and are being monitored to ensure that the child or adolescent has a safe home environment.

In the case of Nick, there were no protective services issues in place. The mother was in firm control of her household and was not engaged in any type of domestic violence or other social deviance that might create an unsafe home environment. In fact, the home was the only safe place Nick experienced, but it became part of his overall isolation and a key trigger for the problems he was suffering at school. In this situation, the clinician would be assured that the child was not experiencing any form of child abuse at home, but having a safe home environment is not always a guarantee that a child is doing well at school.

Step Two: Medical/Psychiatric Diagnosis

The next level to consider is the medical, or psychiatric. It is critical to determine whether all of the diagnostic information has been collected in order to formulate a reasonable diagnostic picture of the child experiencing the problem at school. There are many different psychiatric diagnoses that can reveal themselves at school as aggressive outbursts or that may be the result of being victimized by someone acting out violently at school. It is critical to develop a broad-based understanding of a child in order to design traditional interventions that target symptoms and engage therapeutic interventions, such as individual or family therapy.

In Nick's case, the diagnostic confusion led to a delay in the creation of a treatment plan because of discrepancies in how the child's behavior was viewed from a psychiatric or psychological perspective. There were questions about whether the child was exhibiting symptoms of ADHD or of another type of psychiatric disturbance. This was a point of conflict that resulted in the mother and the school completely disagreeing over the next steps necessary to improve the child's behavior at school. Nick continued to act out aggressively at school, and this was presumed to a symptom of ADHD. The school was not aware of his overall intellectual capacity, nor were they aware that he might have some type of neurodevelopmental disorder (such as Asperger's) that would mimic ADHD, resulting in a misunderstood and frustrated child acting out aggressively at school.

It is critical to ensure that children have had all of their well-child visits with a primary care practitioner. Part of this medical assessment also involves the assessment of their social-emotional needs and the diagnosis of any emotional disturbances or social disruptions. Solving school violence problems is made considerably easier when the psychiatric or psychological needs of children are being addressed in a consistent and coherent fashion. If a child struggling with ADHD is not receiving coordinated care from a psychiatrist or primary care physician, from a therapist, and through school consultations, then it is quite likely that his or her problems at school, at home, and in the community will continue to manifest and to escalate. This approach stresses the broader spectrum of interlocking subsystems, but the nucleus of all interventions is the child. It is imperative that all interventions begin at the nucleus at the center of the subsystems. Successful interventions are constructed and executed with a thorough and accurate understanding of the psychological needs of the child in question.

It is also critical to understand a wide range of potential psychological and developmental issues. In the case of Nick, the school was aware that the child had an average to above-average ability to communicate when not distracted, but that this did not translate into his completing grade-level work. They were attributing this to behavioral disruption, rather than to issues related to intellectual function, as measured with the WISC-IV. This area becomes extremely important when a child has a learning disability related to a language-based problem or a serious emotional disturbance that interferes with his or her attention and concentration. If misunderstood or misdiagnosed, these learning disabilities often create frustration and aggression at school. However, simply knowing that the child has trouble learning is not sufficient to eliminate aggression or seriously disruptive behavior at school. Also, knowing that a child has a language-based problem but not linking this problem to other areas of his or her functioning will not result in a healthier school experience for the child.

Step Three: School Climate

The third level in a multidisciplinary assessment process involves assessing the school climate and how children's individual, psychological, and psychiatric disturbances (including their home lives) influence their roles within a school. Children who are hypersensitive and submissive are likely to fall into patterns that invite victimization (Felix et al. 2009; Reid 2009; Rose et al. 2009). Similarly, children who experience high levels of aggression at home or in their communities may mirror this by taking the role of bully within the school (Brame et al. 2001; Farmer et al. 2007; Wasserman et al. 2003). As we have found, other individuals may be ambivalent and will fall into the role of bystanders and have their overall school experience compromised due to distraction and unhealthy power struggles. A full assessment of a school's climate requires that a clinician be aware of what is happening within any one school without being judgmental. The fact that a therapist knows that a child is being targeted is not sufficient to solve the problem. In our intervention approach, the therapist must be in a position to assess how the school responds to this child and the impact that response has on the child and family. While MHPs may not be in a position to

TABLE 2–2. School climate assessment: common patterns

Principal is active, listens to teachers, mingles with students, and is open to outside help

School is dismissive, with hated, often preoccupied principal and discouraged teachers

School is overly focused on academic achievement or forensics/debate activities and allows social aggression

School overvalues athletics and allows social aggression

School has active social work department

School spends time thinking about climate

change how a school reacts to a child, they may be in a position to work with parents or guardians to approach the school to develop a plan to increase tolerance for children who are different.

We must always remember that school climates are unique to each school. Even schools within the same district are unique social systems. Just like human individuals, every school is different and reflects the overall quality of leadership exhibited by the adults at school. If the school's administration is dismissive and inattentive to climate, then a child experiencing problems "fitting in" will be at increased risk of being a victim or a bully, and thus the cycle of school violence will continue (Twemlow et al. 2002).

During the assessment phase, we advise clinicians to closely examine how the school climate might impact both vulnerable and volatile children. This can be done by visiting the school, meeting the child's teacher, joining the parent in a school meeting, or interviewing the child and parent about his or her school experiences. Children in particular will frequently be rich sources of information about a school climate because they will describe what their daily life is like there. A clinician can ask how teachers respond when certain problems arise at school and also try to understand the way in which the school responds to the troubling behaviors. A suggested format for the school climate assessment is presented in Table 2–2.

Results of the school climate assessment can be used in several ways (this topic is addressed more fully in Chapter 7, "Assessment of At-Risk Children"). There are two major ways of using the information about school climate. First of all, it could be included in the therapeutic treatment plan as an issue to work on with the child and caretakers in both individual and family therapy. The second way to use the information is for the MHP to develop a relationship with the school and offer his or her time and resources to assist them in developing climate-oriented interventions that could help increase tolerance for difference and decrease acceptance of bullying behavior at all levels.

A climate assessment should also include a consideration of what it is like for the child to travel to school. A clinician might assist at the school during transitional times such as recess, lunch, and waiting for the school bus. These transitional periods are frequently the times when children experience the most trouble. Unstructured times offer an opportunity for coercive power dynamics to unfold, requiring that adults be especially vigilant in ensuring that vulnerable children are not pulled into dangerous interactions during nonclassroom times. This is also an opportunity to explore the impact that transportation to and from school has on the overall experience the child has at school. If children in an urban environment are afraid to walk to school because of aggressive older kids or gangs, the intervention needs to address this risk area, developing a strategy to increase the children's sense of safety while going to and from school. Again, the interlocking systems of the community, the school, and the home are the essential ingredients used in understanding school violence problems. Children's experiences while moving through these various interlocking systems will offer the clinician a road map to follow in attempting to reduce violence in schools.

Step Four: Formal and Informal Supports in the Community

The final area of assessment is of the formal and informal supports that exist in a child's community. Many of the new wraparound services[2] (Bruns et al. 2005; Oliver et al. 1998; Pullmann et al. 2006) are based on the identification and engagement of natural supports or helpers in a child's environment and community. We have located both formal and informal supports that exist in *all* communities; when children are disconnected from these supportive resources and protective factors, they are more vulnerable to being lured into destructive activities at school. The formal structures in the community may include YMCAs, Boys and Girls Clubs, youth centers, community centers, faith-based organizations, and organized municipal town athletic or recreation programs. These formal supports offer opportunities for children to engage in adult-supervised social-recreational activities after school and on weekends. After-school

---

[2]Wraparound services are a system of care currently being applied in Massachusetts in response to a federal lawsuit in which a group of parents sued Medicaid and won the right to have their children's residential placement risks reduced by preventive services provided in the home through a wraparound system of care. Wraparound services are covered in greater detail in Chapter 8, "Activating Community Resources Through Therapeutic Mentoring."

activities play a critical role in maintaining a balanced and healthy child who can function in school. When children have nothing structured to do after school, there is a heightened risk that they will engage in unhealthy (and often destructive) behaviors. In fact, the after-school times between 2:00 and 6:00 P.M. are the peak times for adolescents to engage in criminal activities.[3]

Coordination of Resources: Structured Analysis of Current Plan of Care

The next element of school violence assessment involves the evaluation of the overall care and coordination strategies planned for an intervention. In many cases, there are a number of agencies and helpers engaged in independent and fragmented attempts to assist the child and family. There may be someone who is providing counseling from within the school as part of a special educational plan and a therapist working in an outpatient clinic simultaneously involved. There may also be a probation officer and a special needs teacher actively trying to assist the child in his or her daily activities at school. Often, there are competing agencies that work with the same family and deliver services that reflect their specialties, rather than addressing the total needs of the child and his or her family. Thus, an MHP needs to thoroughly evaluate the status of the care coordination efforts so that strategies can be streamlined and targeted to maximize the impact on the child's everyday life at home, at school, and in the community. When these agencies or resources are acting independently and without communicating with one another, they often engage in counterproductive activities that actually become part of the complex school violence problem.

This misguided system of care processes can be detected during clinical interviews, wherever and whenever an MHP enters a school violence case. The clinician is advised to be alert to the resources that have been tried or may be active in a family's life history and current life events. This is an essential piece of information vital to prioritizing and integrating resources, not a "simple" exercise in listing the agency's or provider's names and affiliations of people involved in the family. This assessment is a structural analysis of the care plan being used (or not used) to address the school violence problem. This added process analysis can be

---

[3]After-School All-Stars (ASAS; http://www.afterschoolallstars.org) has a helpful Web site that offers insight into the rationale for after-school programs and provides some references to studies about the incidence of after-school crime and delinquency.

useful in structuring further assessments, as well as in streamlining and linking current formal and informal resources involved with the child and family.

Case Example: Jeremy, a Juvenile Offender at School

A pediatrician referred Jeremy, a 14-year-old white male student who had recently been expelled from school due to his involvement in an attack on a younger female junior high school student, who had accused three boys of raping her in a school bathroom. Jeremy had a history of expulsions due to fighting at school, was on probation for an unrelated drug charge, and had been admitted to multiple private psychiatric hospitals for aggressive behavior. In fact, Jeremy had been involved in psychotherapy ever since his parents' divorce when he was 8. Although he attended regular education classes, Jeremy had been prescribed Ritalin (methylphenidate) for ADHD as a child. Jeremy lived with his mother, who worked as an executive in a financial institution. His parents had very different views of their son's behavior. Jeremy's father was a law enforcement officer who was involved with his son's life but not available to deal with many of the school behavior problems. Jeremy's mother was the primary custodian, while his father had visitation. Jeremy had been attending a substance abuse program as part of his probation agreement and was a participant in a court-ordered child welfare community supervision program.

The MHP in this case was a private practice child psychiatrist recommended by Jeremy's juvenile defense attorney. There was little doubt that Jeremy was struggling with a number of individual psychiatric conditions, including conduct disorder and ADHD, and that his parents' divorce was the triggering event in a series of aggressive behaviors that began with absenteeism and truancy and led eventually to criminal activity (distributing Class A prescription medicines) at school. The MHP undertook a structured analysis of Jeremy's care plan, beginning by requesting separate meetings with each parent. The MHP determined that both parents were concerned about their son, but still competitive and hostile in dealing with one another. They certainly did exhibit very different views: Jeremy's father was authoritarian and his mother permissive. Each seemed to blame the other for Jeremy's problems.

The next step was for the MHP was to obtain releases and to communicate with the various providers, beginning with the probation officer. It was immediately clear to the MHP that the court was ready to sentence Jeremy to mandatory treatment and to recommend that he be tried as an adult in criminal court. Jeremy had failed several drug tests and was not participating in the recommended therapy and medication, although the prior therapist had been effective, according to the probation officer. The school counselor described Jeremy as a "nice kid hanging with the wrong crowd." Jeremy had never displayed aggression himself but was often involved with a group who received punishment for aggressive acts at school. The counselor felt that Jeremy had great academic potential and was very bright and capable. His adjustment to junior high was difficult, however, and Jeremy immediately attached himself (as an "identification with the aggressor"–style bystander; see Chapter 5, "Bullying Is a Process, Not a Person") to a peer group organized around substance abuse and criminal activities, supported by street gangs from a city just outside of his suburban neighborhood. The school counselor reported that Jeremy's probation officer had never contacted the school counselor and only contacted the school principal after eruptions of problem behaviors at school.

The MHP spoke to the case manager from the community supervision program during an hour-long consultation in the MHP's office. The community worker, by virtue of his job, was not allowed to intervene at school or to offer alternatives during the school day. The case manager also added that Jeremy was a talented musician who played the piano and guitar. The MHP determined that the school and the community had drastically different perceptions of Jeremy and also began to see that there was a mirroring of pathology being reflected from the family and enacted by the community agencies. The school principal seemed disconnected from the mother and the community agency. The father, the court system, and the school administrators seemed to believe that all Jeremy needed was more punishment. To make the situation even more complex, Jeremy's father had remained totally uninvolved in any mental health or community agency services.

The serious charges being considered for Jeremy were what united his parents in their desire to protect him from becoming a convicted felon and registered sex offender. The MHP and defense attorney collaborated to offer the court and Jeremy's family an alternative to prosecution. The MHP consulted with the defense attorney, who explained that Jeremy had been a passive participant in the sexual attack. He was present in the bathroom but had no physical contact with the victim. He had simply been there with the wrong crowd, watching them show off their ability to have sex with girls at school. The MHP identified the fact that Jeremy was a passive participant as the "sweet spot" in the case, one that could be used to build and sustain a system of care to help control this sexually predatory form of school violence. The MHP communicated with all parties, including the principal, through brief phone calls; a Health Insurance Portability and Accountability Act (HIPAA)–compliant secure e-mail communication; and a Skype interview with the previous therapist, who was now working at another mental health agency in the area.

The comprehensive plan developed and proposed by the MHP included 1) family therapy alternately with the mother and the father and monthly mediation by family court for the parents; 2) weekly psychotherapy and psychiatric evaluation; 3) strict community monitoring; 4) recovery groups and a substance abuse group weekly; and 5) strictly enforced school attendance and daily monitoring by his father as a condition of being able to remain at home rather than being incarcerated. The defense attorney reached a plea deal that kept the charge in the juvenile court, and Jeremy was placed in a 4-month community residence program for adolescent sex offenders. The charge was continued (without a finding), contingent on 12 months of adherence to the probation plan.

Synchronization of Family, School, and Community Messages

As Jeremy's case illustrates (and as Nick's did earlier), the essential ingredient for conducting successful interventions in the home, school, and community is synchronization of the messages sent to children by adult role models about control, limits, and socially acceptable behavior at home and school. It is the harmonizing of these signals that contains the healing elements needed by children to begin developing internal control and to reduce their confusion when moving between their homes, schools, and communities. When the signals from all these different areas are mixed (as was true for Jeremy), a child becomes anxious and rigid and may engage in stereotypical behaviors that constitute misinterpretations of what is expected of the child in various settings. If the home environment is sending a permissive signal to the child while the school is more restrictive and authoritarian, that child may become confused and is likely to respond in a variety of ways that may be active or passive. In active responses, the child may be disruptive and fight against the rules at school, because at home she or he is allowed to behave in a different way. In more passive forms of response, the child may withdraw when she or he is confused, thus becoming more vulnerable to being targeted by kids at school. The child may be quite gregarious at home but may appear withdrawn in the more socially competitive school climate.

Therapeutic interventions need to begin by the identifying the signals sent to children from the home, school, and community. This establishes the foundation for creating a process or system of care designed to bring those messages together in a coherent and understandable way for the child. When the child receives the same message from school and home, it becomes easier to develop consistent rewards and consequences. When a child is given the same signal from the home, school, and community, that child will experience less conflict when deciphering the messages received at school. Children thrive on predictability and consistency, and this should be the goal of interventions: to unite schools, homes, and communities. The single most important goal of these interventions is to create a harmonious, positive signal for children about self-control, compassion, tolerance, and social interaction.

During the assessment phase, we strongly urge the MHP to pick up what the child in question is hearing from each of these social systems. For example, a child may be receiving messages that breaking the law is okay from his friends in the community. If this is permitted at home, it will surely follow the child to school. Similarly, if the child receives a message from home that listening to authority and following rules is not necessary, it will be difficult for the child to do so at school (or when out in the community), and the child will experience an increased risk of being pulled into criminal peer groups. This multilayered assessment format strives to understand how the child is receiving information from the world and creates strategies to harmonize these messages into a seamless, positive one that creates predictable and safe responses from key figures in the child's home, school, and community. Table 2–3 summarizes a number of typical family patterns seen in family assessment.

TABLE 2–3. Family assessment: common patterns

Seriously disabled but highly focused and motivated
Overinvolved parent, entitled child
Overwhelmed caretaker, little natural support
Traumatized caretaker, no support
Traumatized caretaker, state agency support
Antiauthoritarian parent who blames the school and defends child's aggression
Obsessed and successful parents who demand excellence
Homeless
Children in foster care or adoptive homes
Substance-addicted parent with full, partial, or recurrent pattern
Parent in supervised recovery
Incarcerated father, overwhelmed mother

Portals for Accessing Resources for Children With School Violence Problems

The source of a child's referral to the MHP is a key diagnostic factor that should begin the analysis of a school violence problem. There are a number of entrance points into a care delivery system, and knowing how a child's problem has been presented is critical to developing a multilayered plan. The primary ways a school violence problem can be referred are outlined in Table 2–4.

The entrance points shown in Table 2–4 are the most common origins of mental health referral for children with school violence problems. When a child enters a protective services portal, the MHP must begin planning all assessment or treatment strategies with the state agency case manager, the responsible party who has the legal authority to grant permission for any type of assessment or treatment; this is the state assuming the responsibility that is typically the sole domain of parents. The proactive MHP should begin the assessment by reviewing the needs identified by the child protective services agency and identifying which services are currently in the plan. After that step, the MHP starts to explore the home, school, and community, looking for both problems and resources.

Child protective services is a common portal for referral of children to mental health clinics or individual practitioners such as social workers, psychologists, psychiatric nurse specialists, and psychiatrists. Traditionally, MHPs would accept these referrals and begin a course of psychotherapy that may remain in

TABLE 2–4.   Common portals of mental health professional involvement with violent children

Evaluation requested by child protective services/juvenile justice system

Consultation initiated by family

Referral by school

Referral by primary care physician/pediatrician

Referral as part of stepdown from residential or institutional placement

Referral as part of aftercare for crisis intervention

---

the clinic or may extend into the home or school. The MHP is asked by the state agency case manager to engage the child and family in services as part of a larger plan of service designed to ensure that the child can live safely at home or in a substitute family. These referrals are often more complicated and frequently involve problems associated with school violence. Many children who initiate violence at school or who are targeted as victims, for instance, are already involved with a state agency because of child abuse or neglect. The evaluating clinician needs to understand the relationship between the family and the protective services agency and begin by working collaboratively with the protective services agency in designing school violence interventions. A key error we have observed in designing treatment involves the clinician becoming triangulated against the intervening child protective service agencies. Why? The family may have resentment and anger toward the child protective agency because they feel judged and their powers have been usurped. If clinicians are sucked into this triangle, they will alienate the referring protective services agent and become unable to function as an effective part of the care delivery system for the child.

A family may also refer a child to a clinician working in an outpatient setting because of a school problem. The problem may be that the child presents as either a victim or a perpetrator of violence, and family members are concerned that the child is at risk at home, in the community, or at school. The family in this type of referral is invested in the child's safety and well-being. These referrals may involve families who are already working cooperatively with the school, or they may be in conflict with the school. It is critical for the MHP to understand the status of the family's relationship with other subsystems in the community and to be especially vigilant in assessing the child when he or she is in school. When a family refers a child, the initial stages typically focus on the psychiatric and psychological needs of the child and involve a family consultation. In many cases, these referrals may come as a result of a specific problem, and the clinician must find the reason that the child is experiencing a problem in one of the subsystems. In these types of cases, clinicians are urged to expand their scope and to begin gathering information about what the child's life is like at home, at school, and in the community. It is from this perspective that the clinician can be most helpful to the family. A clinician might suggest strategies to decrease the unhealthy behavior and increase success and achievement at school.

The referral to an MHP may also come directly from a school. School guidance counselors often form relationships with outside providers or with individual practitioners in order to offer traditional clinical services to students exhibiting difficulties in their schools. There are a variety of mechanisms by which this can be achieved within the school, and how this is done often reflects a key element of the relationship between the school and the community. For example, some schools have active and collaborative relationships with outside providers; guidance counselors can be eager partners with outside clinicians, especially during the assessment and treatment phase of a school violence intervention. Other schools, however, may be more closed and may erect unhealthy barriers against outside resources interfering with their school activities. Thus, it is critical for a clinician to understand how the referral was made. When a school makes a referral, the clinician has increased access to the information about how school impacts the child's behavior and how the child impacts the school's climate. The clinician can work closely with the school and then move into the family to assess the harmony (or lack thereof) of the signals between both social systems.

An MHP may also receive a referral from a child's pediatrician or family practitioner because of a specific behavioral disturbance present or reported at the time of physical examination. The primary care physician may attempt a psychopharmacological intervention, such as the use of a stimulant or an antidepressant; he or she may also refer the parent to a mental health clinic or independent practitioner to evaluate the situation and to recommend a treatment strategy. In these cases, it is critical for the clinician to collect as much medication information and history as possible and to begin assessing the psychological and psychiatric needs of the child. The school typically is the third component of the assessment process and can be contacted and involved as soon as the clinician gains a better understanding of the presenting problem as identified by the primary care physician.

MHPs also may be referred a client who is being stepped down from a higher level of care or who is attempting to reenter school. The child may be coming from a residential program or inpatient setting and returning to the same school that he or she left, or the child may be entering a new school from a placement. In either case, this type of referral requires that the clinician assess the overall psychological and psychiatric problems and double-check the existing aftercare plans to ensure that the basic safety and psychological and psychiatric services are in place at the time of release. Many programs will discharge children back into the community with little preparation, and this is a sure way to destroy a child's chance of succeeding in the home, school, or community. Public schools have little choice but to attempt to educate children going through this transition. Aftercare is a critical and often overlooked component of maintaining the success gained in a treatment intervention. Unfortunately, it is often downplayed because of pressures from managed care or state budget cuts to stays in more expensive residential or inpatient settings.

The clinician may also be referred a child who is experiencing a psychiatric crisis and receiving emergency services interventions, either at an emergency room or a clinic. This type of evaluation in a crisis center or emergency department often results in a myopic focus on the crisis symptoms presented in a scattered and fragmented way. The crisis being evaluated is often the result of a poorly coordinated care plan that leaves the child in a disconnected and confusing place within the home, school, and community. This type of referral typically begins with ensuring that the child's psychological and psychiatric needs are being met, especially those involving psychiatric medications, and that therapy includes a crisis management plan. Also, the clinician should determine whether the child is receiving child protective services or is involved in the juvenile court. Once these foundations have been established, the clinician can begin to forge connections to the home and school to evaluate these areas of functioning and to design effective care plans.

Common Barriers to Effective Intervention

It is critical to understand that when developing a process that involves the overlapping of home, school, and community, the responsibility for creating a comprehensive plan is not solely that of the school. Every plan will encounter barriers due to a variety of reasons that need to be incorporated in any treatment plan (see Table 2–5). It is naive to assume that creating this plan is simple. This is a complicated process and requires that clinicians honestly evaluate the barriers and attempt to design strategies to overcome them.

A number of systemic boundaries can prevent the effective implementation of an integrated care plan for a child experiencing a disruption or violence problem at school. There are many competing agencies that often have difficulties working together and thus are unable to be linked in a seamless and coherent care plan. These systemic boundaries are typically historical and may reflect the competitiveness of today's service delivery landscape. Some agencies simply do not get along, and certain schools may feel insulated from the community or threatened by any intervention by outside resources. These systemic boundaries create barriers to effective care planning and need to be addressed in a positive and therapeutic fashion in order for an intervention to have its maximum impact.

TABLE 2–5.   Seven common barriers to sustained intervention

Systemic boundaries

Financial resources

Professional time

Transportation

Access to natural supports

Availability of community resources

Degree of motivation on the part of home or school

Of course, interventions cost money. It is critical for the clinician to become aware of financial resources that can be accessed within any family or community. The clinician has an expanded role in being challenged to overcome these barriers, making suggestions that might include having a child apply for Social Security, WIC, transitional assistance, or scholarships for community activities.[4] The clinician would be well advised to develop an ongoing repertoire of resource acquisition techniques. This becomes part of the care plan for any child involved in a school violence scenario. Overcoming financial barriers is not easy but is often possible, depending on the motivation of all parties. If the resource needed is not affordable, an alternative resource system may be constructed, with natural supports—such as aunts, uncles, and extended family members—providing some of the activities or resources needed.

Another key barrier to developing and implementing an effective care plan is the lack of availability of professional time to oversee care plans or to provide specific services in a coordinated fashion. In order to offer the most focused intervention, there needs to be a communication and service delivery processing mechanism that requires and obtains regular updates. Providers must be able to communicate with each other and must be in touch with formal and informal supports in the community in order to maximize the effectiveness of interventions within the home, school, and community. The limitation of professional time is a barrier that often interrupts the ability of a care plan to be implemented.

Transportation is probably the most formidable of all barriers to community activities. Often the child and family have the interest level and may be able to afford the fee to participate in a community activity, but they encounter difficulty in transporting the child to such activities. Transportation may be a very

---

[4]See Chapter 9, "Role of Medical Leadership in Unlocking Resources to Address School Violence," for more information on accessing resources such as the Women, Infants, and Children (WIC) nutrition program and disability benefits.

difficult hurdle to leap in any type of environment—urban, suburban, rural/industrialized, or rural. Many times the parents are busy at work, or they may simply lack the vehicles or finances to afford transportation. Public transportation is not typically an effective or universally reliable way for children to regularly participate in community activities or services.

Every family, however, has a network of "natural helpers" in the community or extended family. These supportive individuals are positive people who are involved with the child and family; they may be real assets in enhancing the child's adjustment to school. The family may be too proud to make contact with and work with natural helpers, or they may feel that they will be rejected if they express a need. The disconnection of natural supports from the needy child is a barrier to building strong and resilient plans within the community. Natural helpers are powerful resources in containing aggression, as well as in creating activities within the community and at home. When a child is enrolled in a program or activity that is supported by a natural helper, the child's resilience is enhanced. The motivation of a natural helper is altruism, and this adds a certain spiritual dimension to the power of the resource.

The availability of community resources may also be an issue. This is a greater problem in rural or rural/industrial areas. Within urban areas, there may be resources, but they may not be available for children with psychiatric and emotional problems. In these cases, specialized programs are required, but they may not be available to families because of a disconnection from agencies that supply funding, or because there is simply not enough funding to support these programs in general within the community. When budgets are tight, prevention and recreation programs are typically the first to be cut in municipal, state, and federal budgets.

The largest barrier that exists in coordinating home, school, and community is a lack of motivation on the part of any of the three subsystems. When a parent is not motivated to work with the school, or a school is defensive and not motivated to work with a parent, the ability to build a multilayered plan is blocked. Motivation is crucial in order to begin to build alliances that can focus on the children and begin to help them.

Conclusion

Interventions addressing school violence are not simple. They require a coordinated strategy involving different disciplines, state agencies, the family, and the school. The goal is for the student to receive a clear signal from all adults that self-control is critical, trying hard is important, and respecting oneself and others is necessary. Effective treatment plans require the MHP to thoroughly assess the school violence problem from a multidimensional perspective with a coordinated focus.

KEY CLINICAL CONCEPTS

- Therapeutic interventions target the interlocking systems of family, school, and community.

- The MHP should begin with the identified school problem experienced by a child.

- Effective assessment is multilayered and takes place in the community, the school, the home, and the clinician's office.

- Treatment plans require care, coordination, and supervision in order to be sustained and helpful in the various subsystems surrounding the child.

- There is a hierarchy of treatment needs, requiring a multidisciplinary assessment.

- A child needs to receive consistent signals that are synchronized among the key subsystems of home, school, and community.

- There are multiple entry points from which a child with a school violence problem may come to the attention of an MHP.

- All care coordination plans should incorporate strategies designed to overcome barriers that will interfere with sustained interventions.

References

American Psychiatric Association: Diagnostic and Statistical Manual of Mental Disorders, 4th Edition, Text Revision. Washington, DC, American Psychiatric Association, 2000

Brame B, Nagin DS, Tremblay RE: Developmental trajectories of physical aggression from school entry to late adolescence. J Child Psychol Psychiatry 42:503–512, 2001

Bruns EJ, Suter JC, Force MM, et al: Adherence to wraparound principles and association with outcomes. J Child Fam Stud 14:521–534, 2005

Farmer TW, Farmer EM, Estell DB, et al: The developmental dynamics of aggression and the prevention of school violence. J Emot Behav Disord 15:197–208, 2007

Felix ED, Furlong MJ, Austin G: The cluster analytic investigation of school violence victimization among diverse students. J Interpers Dynamics 24:1673–1695, 2009

Goldstein AJ, Solnit AJ, Goldstein, S, et al: The Best Interests of the Child: The Least Detrimental Alternative. New York, Free Press, 1996

Hirte C: The relationship between socioeconomic status and child abuse and neglect in South Australia. Research Unit presentation at the Australian Institute of Family Studies (AIFS) Conference, 2010. Available at: http://www.aifs.gov.au/conferences/aifs11/docs/hirte.pdf. Accessed March 20, 2011.

Oliver RD, Nims DR, Hughey AW, et al: Case management wraparound expenses: five-year study. Adm Policy Ment Health 25:477–491, 1998

Praed Foundation: Child and Adolescent Needs and Strengths (CANS) Comprehensive Multisystem Assessment Manual. Chicago, IL, The Praed Foundation, 1999. Available at: http://www.praedfoundation.org/CANS%20Comprehensive%20Manual.pdf. Accessed March 20, 2011.

Pullmann MD, Kerbs K, Koroloff N, et al: Juvenile offenders with mental health needs: reducing recidivism using wraparound. Crime Delinq 52:375–397, 2006

Reid JA: The latent class typology of juvenile victims and exploration of risk factors and outcomes of victimization. Crim Justice Behav 36:1001–1024, 2009

Rose CA, Espelage DL, Monda-Amaya LE: Bullying and victimization rates among students in general and special education: a comparative analysis. Educational Psychology 29:761–776, 2009

Trickett PK, Aber JL, Carlson V, et al: Relationship of socioeconomic status to the etiology and developmental sequelae of child abuse. Dev Psychol 27:148–158, 1991

Twemlow SW, Fonagy P, Sacco FC: Feeling safe in school. Smith Coll Stud Soc Work 72:303–326, 2002

Wasserman GA, Keenan K, Tremblay RE, et al: Risk and protective factors of child delinquency. Office of Juvenile Justice Prevention Bulletin, April 2003. Available at: http://www.ncjrs.gov/pdffiles1/ojjdp/193409.pdf. Accessed December 3, 2010.

Wechsler D: Wechsler Intelligence Scale for Children—Fourth Edition (WISC-IV). London, Pearson Assessment, 2004

3

Providing Mental Health Consultation to Agencies Intervening With Violent Children

SCHOOLS are always faced with the difficult choices of whom to educate and in what fashion. When resources are scarce, education becomes a privilege and not an absolute right. The more developed countries have a more complex problem than their less developed counterparts. In the United States, for instance, there are very complicated structures and processes that direct how a school district handles "difficult" (mostly violent and disruptive) students. There are also complex systems of care that exist in the community, funded by the government or community, to assist in the care of violent and disruptive students. The mental health professional (MHP) in this type of environment has a different set of steps to take when managing a violent or disruptive student. Countries where no such formal structures and processes exist run the risk of creating a permanent, oppressed underclass that will begin to disconnect from civil society, emerging later as the community's "young guns" or violent young recruits, often inaccessible to reason. These countries share the same initial processes with their more resource-rich counterparts, but the less formal the systems and processes are, the more the MHP has to adapt to working with natural social supports. In both cases, the successful intervention involves reaching out to the community for help. The violent or disruptive student often either has a medical condition or lives in a social system that blocks his or her ability to function in a school setting.

There are many good reasons to either expel or educate certain students in public schools. The decision for administrators in schools is whether potential harm is clearly presented to the general safety and education of the other students by allowing the violent or disruptive student in that school. The MHP plays a special role in advising the school's leaders about the risks and threats presented by a student's behavior. This assessment will require the development of a risk and protective factor equation. If the risks cannot be balanced, then the ability of the school to educate violent or disruptive students is reduced. (For a more detailed discussion regarding risk and threat assessment, see Chapters 6, "Children Need to Feel Safe to Learn," and 10, "Risk and Threat Assessment of Violent Children.") The more support that can be activated within the school and community, the greater the likelihood of successful education becomes for the general student population.

The Consultation Process: Working With Interagency Teams and Schools

Before directly examining the MHP's role in working with health service agencies and schools, it will be useful to take a careful look at how the process of consultation works in an interagency setting. The work of Goodstein (1983) and of Petti and Salguero (2005), as well as our own work (Sklarew et al. 2004; Twemlow and Sacco 2003), suggests a number of characteristics of health service agencies that the MHP should be well aware of before beginning. First of all, each agency will tend to operate as if its patients have a single isolated problem that can be solved by the agency autonomously. This may be a result of the type of leadership within the agency that tries to keep morale up by exaggerating the importance of its own role in the community. It is important to remember that the agency's shortcomings are problem- rather than person-oriented. Today's dehumanized business-style model has caused many difficulties because people respond to problems in a variety of idiosyncratic ways. When there are charismatic leaders and a cohesive element within the organization, an individual may be forced into a model that does not suit the employees.

TABLE 3–1. Rating mentalization

Mentalization item	Description	Rating (1–10)
Reflectiveness	Think before you act	—
Empathy	For self and others and with feeling	—
Affect	Control storms of affect—be aware	—
Reestablish self-agency	Assertively stand up for yourself	—
Put boundaries in place	Reestablish your independent self	—

Facilitating Mentalization

In a violent setting, many of the responsibilities of the leader role must be taken over by a competent MHP, especially since the adults who care for the child or the children may themselves be so overwhelmed with trauma that their mental processes are exhausted or irrational. We call this "the collapse of mentalization" (Fonagy et al. 2002). *Mentalization* refers to the process in which the individual is *not* operating under the "freeze, flight, fight, or fright" (Bracha 2004) fear-based stress reaction first described by Cannon (1915) and thus can make logical choices based on an interpersonal perception of reality rather than on fear-based personal choices. The mind of a nonmentalizing person has trouble organizing itself.

Therefore, the MHP must be able to quickly assess the degree to which an individual is able to mentalize and whether that individual will be able to create the necessary links to the services he or she needs. The checklist in Table 3–1 can be helpful in conducting a quick assessment of mentalization skills. Patients can also use this rating scale to monitor themselves.

Improving Interagency Communication

The MHP must also become acutely aware that there is a lack of interdependence between agencies. He or she will also find that conflict is managed by smoothing over—rather than resolving—differences, even avoiding them to preserve the status quo of the workplace. It is crucial to avoid having employees of the agency feel they are entering situations where their jobs may be jeopardized. The damage that may have resulted from earlier failures in interagency communication is best confronted by putting aside the present and going forward into the future with a stronger model designed to improve communication and efficiency. What tends to happen if MHPs are not aware of these issues is that they will personalize problems and become angry and fairly useless advocates for their clients and patients.

Fostering Awareness of Countertransference

Like it or not, MHPs must have awareness of their own unconscious processes in order to be effective. The MHP often has to participate in and absorb the (often disturbingly chaotic) experiences of both sides, searching for a common psychological ground. This process can sometimes lead to a temporary loss of contact with a neutral perspective as the MHP moves in and out of the advocacy role.

Without an awareness of countertransference, the MHP may be pulled into an advocacy role for one side only. Personal consultation is very important for MHPs in such situations, and supervision, including psychoanalytically informed psychotherapeutic treatment for the MHP, is often tremendously valuable.

Psychological Aspects of Mental Health Consultation

We are not the first researchers to note how a mental health consultant's role is often blurred, especially when dealing with situations that can lead to school violence (Petti and Salguero 2005). The consultation can focus on the individual, on the case, on the program, or on the leader. When the consultant finishes, there is no obligation on the school to use any of the information from that consultation. The MHP has two main challenges: problem solving and the transformation of the participants through the development of mutual trust, defined as the knowledge that employers and co-workers will not harm you (Jacques 1998). The true essence of transformation is that each side becomes able to see and appreciate—or *mentalize*—the other's point of view. The key negotiation principles as enumerated by Sklarew et al. (2004) in their Introduction are as follows:

1. To establish a point of similarity between participants that allows for tolerance of differences in others and acceptance of negatives.
2. To develop the habit of initially discussing nonconflictual issues to help establish a common ground and agreement before addressing complex problems.
3. To develop personal relationships and perceptions of each other so that the people and the process become humanized.
4. To establish mutual respect for differences with the potential to trigger racial, religious, gender, or ethnic stereotypes.
5. To develop an agreed-upon common language to communicate ideas.
6. To understand that the process will require continued maintenance.
7. To recognize that only a collaborative nonblaming rather than competitive partnership will result in change.

Development of a Collaborative Plan

Step One: Making Contact and Respecting Boundaries

The first step in a collaborative plan is to understand the relative roles of certain individuals within the various social systems at home, school, and community. It would be difficult, for instance, for an outside clinician to enter a school and act as a school counselor. An outside clinician is ordinarily viewed as just that: someone outside of the school's social system with no ongoing contact with the frontline teachers and administrators. Even when the outside clinician is associated with child protective services, there is a limit to what that clinician can do within the school system without the cooperation of a clinical partner within the school, one deeply committed to the same treatment goals.

It is also true that clinicians who work within a school are not able to develop as many resources as may be needed to respond to the child's problem. For example, the school's psychologist will not necessarily have access to a psychiatrist or a prescribing nurse practitioner. Not only is it important to find a resource, but the school's clinician needs to get permission from parents or guardians in order to connect the child or young adult to some type of program or intervention resource before, during, and after school. School clinicians need to be aware that often schools have to pay for the care if they make the direct referral.

The clinician working outside of the school must forge connections within the school with a clinician or school administrator in order to begin to understand and respond to a problem that is expressed at school, in the home, or the community. Many clinicians may try to diagnose and treat a problem that is acted out within the school solely in their clinics or treatment rooms. This approach is one that will quickly lead to an abstraction of the problem and will not offer the clinician the power of accessing real-time information concerning the impact of their intervention within the school system. Again, a clinician working in the community will need to seek permission and obtain signed releases to communicate with the school concerning the strategies that are being designed to respond to the problem of violence within the school.

Case Example: Tony, Family Caretaker and Bullying Victim at School

Tony, an eighth-grade student, had missed 92 days of a 180-day school year. Child protective services were contacted by the school, and the family received visits from a state case worker. The case worker then referred the family to a community mental health clinic in order to intervene with this problem. Tony was allowed to stay in school, and the family was referred to a home-based mental health clinic in order to assess why this child did not go to school, as well as to create strategies that would reduce the absenteeism.

Initially, the assessment pointed to a pathological family dynamic that included a chronically ill mother relying on the support of her only son in managing her illness. The net result of this problem was a year in which the student missed a considerable amount of school. Earlier in the year, it was reported that Tony experienced a great deal of bullying because of his lack of social skills, his unkempt appearance, and his difficulty in learning. It was easy for this student to remain at home, since when he did go to school he was frequently attacked both verbally and physically.

The mental health intervention began with several home visits in which the dynamics of keeping Tony home from school were explored, with his two sisters and his mother participating in a family therapy plan. At the same time, the community clinician sought permission from the intervening child welfare workers who had gained custody through the court to communicate with the school. The community clinician quickly realized that there were no active social workers in that particular school and that the vice principal was unmotivated to participate in a community-focused plan. At this point, the community clinician was working regularly with the family members in their home twice a week in order to stabilize the crisis that had precipitated the referral. Family therapy alone was not enough to improve Tony's attendance record. The community clinicians also sought the help of the child protective agency case worker, who had experienced a similar roadblock in accessing an internal social worker or guidance counselor to assist in developing a strategy to increase attendance.

Tony was eventually removed from his parents' custody and placed in a residential school. There were notably few opportunities to reintegrate him into the community school due to the inability of the community clinicians to latch onto a partner within the school to begin a collaborative effort to motivate Tony to attend school. The clinicians were very active in confronting the student's mother. While Tony's mother became aware of her unconscious demands to keep the child at home, there was no change in the overall treatment the child felt at the school. The net result was that the overall intervention was a failure and did not result in the child being able to remain in the community and be educated.

After the 45-day diagnostic assessment at the residential school, Tony was returned home and the therapy began again. The diagnostic assessment recommended placement in a different community school. Once this shift in school occurred, the community clinicians collaborated with the school social worker and began a plan that involved Tony in an extracurricular school activity. Tony had a passionate interest in computers, and the school was able to place him in programs of high interest. This was followed up when a member of the community team identified an after-school apprenticeship in a local computer store. The students developed a relationship with the repair person at the computer shop and also earned a small amount of money. The net effect of the intervention was then that the student began to go back to school, asserted himself, did not fall into the role of victim at the school, and had high-interest activities that stabilized him both at home and in the community.

The outside community team was able to focus on assisting Tony's mother to obtain personal care assistance so that she had a professional caretaker to replace the help that her son had given her over the course of the year. While the student in this case was a victim and did not act violently within the school, the principles of approaching the intervention illustrate the value of the MHP's role, both inside the school and in the community. When those two parts of the intervention are synchronized, the net result is a more comprehensive strategy that will improve stabilization both in the school and in the home. The student in this example was targeted by students who were being bullies and disrupting social activities at school. This made it easy for the victim to be pulled into a family dynamic that led to his missing school.

We recommend using instruments capable of assessing the family's strengths and weaknesses in a variety of domains. One such instrument that is widely used is the Child and Adolescent Needs and Strengths (CANS) Comprehensive Multisystem Assessment (Praed Foundation 1999), which Massachusetts adopted as part of its Children's Behavioral Health Initiative remedy in settlement of a class action lawsuit over Early Periodic Screening, Diagnosis, and Treatment (EPSDT) services to Medicaid-eligible children with serious emotional disturbances (Massachusetts Behavioral Health Partnership 2010). The Massachusetts initiative, grounded in a comprehensive multidimensional CANS assessment, embodies the spirit of EPSDT for young people exhibiting school violence problems. Similar federal court initiatives are active in at least seven other states, and new litigation in this area is spreading rapidly across the country (Perkins 2009). In fact, this model is likely to soon become the standard used by states when they create systems of care for children with serious emotional disturbances.

Step Two: Defining the Problem

Regardless of the MHP's entrance point into a school violence problem, there needs to be some assessment of why violence is erupting at school. One approach to assessing the nature of a school violence problem is to search for the areas in which shame may be fueling a school violence problem. This approach is valuable because it can be applied to both the individuals and groups who make up the populations of schools. When a school system "allows" children to be bullied, but adults see it as a normal part of childhood, a situation is created in which violence is condoned by the adults. As a result, children are victimized by bullying with repetitive public shaming in the school setting. Assisting someone who is either a bully or a victim in this type of school would be difficult if the school was not willing to address some of the climate issues that impact how the child experiences every day at school. It may seem grandiose for outside clinicians to hope that they will be able to convince an entire school to change the way children behave on a daily basis. Nevertheless, the points of shame often become clear pressure points that must be relieved. A child may show aggressive behavior at home and the parent experiences trouble controlling that child's behavior with younger siblings. This might be a reenactment of a situation that begin at school and unfolds once the student comes home. Simply applying family therapy to solve the problems at home will not change the fact that the student has to go to school every day. Once there, he or she will continue to experience humiliation and may either explode or withdraw.

A recent research experiment in Jamaica (Twemlow et al., in press) described how a humiliation "pressure point" was identified and a program targeted the genesis of the coercive behavior. We identified shame originating from the placement of older students who had failed the sixth-grade streaming exam. The older students had lost hope, were perceived as worthless, and engaged in aggressive behaviors with themselves and the younger children as a result. The intervention in this Jamaican school was designed based on an understanding that the shame began during seventh grade because of academic failure. The intervention specifically targeted the older students in seventh, eighth, and ninth grades and involved creating arts and crafts under the careful supervision of supportive adults. The net effect of this intervention over 3 years was a large reduction in violence within the social system. In fact, the younger children in the school experienced significant benefits without having had any exposure to any content of the intervention. Intervening in a social system at a point of shame will create positive results by reducing the humiliation experience and thus removing some of the fuel involved in the school violence. There was a "trickle down" effect of positive energy by reducing shame and creating a sense of value in the older youth.

An MHP must remember that it is virtually impossible for children who live in homes that are unstable, chaotic, and unsafe to come to school and not become either bullies or victims. This again seems rather commonsensical, but often is ignored or overlooked in terms of specific interventions within a school system. Most school counselors are aware of the nuances of a student's violent behavior within the schools, but they may be blind to or uninformed about the nature of the child's experience living at home. The child may be a victim of child abuse or domestic violence, may often be left unsupervised with his or her basic needs neglected, or may be the victim of a sibling or predator living within the home.

All of these circumstances are sufficient to create a high-risk situation for a child that can, in turn, become the catalyst for school violence. In the United States, schools are among the primary reporters of child abuse to state agencies. This is a clear example of how the community and the school are linked in a process that has as its primary target the identification of child abuse in the home. Children who are abused at home frequently will act out this abuse in school. When someone from the school initiates a child abuse report, an outside investigator will be assigned to visit the child's home and to look into the concerns expressed by the school about the child's behavior.

Once the child protective services agency investigates a case and identifies a chaotic home, a series of steps is taken to protect the child. The family may be required to develop an individual service plan, monitored by the state and courts, providing an opportunity to deal with the problems that have led to the child's aggressive, disruptive, or violent behavior. This generally involves a referral to a community agency that will intervene with the family to reduce the impact of the chaotic home life on the child. Once again, this is a point at which the idea of collaboration between MHPs within and outside of the school becomes critical to the development of a comprehensive and sustainable intervention that will decrease school violence. If the community intervention consists of a referral to a psychiatrist who then provides medication to the parent and/or child, this may result in a temporary improvement of behavior with little sustained growth and improvement in how the child functions at school. In other words, the child may be less aggressive because of a psychopharmacological intervention, but the prescribing physician will not have access to vital real-time information about the impact of the medication on the child's performance at school. Additionally, the school will not be kept regularly informed about the variety of interventions or strategies used in approaching the family to solve problems in a less aggressive and dysfunctional way.

Students who act aggressively at school may be experiencing a serious emotional disorder that is a result of trauma experienced in the community or home. Children who live in violent neighborhoods and are required to traverse dangerous territory to get to school, for example, may be hypersensitive to risk and may act aggressively at school in response to this sensitivity. Children with anxiety conditions who enter school worrying about every aspect of their behavior will become easy targets for bullies and aggressive students. One of the key premises in this approach is built on the idea that the co-created roles of bully, victim, and bystander are involved in the evolution of violence at school. Responding to aggressive children must include a consideration of the role of the victim and how his or her behavioral or mental health problems impact the school climate.

Step Three: Synchronizing Community Agencies Involved in Managing School Violence

As we have mentioned, children who are violent at school are frequently connected to a variety of community agencies. There are three main areas of connection that need to be synchronized for children experiencing violence who are also aggressive at school (see Table 3–2).

Child Protective Services

The first main area often involved in cases of school violence is child protective services. In the United States, this is a very complicated system composed of

TABLE 3–2. Community agencies involved in managing school violence

Service category	Area of responsibility	School violence impact
Child protective services	Home safety and basic caretaking	Reenactments of home trauma, oppositionalism, absenteeism
Juvenile justice system	Criminal activities at home, at school, or in the community	Fighting, assault, gangs, drug distribution, extortion
Mental health and human services	Support for families with mental impairments	Disruption, impulsivity, explosiveness, being a victim

partnerships between the federal government and individual states. Each state develops a plan and regulations concerning how child abuse and neglect investigations and case management will be handled. This function is very well developed and is part of the state agency structure. The child protective agencies act as a backup for the parental responsibility to protect children. In many cases, the state intervenes through a child protective services agency and removes the child from the biological parents' custody, thereby assuming responsibility for the care and safety of the child. In these cases, the state becomes the child's legal guardian and the child may live in a variety of different settings, including private or state-run foster homes.

The children in this category are also frequently connected to a wide range of services within the mental health and human services systems. These services often are part of an individualized service plan designed by the state as an attempt to enhance safety and basic caretaking skills within the biological home. The child protective agency is typically represented by a case worker who is part of a larger agency structure responsible for the management of children who go to school. In many urban public schools within the United States, a significant percentage of students are in this situation. A child protective agency may be involved in a supportive fashion—meaning that they are providing services and support for parents who are struggling to care for their children—or may have full legal custody of the children. It is critical in designing strategies from either inside the school or out in the community to know who is legally responsible for the child and to begin any intervention strategy by contacting the responsible party. If this party is a parent, then he or she needs to be the first person contacted by the MHP. If the state agency has had custody granted to it by the court, then this is the first phone call that needs to be made in order to establish both permission and the critical involvement of the responsible party. This is especially true as the aggression increases in school and the violent behaviors escalate to a life-threatening point.

Child protective agencies frequently are held responsible for child behaviors that can be seen as reenactments of the trauma experienced in either the home or the community. These reenactments may be highly sexualized in cases of children who are sexually abused over long periods of time. The chaotic home can also be reflected in school through bullying behavior, which is then modeled by a child who has lived in a home impacted by domestic violence. Children raised in such homes see dominance and aggression as the way in which people relate to each other. The child often identifies with either the bully or the victim role. In these cases, the child's reenactment at school is the direct result of the trauma experienced in his or her home life.

Our experience is that boys who have been abused will often become abusers when grown up, whereas girls tend to direct the rage at themselves with self-destructive actions like eating disorders, self-cutting and suicide attempts.

In addition, we have noticed a behavioral pattern in chaotic homes consisting of either overly active or overly passive styles of responding. In other words, children will tend toward the extremes of being either a bully or a victim. Although many children attempt to hang back and play the role of bystander, the intensity of the trauma makes it virtually impossible for them to resist being sucked into one of these pathological roles in school. Children who are living in traumatic multicrisis homes with marginal caretakers frequently stay home from school. Such absenteeism can be seen at one end of the continuum of acting out the problems in their homes at school. Being trapped at home with caretakers who disregard the value of the child's education is a passive form of school violence. When these children do return to school, they either become fodder for a bully's ongoing patterns of humiliating others or become bullies themselves, aggressively asserting dominance at school.

Juvenile Justice System

The second major agency that a child with violence problems is likely to be attached to is the juvenile justice system. This occurs in countries that differentiate between crimes committed by youth under a certain age and adults. This is a highly variable protocol, one that reflects the basic values of the culture within which a school exists. In the United States, for example, a separation exists between the juvenile justice system and child protective services. This split in state agency responsibility reflects an overall attempt to separate the oppositional and defiant child from the more impulsive and aggressive criminal youth. The juvenile justice system is typically engaged when a young person commits a crime. In the child protective services agencies, the offenders are typically exhibiting oppositional and defiant behaviors rather than violating the rights or property of others. When a student's behavior rises to the level of criminality, the court will adjudicate the child a delinquent and typically attach him or her to a probation officer or case manager.

MHPs are well advised to understand how the community in question handles situations. The MHP needs to discover whether or not the community understands the difference between an oppositional offense and a criminal offense or conduct disorder. Once this *is* understood, the MHP needs to involve the representative from the juvenile justice system in any and all planning of interventions. In some cases, young people who are found to be delinquent and are managed by the juvenile justice system still live in the community and attend public schools. If the severity of their aggression or the repetitions of their crimes increase, these children are typically separated from the community. Such offenders are often referred to secure facilities and are often connected to programs such as community monitoring and day reporting. The more violent the crime, the less access to the community the student will have.

Mental Health and Human Services

The third major system critical to all school interventions is mental health and human services. In the United States, these services can be financed by local government; state, federal, and local partnerships such as Medicaid; and private foundations. Some communities may rely on natural helpers who exist in the school or the community. Family physicians may also be key players in the management of school violence problems. There are considerable differences among states and within states; some are highly resourced, with services delivered in myriad ways. The typical school violence problem referred to MHPs involves impulsivity associated with attention-deficit/hyperactivity disorder (ADHD) or other mental impairments, explosiveness, and associated psychiatric disturbances resulting from exposure to trauma. The MHP may be trying to assist the family in solving this problem, or may be asked by a school to help in assessing a specific problem within a school.

Some children need to be protected and their basic needs supplied by substitute caretakers. These children will reenact their trauma at home actively or passively. In the active form, this reenactment typically involves oppositional and defiant behavior. The passive form is likely to be absenteeism or an abrupt, chronic discontinuation of efforts toward achievement goals. In the juvenile justice system, the behaviors that children exhibit in school are more easily addressed, since they involve clear crimes. It is not bullying when somebody physically assaults someone else in a hallway, regardless of their age. Once that line has been crossed, bullying behaviors clearly become criminal actions. In the middle school and high school years, criminal behavior begins exhibiting itself

TABLE 3–3. Process for connecting and managing community resources

Assess nature and locus of problem	Home
	School
	Community
	Child protection, juvenile justice, mental health
Join the social system	Connect with in-school or community contact
	Understand the family's view
	Create buy-in from within school and family
Identify supports	Seek out formal services and programs
	Identify natural helpers
	Discover community resources and activities
Create strategies to access support	Identify barriers
	Make contact
	Manage involvement from inside and outside

at the school in the form of gang initiation, drug distribution, extortion, and threats of violence.

Step Four: Coordinating and Managing Community Resources

Once an MHP understands the custodial landscape, regardless of levels of affluence, and understands who is legally and physically responsible for the child exhibiting the aggressive behavior, the process of coordinating and managing community resources can begin (see Table 3–3). An MHP is not always responsible for being the primary case manager or the individual in charge of decision making; the MHP may also function in a supporting role. The key point for the MHP is to understand who the leader is and what the overall nature of the intervention plan is, in order to be able to make suggestions, offer support and services, or deliver direct or indirect services.

The first step in creating the process summarized in Table 3–3 is to assess the nature and locus of the problem behavior. This assessment is designed to identify areas of weaknesses and strengths that can be used to create a more harmonious signal, helping the child build internal self control. The intervention is designed to create a unified front in the adult-authority world that will increase a child's ability to internalize and exercise self-restraint.

The question that needs to be asked is whether the aggressive behavior occurs in one setting or in multiple settings. When a child behaves aggressively only at school and not at home or in the community, the probability is that the child is receiving signals from the school—most often unwittingly—that encourage dysregulation and do not offer opportunities for attachment to supportive adult/peer figures or activities. It may be clear through the clinical interventions that a child is experiencing bullying, being a bully, or observing considerable amounts of disturbing bullying or violence at school. This may be a primary factor in the child's aggression at school. When a behavior occurs in all three settings, there is a strong likelihood of a biological basis (e.g., autism spectrum disorders) that needs to be ruled out prior to creating more sophisticated psychosocial interventions. Children with intermittent explosive disorder or with some forms of temporal lobe epilepsy will erupt in any setting and will require medication to regain self-control.

If a child's parents have custody, they must be the first point of contact for any intervention into aggressive behaviors at school. Often, in more active situations, parents are involved in school aggression only through disciplinary dialogue. The student will act out at school, the teacher will expel him or her from class, someone from the school administration will be responsible for managing discipline, and then the parent is called either to pick up the child or to somehow respond to the problem at school. Parents need to be involved at two other levels: first, as partners in collaborating on a solution to the specific problem presented by their child, and second, in any and all processes that are designed to improve the climate of the school. Parents of children who exhibit either active or passive school violence difficulties are excellent candidates for involvement in school climate improvement campaigns. They can be encouraged to cooperate with the school through involvement in activities that promote positive school climates, rather than blaming the school for their child's unruliness.

The second step in managing community resources is to "join the social system." This phase is something that MHPs are trained to do when dealing with families. The principles of family therapy stress the ongoing need to ensure that the therapist is in step with the family before making recommendations to change any direction or approach to a problem within a family. Minuchin (1974) referred to this process as "joining" a family system. Therapists look for the "sweet spot" in the family that allows them to be included in the flow of the family social system. The same principle is true in dealing with management of multiple agencies for the child experiencing aggression at school. The "sweet spot" in a family can be viewed by everyone as supportive of the family as a whole without being against anyone else. A family might be powered by an aggressive child, a rebellious or criminal adolescent, or an impaired parent. The MHP, like the family therapist, must first "hook" or create therapeutic "buy in" with the power source.

Case Example: The Gibsons, a Troubled Family Helped Through Interagency Collaboration

The Gibson family consists of a single mother and three children. The oldest child, a 14-year-old male, was referred for chronic truancy and was expelled from school for fighting and for destruction of property. The middle child was a 10-year-old female honor student, and the youngest child was a 5-year-old female just beginning kindergarten. She was very shy and the favorite of the older brother when he was at home. The therapist quickly realized that the "sweet spot" was between the youngest child and the oldest boy. The mother was an overwhelmed and depressed woman of 42 working as an assistant in a nursing home. After the oldest child was referred to the juvenile court for truancy, the family was visited at home, with all members attending the session. A limited release was signed between the family and the juvenile probation department. Another "sweet spot" was between the school, client, and probation officer.

With school attendance in mind as the desired outcome, the therapist developed a relationship with the youngest child with the mother's assistance. Eventually, the troubled brother was drawn into the family discussions. A meeting was scheduled between the probation officer, therapist, and mother. The clinician made an arrangement with the probation department to ease restrictions based on increasingly successful days at school. The therapist followed up with a meeting at school to create a special arrangement. The special education department created a plan that was very flexible, allowing the student to attend only high interest classes and to come and leave school early. His mother agreed to provide special transportation.

The MHP must develop a clear understanding of the problem from the school's perspective without becoming trapped in a power struggle with any distinct social system. This particular obstacle is referred to by Bowen (Kerr and Bowen 1988) as "triangulation," or a process of systems being played against one another. The MHP needs to be sensitive to power issues and boundaries and needs to maintain the focus of the intervention on one clear message to the student. This starts by building the "buy in"—that is, a shared feeling among all staff, students, and family members that the school needs to change. School violence is a direct result of a failure in one of this key system's responses to a particular child at a crucial time in his or her educational development.

The third step in this management process is to identify community supports. This is an area in which the MHP can be extremely helpful to both the home and the school. Whether the resources are formal or informal, the MHP is responsible for searching the community to find sources of help. This may be a formal process with many organized agencies delivering a variety of services, or it might involve searching the community for an internship or other outlet for a student whose misdirected energy is leading to aggression at school. Identifying supports is the role of the MHPs, regardless of where they are positioned in the school or the community. Community clinicians have more expertise in reaching out into their respective service landscapes to identify and engage available services. In some more informal settings, school counselors or natural helpers within the community can be contacted to request their involvement in providing needed support to a child who may be acting aggressively in the community. Most communities have private agencies through churches, social activities, and other groups that offer many helping opportunities for needy young people.

The fourth step is to create strategies for accessing these supports. This is a process involving identification of a resource, followed by targeting any barriers to accessing those resources. In all cases, strategies need to be developed by adults to look for and engage natural supports in the community. This is also true within the school itself. Schools need to be challenged to examine their own formal and informal structures to develop supports that could be woven into any intervention designed to reduce the types of aggression that occur at school. Creating databases on resources would be one obvious example, and can lead to more effective future interventions to assist students and to create a safe overall environment for the general population.

Step Five: Creating a Goal-Focused Action Plan

Once the MHP is satisfied that everything possible has been done to understand the aggressive behavior exhibited at school, he or she needs to develop an action plan with certain goals that can be accomplished by activating the various elements identified in the community, home, and school. These interventions have a set of goals specifically designed to cope with the evolution of aggression in the school and are what MHPs work toward achieving in their treatment plans (see Table 3–4).

Contain Aggression

The first intervention goal is containment of the aggression, meaning the MHP must design concrete ways in which school personnel, transportation workers, and other school employees can be protected from the eruption of aggression during the school day or during transportation to and from school. Containment is a strategy in which the behavior is clearly identified and a pattern established regarding how the aggression may unfold in the course of a school day (see also Chapter 5, "Bullying is a Process, Not a Person"). Containment strategies specifically target these behaviors and use prevention to quickly smother

TABLE 3–4. Creating an action plan: intervention goals

Strategy	Goal
Contain aggression	Home and school discouraging coercion
	Parents supporting teachers
	Teachers modeling socially desirable behavior
	In-school detention
Redirect focus	Creating positive adult mentors
	Identifying positive, high-interest activities
	Rewarding positive behavior
Reduce pressure	Changing schedules
	Offering breaks
	Eliminating frustration-inducing activities
	Promoting involvement in extracurricular or after-school activity
Prevent shame	Learning and assessment accommodations
	Eliminating public discipline
	Active bullying prevention
	Managing cyberbullying
Value nonviolence	Public awards for compassion
	Art and theater with positive, nonviolent messages
	Climate campaigns that focus on nonviolence and character building

any bullying or aggression that may be occurring at any time during the school day or when a child is going to and from school. It is these strategies that strive to eliminate aggressive behavior through quick response and coordinated efforts to send a very clear signal to the child that out-of-control behavior will not be tolerated and that internal controls are necessary. This can be a very complex plan involving many different parties, or it could simply be the work of a single classroom teacher with the help of an outside MHP.

In order to contain aggressive and disruptive behavior, it is critical that the home and school be on the same page regarding tolerable levels of aggression during the school day. If a parent has a different set of values than the school does, the child receives a mixed signal, and containing aggression at school will become increasingly difficult. If the school points a finger at the family as the sole source of the problem, it will be more difficult to help the school and home work together regarding the student's behavior. This process can be understood as a dialectic of victim/victimizer in which the school and the home engage in unconscious power struggles that will determine the responses to the student's aggression at school. It is essential that both home and school send the child the same message about assuming responsibility for the student's control of his or her behavior at school. Interventions that promote the harmony of the signal from both parent and school will have the best chance of reducing aggression or disruption at school, and that includes awareness of countertransference by the MHP.

One concrete way of achieving a coordination of home and school signals about aggression is to have the parents available to support the teachers in their struggle to maintain control of the classroom. When a parent works directly with a teacher concerning specific behaviors, then the child receives a clear and direct limit that is essential for preventing the evolution of aggression in school. Parents can also show support for the teacher by participating in climate interventions that model positive adult behavior. When a child sees his or her mother or father working with teachers in a collaborative way to improve the quality of the school environment, the child receives an unmistakable message that coercion is unacceptable and that working for the common good is a way to receive positive attention. Another strategy that fosters containment in the schools is to create programs in which teachers are provided with rewards and incentives for encouraging prosocial behavior in children. When teachers are seen in this natural leadership role, the children are more likely to follow the model.

Schools can also develop ways to contain eruptions of aggression; each school may have an entire program dedicated to discipline and the implantation of school and classroom rules. These systems may or may not be of assistance in containing aggressive behaviors. Many school protocols and procedures may, in fact, unwittingly provoke and sustain the evolution of aggression within the school settings. Schools are advised to develop containment strategies that do not offer the child the opportunity to leave school as a punishment for disruption and/or small amounts of aggression. When a student crosses the line and engages in criminal activity, the school is advised to involve law enforcement and to create protective barriers between the youth committing the criminal activity and the overall school population.

How this violent student is reintegrated back into the school, however, is another question. The principle of containment concerns how a school manages small eruptions of aggression and disruption through use of programs such as in-school suspension, after-school disciplinary activities, or other approaches. One such strategy uses an approach that emphasizes insight and shared responsibility rather than punishment, focusing on classmates managing each other to some extent. For example, the classroom may be quiet when the teacher is there but erupt into chaos when he or she leaves (punishment focused). Discipline is an internalized state a child learns by modeling, mainly through teachers and other members of the classroom (insight focused). We have seen students impose their own limitations on their impulsive actions. Even though it is true that children—probably even as high as twelfth grade—are primarily in school to have fun, teachers and parents may instead wrongly assume that the child is there to work. In fact, teachers who make schoolwork fun are usually the teachers with the best class academic performance and (certainly in our experience) are the ones students remember for the rest of their lives.

The following example illustrates two ways of dealing with small eruptions of aggression or disruption in the classroom. A spitball hits a teacher as she is writing on the blackboard. She turns around furiously, picks out "Billy" immediately (since he has done this before), and sends him off to the principal. This would be a punishment-focused event that "scapegoats" Billy. A more peaceful way of managing this situation might play out as follows: As the spitball hits the teacher, she puts down her marker, turns to the classroom and says, "Everybody stop working. What went on here?" There is almost always a child who volunteers that the teacher was the victim of bullying and aggression; a general murmur will affirm that. The bully will look downcast, and quiet will descend on the classroom until some child asks, "Where are the bystanders?" After another moment of quiet, finally somebody says, "We all were, we laughed." In this essence the "blame for the event" is quietly distributed to every child in the classroom, creating a teaching and learning moment for everyone present. Billy is no longer the scapegoat for the group's aggression, and he settles down into a more peaceful role.

An MHP can help introduce this insight-oriented classroom management plan. Of course, this type of plan has its limits. If Billy continues to reoffend, the classroom can create a "power struggle referral alert," as shown in Table 3–5. The referral is made to a counselor or a social worker who uses it as a point of discussion with the child and not as a punishment. Our research has shown that while the MHP may be initially overwhelmed with referrals, the number of referrals declines significantly after about 3 months, and classes settle into a new and much less rowdy format. In this approach, Billy only becomes a problem for the principal when some major school behavioral rule or criminal action has occurred. This approach was successfully initiated in—and very quickly brought peace to—a number of classrooms.

Redirect Focus

The second main goal of intervening in school aggression is redirection. In a redirection strategy, the operating idea is that aggression is actually misplaced leadership and that fun can interrupt the aggressive mind-set. Many aggressive children have strong social skills and may impose their dominance, losing control of their aggression as part of feeling out of control. Redirection strategies do not simply block or contain; they are essentially active strategies that attempt to take aggression as a misguided form of assertiveness and view it as a potential leadership quality. Redirection strategies see aggression as unsublimated creativity rather than as isolated psychopathological events.

TABLE 3–5. Power struggle referral alert (sample)

CHILD'S NAME _____

TEACHER MAKING REFERRAL _____

DATE _____ TIME OF DAY _____

Check off all behavior to be disciplined

Adult disrespect

Talking back to a teacher

Refusing to follow a teacher's directive

Swearing in the presence of a teacher

Calling a teacher a name

Threatening a teacher verbally

Using a loud or rude tone with a teacher

Failing to complete assignments

School bus disrespect

Instigating power struggles

Engaging in horseplay

Threatening and putting down others

Minor pushing and shoving

Making excessive noise

Throwing others' property around

Making fun of or ridiculing another student

Classroom disrespect

Not sitting with someone—Urging others not to sit with a child

Clowning and distracting the class

Interrupting the teacher

Inappropriate touching, pulling hair, or poking

Cheating

Disrupting other children while they try to do their work

Defying a teacher

Refusing to work

Making fun of classmates' mistakes or wrong answers

Making noise

Talking without permission

Peer disrespect

Teasing

Name calling

Spreading rumors

TABLE 3–5.   Power struggle referral alert (sample) *(continued)*

CHILD'S NAME _____

TEACHER MAKING REFERRAL _____

DATE _____ TIME OF DAY _____

Check off all behavior to be disciplined

Peer disrespect *(continued)*

Being overly aggressive in a game

Playing mean tricks on other students

Ostracizing others and forming cliques

Extorting lunch, money, or other valuables

Taunting or group teasing

Victim behavior

Complaining or tattling a lot

Provoking trouble and then tattling and complaining

Giving in easily when pressured

Frequently being by him-/herself

Being easily led and manipulated

Corridor and schoolyard disrespect

Pushing

Making loud noise

Playing mean games

Engaging in social games that exclude others

Intimidating others

Threatening others

Engaging in group ridicule

Changing the rules of a game in the middle

Pushing to be first in line

Unwanted touching

Name calling

Destroying school property

Dominating a game at the expense of others

Bystander behavior

Instigating power struggles

Appearing to enjoy classroom or playground disruptions

Not helping with classroom or playground fights

Assisting bullies in bullying behavior

Comments of teacher (including behaviors not listed above):

Redirection strategies often rely on locating or assigning positive adult or older peer mentors. These programs serve both an individual and a larger climate purpose. When a youth is acting aggressively, this may indicate that there is a lack of connection to a positive adult model that could provide appropriate positive feedback for nonaggressive behaviors. One such adult playground mentor would expertly use sleight of hand to make kids laugh and be curious. Many young people today are bombarded by aggressive virtual role models portrayed in video games masquerading as real human relationships. This lack of attachment to real relationships (discussed in greater detail in Chapter 10, "Risk and Threat Assessment of Violent Children") is a critical component of this particular intervention goal; attaching an aggressive youth to a positive adult or older role model can have a calming and soothing effect on insecurely attached individuals.

Redirection can also be accomplished by identifying and connecting a youth to high-interest activities. Many times we have seen frustration, boredom, and lack of stimulation lead to aggression. Young people with nothing to do can constitute a clear risk factor. Redirection strategies offer young people the chance to explore and participate in activities such as computer design, music, theater, martial arts, sports, or drama. Most young people have an avid interest of some sort and will be strongly influenced by how this interest is encouraged and allowed to be exercised.

These strategies should be complemented by offering clear alternatives that provide opportunities for young people to be rewarded for positive behavior. Many wise, experienced teachers have put their classroom bullies in charge of classroom maintenance chores, delivering lunch, or otherwise contributing to the larger good. The bully may initially view this treatment as an opportunity to get out of class, but eventually the skilled teacher uses this redirection to control the aggressive and provocative behavior of the bully. A basic principle of discipline is to reward at least twice as much as you punish; otherwise punishment, however severe, will not work.

Reduce Pressure

The third goal in intervention strategy is pressure reduction. When young people feel pressured, they also feel raw and vulnerable to their social environments. When they encounter experiences during the school day that are frustrating, the pressure increases. This pressure may come from teachers who are trying to motivate increased participation, or it may come from peer networks that exert social pressure on the student directly or through cyber- and digital communication. Highly sensitive youth may be especially vulnerable such pressures, which can be the triggers that lead to an eruption of violence. Concrete pressure-reduction strategies might include changing schedules. Many aggressive children have extreme difficulty with transitions. Simply put, changing the arrival or departure time to class and/or school can be a simple way to reduce pressure. These adjustments in the school schedule can act as pressure relief valves for young people trying to adapt to a public or private school setting and its social demands. This is particularly true for students who may be entering a new school after a residential placement or children known to have been exposed to high levels of trauma either at home or in their communities.

Pressure relief can also be achieved by identifying a special place within the school that can be viewed by students as an oasis from the mounting pressure from teachers or peers—a safe haven. Another approach to pressure reduction is elimination of frustrating activities within the school schedule. Teachers need to be aware of students who have learning disabilities and be mindful not to create situations where public humiliation can result (e.g., a demand to perform weak or absent skills in front of the class). The MHP can assist in brainstorming ways in which a schedule can be adjusted to reduce the amount of frustration in the student's schedule. The less frustration, the less likelihood that pressure will build for both student and teacher, and the net result will be fewer incidents of school violence.

Pressure reduction can also be directly accomplished within the school setting through classes that involve high levels of physical activity, such as a gym, martial arts, or sports, which can sublimate frustration and absorb excess energy. Vocational activities like woodworking, domestic arts, mechanical engineering, and computer graphics are examples of potentially high-interest pursuits that will serve to reduce pressure during the course of the school day. Alternative schools are quite familiar with the use of high-interest activities that burn energy and present minimal frustrations. This approach can be applied in public or private settings, can be customized, and often involves virtually no additional expenses.

Prevent Shame

The fourth goal of interventions in school violence is the prevention of shame (Gilligan 1996, 2001; see also Chapter 5, "Bullying Is a Process, Not a Person"). As we have explained, the relationship between shame and the eruption of violence is a key guiding principle behind an intervention. An MHP may be uniquely positioned to understand how a child may experience various activities in his or her varied social systems as shameful. If this shaming is occurring at home, then strategies need to target this. If this student is experiencing community difficulties and shame is a constant part of his community life, then resources need to be applied to reduce the shame in that specific area. If the shaming is occurring as part of school bullying, either during the school day or in cyberspace, there need to be ways to intervene.

A considerable amount of shame is generated when a student has a learning disability that is not well understand by his teachers, parents, or the world in general. On an individual level, teachers who are aware that students have learning disabilities need to establish a way to reward the students for developing compensatory strategies or for using high levels of motivation to achieve a task. Individual rewards for effort will go a long way in inoculating students against an overall and pervasive sense of shame. Learning accommodations are part of many countries' laws and will follow students throughout their educational life cycles.

Public discipline is another common source of shaming. When students are confronted publicly about misbehavior, there is a strong likelihood that violence will escalate. This is particularly true in older grades, when students may be armed, aggressive, or involved in criminal gangs. Public discipline is an activity that often occurs during transitional periods of time, when at-risk youth are at their most vulnerable. Public discipline might include demands to remove clothing or iPods or to show identification. All of these activities may be critical for the school to target as disciplinary activities, but the use of public discipline needs to be as limited as possible. Teachers need to be trained to avoid public disciplining, and if they must use it, to do so minimally and with clear reasons given to the whole class. Bullying is also a primary source of shame throughout the educational life cycle. All levels of education need to be aware that bullying, especially the use of repetitive nonphysical shaming, is a source of both active and passive violence. The creation of antibullying programs or activities is an area in which skillful management of community resources is critical. Good bullying prevention programs rely on active partnerships between home, school, and community.

An MHP must take special steps to ensure that cyberbullying (see Chapter 10, "Risk and Threat Assessment of Violent Children") is included in any discussion of shaming in any school. The increased use of texting, social networking, and other means of cybercommunication has dissolved the boundaries between home and school. The young person exists in both home and school social systems; this cyberworld connects both and has created a seamless and inescapable mental environment, with dangerous reductions in personal space and time for privacy and reflection.

Overworked schools in the public, private, or charter sector often have child turnover of 20%–30% and very high teacher turnover in the course of a school year. Orientation of staff and students, especially ones who arrive in the middle of the semester, is often left out of the process of pressure reduction. Part of an MHP's role is to establish a plan for orienting new students and staff. Central pieces of such a plan might include the following:

1. Basic information about the school and where its Web site is located.
2. Informal discussion of racial prejudice, religious prejudice, gender bias, and other tensions that may make it difficult for students or staff members to integrate, and what the school is doing about this.

3. Assignment of a peer mentor to the child and a staff mentor to the staff to troubleshoot problems over time. Interpreting the informal processes of the school is far more difficult than setting school rules and following procedures. Human contact with a more senior individual staff member or student, one who understands the school, can help greatly.

Value Nonviolence

The fifth goal in intervention strategies focuses on creating ways to value nonviolence in the community. This is an especially rich area in which MHPs can utilize their skills in managing relationships with outside agencies involved with violent youth. Programs in this area may be in the community or may present themselves as logical partners with schools, both after school or during the actual school day. This goal would require designing and running programs in which individuals have the opportunity to be publicly rewarded and recognized for their contributions to the community. Such programs are relatively simple and direct if and when the correct people are involved.

Younger children seek praise from their parents and teachers, while older students are more interested in peer acceptance and public recognition. The older the students, the more future-oriented they are and the more likely it is that they can be motivated to participate in activities where they will be recognized for their public service.

Art and theater programs are excellent arenas in which to develop public events that support nonviolence. There are a number of different plays, written and performed by young people, that extol the virtues of friendship, compassion, and caring for the vulnerable. There are antibullying plays, as well as movies and events that have as their primary concern a public acknowledgment of the value of nonviolence. We have successfully invoked rock stars and bands to carry this message.

Conclusion

The structures and strategies discussed in this chapter are useful in the hands of MHPs who are open to working outside their traditional roles. Having an aggressive child adjust to a community school and resocialize greatly benefits the entire community. Public education is challenged to accept all students who can function in the community, but resources can be quickly exhausted if young people with aggressive tendencies are not properly managed in the school, at home, and in the community. Our approach stresses the role of the MHP in a variety of social contexts. It is this skillful management of resources that creates the safety net that allows youth who have violent tendencies to be educated in the community.

KEY CLINICAL CONCEPTS

- In order to play an effective role, the MHP must understand the following dynamics of the community consultation process:
  - Agencies tend to operate as if they can/should be able to solve all problems alone.
  - Agencies' shortcomings are problem-focused rather than person-focused.
  - An agency's leadership model may not fit all of its employees, who might hold very different views of how the agency functions.
- Key negotiation principles include
  - Facilitating mentalization.
  - Establishing a point of similarity with the agency, school, child, and family.
  - Being aware of your countertransferences.
- Development of a collaborative plan involves
  - Respecting boundaries and roles of those outside your discipline.
  - Defining why violence is erupting in the school.
  - Synchronizing community agencies: child protective services, juvenile justice system, and mental health and human services.
  - Coordinating these services by creating strategies to access them.
- Address intervention goals:
  - Containment of aggression
  - Redirection of focus
  - Reduction of pressure
  - Prevention of shame
  - Promotion of a climate valuing nonviolence

References

Bracha HS: Freeze, flight, fight, fright, faint: adaptationist perspectives on the acute stress response spectrum. CNS Spectr 9:679–685, 2004

Cannon WB: Bodily Changes in Pain, Hunger, Fear and Rage: An Account of Recent Research Into the Function of Emotional Excitement. New York, D. Appleton & Co., 1915 (see http://www.archive.org/details/cu31924022542470)

Fonagy P, Gyorgy G, Jurist EL, et al: Affect Regulation, Mentalization, and the Development of the Self. New York, Other Press, 2002

Gilligan J: Violence: Reflections on a National Epidemic. New York, Vintage Books, 1996

Gilligan J: Preventing Violence. New York, Thames & Hudson, 2001

Goodstein L: Consultation to human service networks, in The Mental Health Consultation Field. Edited by Cooper S, Hodges W. New York, Human Sciences Press, 1983, pp 267–287

Jacques E: Requisite Organization: A Total System for Effective Managerial Organization and Managerial Leadership for the 21st Century. Arlington, VA, Cason Hall, 1998

Kerr ME, Bowen M: Family Evaluation. New York, WW Norton, 1988

Massachusetts Behavioral Health Partnership: Children's Behavioral Health Initiative (CBHI) Information. Available at: http://www.masspartnership.com/provider/index.aspx?lnkID=CBHI.ascx. Accessed June 2010.

Minuchin S: Families and Family Therapy. Cambridge, MA, Harvard University Press, 1974

Perkins J: Medicaid EPSDT litigation. National Health Law Program, October 2, 2009. Available at: http://www.healthlaw.org/images/stories/epsdt/1-EPSDT-Docket.pdf. Accessed December 7, 2010.

Petti TA, Salguero C: Community Child and Adolescent Psychiatry: A Manual of Clinical Practice and Consultation. Washington, DC, American Psychiatric Publishing, 2005

Praed Foundation: Child and Adolescent Needs and Strengths (CANS) Comprehensive Multisystem Assessment Manual. Chicago, IL, The Praed Foundation, 1999. Available at: http://www.praedfoundation.org/CANS%20Comprehensive%20Manual.pdf. Accessed March 20, 2011.

Sklarew B, Twemlow SW, Wilkinson S (eds): Analysts in the Trenches: Streets, Schools, and War Zones. Hillsdale, NJ, Analytic Press, 2004

Twemlow SW, Sacco FC: The management of power in municipalities: psychoanalytically informed negotiation. Negotiation Journal 19:369–388, 2003

Twemlow SW, Fonagy P, Sacco FC, et al: Reducing violence and prejudice in a Jamaican all-age school using attachment and mentalization approaches. Psychoanal Psychol (in press)

4

Case Studies in School Violence

A Staging Paradigm

ANNA Freud was clear in her approach to understanding the development of children (A. Freud 1965, 1966). She understood the need to predict the developmental pathways a child might take and the value of prevention and early intervention concerning psychiatric illness. Karl Menninger (1952), in his early manuals of psychiatric interviewing, recognized the need for a multiple systems perspective in creating an accurate psychiatric history. Although much has changed since these solid ideas were expressed, children still go to school, have problems, and exist in multiple social contexts. What has also not changed is that school is where children's problems are most likely to be identified and is the most logical platform for early intervention for problems that lead to violence within a school and ultimately spill into the community. This makes the school, in a sense, a clinical hub for service delivery. Schools are not just houses of learning, but have become villages for the socialization of a community's young people.

The family and school stand alone as the arenas within which a child develops. They are interlocked within a community wrapped in the virtual reality of the Internet that connects all the best and worst parts of the world in a network of constant communication. When a child has a problem at home or school, it forms a ripple effect that extends through the home, school, and community. The Internet has collapsed the boundaries between a child's life and, ultimately, his or her consciousness. When a school violence intervention is designed, the same ripple effect must be included in the service elements. Effective solutions can follow from any of the points that begin within the home, school, or community. The intervention can begin anywhere, but the road map must be comprehensive and must include the necessary elements for offering each child the best chance to go to school safely, learn, and live a balanced life. In our model, school violence is viewed as a signal of a nonmentalizing social system with unregulated power dynamics that impact at-risk children.

A mental health professional (MHP) begins treatment by dutifully understanding the nature of the problem and how it has been amplified throughout the home, school, and community. The goal is to keep as wide a perspective as possible while still guiding children through the various social systems. This treatment objective requires that the aggressive behavior at school be considered as a reflection of a larger social context: the home and community. DeRosier et al. (1994) studied children's aggressive behavior in playgroups, reporting that group context influences how children reacted to aggression in the group. The location of the intervention is applied as part of this assessment. Treatment begins by working with what is available and should always be anchored in a wider vision of factors. Effective interventions that promote mentalizing result in the harmonizing of signals with the goal of creating winners all around rather than adversaries wagging fingers and defending what they may consider "their" turf. This clinical task could be accomplished with a full oversight committee, or it may be the work of a single MHP in a community setting who uses therapy, medication, and consultations to build solid relationships with the school and family. A school social worker could also refer the family to an outside resource or work actively with outside resources already working with the student.

The treatment is seen as a family-driven process in which a blend of formal and informal resources is coordinated within the community. States have committed to the use of wraparound treatment strategies in remedies to class action lawsuits against Medicaid (Perkins 2009). Sacco et al. (2007) outlined a mental health intervention that offers cost containment and keeps children home and out of hospitals. This approach emphasizes the use of a containing agency relationship developed through long-term, mentalization-based psychotherapy in the family's home, which is also followed by a multidisciplinary team, including a psychiatrist, psychologist, and nurse practitioners. Ultimately, the goal of these treatments is to co-create solutions that empower families to care for their children. When clinicians empower families to solve problems, the main players in the evolution of school violence disappear slowly and are replaced with men-

---

TABLE 4–1.   Treatment philosophy for school violence interventions

All interventions seek to send the same positive signal to the developing child at home, in school, and in the community.

Interventions must create a sustained care plan that can follow a child through all levels of education.

Children need to learn how to contain aggression, including an understanding of power issues and power struggles.

Social systems need to be mentalizing and nourish the best interests of the child.

A child advocate is needed to drive the care plan and keep the signals straight.

Both physical and mental health must be considered in all solutions.

The community is a rich source of protective factors and natural helpers.

Risk and threat need to be assessed in a coordinated and clear-minded fashion.

---

talizing, compassionate role models. Table 4–1 summarizes the essentials of this approach to school violence.

Synchronizing the signal to the child is the crucial key element to all interventions in school violence. Children will act out when they do not receive clear signals from the outside world that direct them in positive ways. Blos (1974) described the process of an adolescent using action as denial of early trauma and posited that teenagers slowly lose the ability to symbolize and use words. Instead, they are more likely to "act out" their unresolved tensions. The following case example illustrates how a child confused by mixed signals might present to an MHP and demonstrates an intervention focused on synchronizing signals from the home and school.

Case Example: Bernardo, a Child Lacking Consistent Role Models and Clear Signals About Behavior

Bernardo was a 9-year-old Puerto Rican boy in foster care. He had experienced significant early childhood trauma, requiring the state to remove him from his biological home. Bernardo's father was incarcerated for drug distribution, and his mother was addicted to heroin. Bernardo was only 5 years old, just beginning preschool, when he was placed in his first foster home. He was already displaying very aggressive behavior at school, literally from his first day. He did not share, and he became very upset with any child or teacher who interfered with what he wanted to do. Reaching the boy's mother was virtually impossible, as the phone service was often disconnected, or else the calls were simply met with angry dismissal. The school filed a child neglect complaint that resulted in Bernardo's removal from his mother's custody and placement with his paternal grandmother, who was also caring for several of his cousins. Bernardo remained in the same school system, but his behavior escalated. When Bernardo was home with his grandmother, he did not display this aggression; consequently, when the school contacted the grandmother, she was dismissive of their concerns because he behaved well at her house.

Eventually, Bernardo attacked another child with scissors and was referred to a local inpatient child unit. Bernardo was discharged to a step-down program and eventually returned to his grandmother's home, reentering the community when he was in the latter part of first grade. Although he had done well in the small special school in the residential program, Bernardo almost immediately became aggressive when he returned to public school. The school counselors reached out to his grandmother and to local state agency case workers. A referral was made by the state agency case worker to a local mental health clinic. Bernardo's grandmother had limited English ability and was becoming resistant to the school's attempts to intervene. Bernardo's aunt acted as an interpreter, but began blaming the school for not doing its job. Bernardo's family did not take him to his appointments at the clinic, and no treatment was ever successfully initiated. Bernardo was in real danger of being placed in a residential program.

This case illustrates what can happen when the school and home are not sending the same signal. Bernardo received a mixed message; his role models were unintentionally reinforcing an antiauthority position, as well as giving him tacit permission to be aggressive at school. The clinic could not use a traditional office therapy approach, and cultural and linguistic issues further complicated the problem.

The first step in synchronizing the signals is to use a home-based approach with a resource person who is culturally suited to build the trust needed with the family. Next, the therapist should make contact with the school and attempt to discover what is happening behaviorally when the child is there. While observation might be ideal, it is often impractical. Case consultations (often by telephone) with the school counselor can offer an MHP the information necessary to conduct a thorough assessment of a school violence problem. Table 4–2 presents a sample checklist for use in interviewing the school counselor.

Bernardo *(continued)*

The therapy progressed by fine-tuning the ways in which Bernardo could be rewarded for being nonaggressive at school. Through a therapeutic mentor, Bernardo became involved in a basketball league at a local community center. His coach provided rides to practice and games. Eventually, a very sports-minded maternal uncle emerged, taking interest in Bernardo's playing in a local Catholic Youth Organization (CYO) league. During consultations with the school, the therapist and the counselor worked on a bullying prevention program that had a leadership role for Bernardo.

Bernardo benefited from this intervention initiated at the end of his first year in school and the beginning of the second year. We followed his case until he graduated from high school with a National Collegiate Athletic Association

TABLE 4–2. Sample checklist for interviewing the school counselor

Exactly when and where does the aggression show itself—at both home and
school, or just one of these places?

What is the nature of the classroom?

What is the nature of the child's relationship to the teacher(s) and principal?

Are there efforts to monitor school climate? antibullying programs?

Are there natural supports that seem to calm the child during the school day?

What specific help can the home provide to the school?
• Academic
• Disciplinary
• Recreational

Is there a role for the family in the school?

Are family resources being used?

Who is the main school contact from the family?

What are the most efficient communication channels?

Are there after-school or extracurricular opportunities?

Is the school open to an outside provider of clinical services?

Is the child involved in special education, or should he or she be referred for
such services?

(NCAA) Division II scholarship in basketball. His uncle enrolled Bernardo in an
American Association of Universities (AAU) basketball team through their local
community center. This required that Bernardo travel on weekends with the team
to play in tournaments. Bernardo was athletic, and this strength created a regular
way to discharge energy through sport, conditioning, and competitive sports.

Bernardo's case illustrates how an effective school violence intervention requires coordination of resources among the school, family, and community.

Learning to Contain Aggression

There are two keys to containing aggression. The first involves having a well-
supervised way to release tension. It is cruel to leave a child without a way to
"blow off steam." This buildup of tension is a universal part of the developing
child, regardless of socioeconomic status (SES), race, religion, or culture. When
a child from a wealthy family attending a private school feels disconnected and
pressured to succeed, the tension that accumulates in the child will be the same
as for Bernardo, whose life could not appear more different, at least on a superficial level. The second key is to offer a positive signal through important role
models. In Bernardo's case, the release came through basketball, and the role
models became coaches and his uncle. There are an infinite variety of combina-

tions of this principle, and a wide variety of approaches using martial arts, sports, drama, and a number of other outlets to release tension and contain aggression. We have posited that physical exertion can help contain aggression if directed in the proper fashion, in this case by the use of traditional martial arts (Twemlow and Sacco 1998; Twemlow et al. 2008). Table 4–3 highlights strategies for containing aggression.

Within schools, homes, and the community at large, we have observed a need to foster mentalizing as a way to contribute to containment and self-regulation of small groups. While many of the elements impacting social systems may be out of the sphere of influence of the MHP, there remains a need for the MHP to be aware of the social dynamics and how they interact with the individual psychology and development of the child. In Bernardo's case, the school was very cooperative and the counselor was the school's interface with the outside agencies. There was openness toward working with the family and there were no unhealthy dynamics that protected Bernardo's status as a bully when he was at school. This type of behavior was noticed quickly, and as he grew older and entered later grades, the schools were equipped with programs that helped contain aggression by offering peer mediation and other programs that fostered altruism and friendship. The schools in this particular case were not dismissive and definitely involved mentalizing. They regulated the aggression by sending a positive and firm signal about the intolerance of bullying at every grade.

The involvement of a male relative also served to mitigate the buildup of aggression by offering Bernardo positive role models. The home and community can provide rich sources of natural supports that can be effective in containing aggression at home.

Managing Psychiatric Conditions at School

School violence problems may also result from a psychiatric impairment that is best treated with the combination of medication and psychotherapy. This treatment needs to be evaluated using real-time feedback from the home and school.

Case Example: Jason, a Child With Attention-Deficit/Hyperactivity Disorder

Jason was a third grader repeatedly being suspended from class and who spent a great deal of time in the principal's office. Jason attended play therapy at a local clinic because of his impulsivity and his parent's difficulty controlling him at home. He hit his brothers and frequently picked fights with his classmates. Jason

TABLE 4–3. Strategies to contain aggression in the school

Reduce academic pressures through decreased demands and accommodated learning strategies.

Use psychopharmacology with mood-regulating medications where appropriate.

Schedule after-school activities that stress physical exertion.

Offer mediation and peer mentoring programs.

Provide adult mentoring with community involvement.

Identify and eliminate consistent sources of humiliation for individuals and within social systems.

Create safe and secure places and relationships within the school and community.

Reward altruism, compassion, and friendship among peers.

Reduce the victim pool by teaching assertiveness.

Seek participation of invested school leaders who are intolerant of coercion at any level.

was inattentive and hard to motivate in his classroom. His mother contacted a therapist when the school suggested that Jason might be expelled to a 30-day class for behavior disorders within the school system.

The therapist was aware of Jason's symptoms and that he had been diagnosed with attention-deficit/hyperactivity disorder (ADHD). His mother was unwilling to consider a referral for medication, however. The therapist communicated with the school, and with Jason's mother, making a referral to a consulting psychiatrist. The therapist encouraged the school to fill out the survey to assist the psychiatrist in making an evaluation. Jason eventually was placed on Strattera (atomoxetine) and began to behave less impulsively, according to both his mother and the school. The therapist and school remained in touch, and feedback was regularly provided to the prescribing psychiatrist.

This case illustrates the traditional therapy role in intervening in the eruption of early violence in the form of school disruption. Jason represents the type of child that can easily become involved in violence at the school or in the home. Early intervention offered him a chance to stay with his classmates instead of being placed in programs that would expose him to more negative peers. Sacco and Larsen (2003) described how a therapist became involved in the case of a high school student who had threatened to shoot the superintendent of schools. Although the student was expelled, the therapist remained involved, providing home-based family therapy with the youth and his aunt. The psychotherapy facilitated the student's return to school; he eventually graduated and entered community college. This approach used psychotherapy; while the intensity of the problem may vary, the goal is to use psychotherapy as a protective factor in managing a school violence problem involving the home, school, and community.

TABLE 4–4.   Interventions to assist in working in the child's macrosystem

Repairing burnt bridges between families and schools
Teaching negotiation skills in the system
Finding resources and building new connections
Humanizing the system: putting a face on bureaucracy
Draining authority conflict:
• Encourage assertiveness rather than aggression
• Avoid triangles
Understanding other professionals' problems with patient: knowing the other
Validating difficulties without blaming patient: being straight
Derailing blame: decreasing targeting of victim
Educational advocacy: using special education laws
Parent–school signal resonance: setting common goals

Table 4–4 outlines general objectives that may help guide the MHP in creating specific, family-tailored strategies that can reduce the impact of school violence.

Affluent At-Risk Children

The phrase "failure to launch" describes adolescents who (for a wide variety of reasons) lack the social skills to enter life and to launch themselves into Erikson's (1963) psychosocial moratorium of young adulthood, in which they experiment with jobs, interests, relationships, and other conventional features of adult life. When children from affluent families learn to feel privileged and contemptuous of others at home, they may feel protected and entitled to act violently at school.

Failure to launch appears to stem from several different elements in a number of more affluent families. One is the amount of money available, which allows these children to indulge their desires without the need to leave their home. There is often not sufficient supervision of the child. Such homes may also be dismissive, in that they avoid anxiety and the children are "paid" to remain out of the way of the busy parents, who are both pursuing their professional lives. Second, the children have often been brought up with their own television sets and video games in their rooms, accustomed to the passive feeding of information into their brains that does not encourage their capacity to imagine, self-regulate, or apprehend reality. These problems are also aggravated by the extraordinary growth of cybertechnology and the effortless attainment of information. In other words, the active roles of pursuing and finding ways to obtain what one needs to survive are underdeveloped in these entitled children. Third, they may become involved in a variety of peer-supported self-destructive activities, such as compulsive Internet pornography viewing, online gambling, and illicit substance use.

Sometimes these problems can reach dangerous proportions before the parents become aware of them. The outcome depends on how clever the young person is in hiding such activities and how much money is freely available for him or her to devise ways to hide behaviors. Many young people have told us that their lack of respect for parents was generated by what they feel is a parent's stupidity in not seeing what was going on. A fourth element contributing to failure to launch—frequently seen in professional families—is that parents may be preoccupied with their jobs or with social or volunteer activities. Preoccupied parents have not developed parenting skills with their children, and they may receive little guidance and assistance from the grandparents or great-grandparents. The extended and nuclear family units are slowly disappearing. Corporate CEOs tend to bring up their children as though they were employees in their businesses, with accountability and productivity as their guiding principles. One young man offhandedly stated that he regularly made appointments at his father's office to discuss personal issues, because his father was so busy. Most importantly, the atmosphere within the home may be very adversarial and competitive. A child is not encouraged to expose weaknesses and difficulties and instead receives reinforcement primarily for academic and athletic performance.

The following case example illustrates the deeper dynamics of a higher-SES family as observed in psychoanalytic psychotherapy. This analysis is to reinforce the idea that higher-SES families also have struggles that involve violence. School violence does not happen just in disadvantaged communities and families. The processes that create at-risk children operate without regard to race, culture, or income status.

Case Example: Adam, a College Student From an Affluent Family Who Needs Medicaid Help

Adam was a 25-year-old young man from an extremely wealthy family who was admitted to an inpatient unit for diagnostic assessment following the failure of six treatment programs that had focused on alcohol and substance abuse rehabilitation. His parents had divorced during his latency years but lived only a short distance from each other. During this period, Adam was seriously bullied at school and became depressed and suicidal, which led him to self-cutting to gain relief through counterirritant pain.

Although Adam's parents were not aware of his self-injurious behavior, his reaction in the family was to become an extraordinarily compliant shadow for his mother. However, because he described his current relationship with his mother as hateful and his mother as abusive to him on a regular basis, the social worker initially insisted on excluding Adam's mother from family consultation, believing that her presence would prevent further good work. Adam's father was a very passive man who gave in to his ex-wife's wishes and in fact openly declared his inability to deal with Adam's struggles. Both Adam and his mother would tongue-lash each other with his father and social worker as their audience.

Adam was a good-looking young man who nevertheless had a number of concerns about his body. He had mild acne that he saw as severe, worrying that he would not appear as competent, strong, and in control, yet at the same time he could not control the stream of contempt that came from his mouth whenever he felt somebody was caught "being stupid," which then alienated him from his peers. He had chronic suicidal thoughts with no serious attempts, except through boastful experimenting with massive doses of drugs, establishing himself as a drug kingpin. He also enjoyed experiencing pain through torturous punching of holes in his ears and allowing friends to beat him up.

During psychoanalytic psychotherapy, Adam first developed an idealizing transference to a mentoring older male therapist who assisted him in seeing himself as worth something and capable of living without his parents' money. Adam then participated in family sessions with his mother included and was much more communicative with her; sessions often ended with everybody on good terms. Adam's chronic suicidal thinking disappeared, and he began making plans to go to college. At one time, early in his therapy, he said that he was only about halfway through spending his parents' money, but by the end of therapy he was very clear and pleased to be engaging in a plan that would help him succeed without remaining dependent upon his parents.

In this instance, Adam's parents bought a very intensive set of therapies, including family therapy, dialectical behavior therapy (DBT), group psychotherapy, a mentalizing power issues group, together with creative expression, relaxation, self-regulating social skills training, and a twelve-step recovery program, in addition to individual therapy. Adam also received 24-hour nursing care and peer interaction in the milieu in which he repeated in microcosm the problems of his life. Ironically, what he did not receive as part of aftercare, his parents could not buy. One example was a careful therapeutic mentoring program with family, school, and community wraparound (see Chapter 8, "Activating Community Resources Through Therapeutic Mentoring"), now available to children through programs such as Medicaid; these programs are expensive, and their availability is limited. Adam needed additional services that were not easily funded through traditional insurance coverage. However, his family could have approached the court, and they would have been able to access Medicaid but lose temporary custody of their son. Special education was another option, but Adam's problems were too diverse to be addressed by an Individualized Education Program (IEP).

Poverty and Multistressed Families

Parents are usually very close to the problems of their children; it is difficult for them to develop a strategic mind-set if they are personally overinvolved in the difficulties of the situation. The MHP is advised to focus on teaching families how to go with resistance, rather than to fight against it. "Going with resistance" is a rather delicate skill that will require a therapeutic relationship to begin enlisting and earning the trust of the family, and then transferring that trust to other agencies in the community and the school.

Case Example: The Quincys, a Multiproblem Family With an Overwhelmed Parent

The Quincy family had three children enrolled in the same elementary school. Ms. Quincy was a single mother with two children diagnosed with ADHD; one boy (in second grade) had serious learning and language disabilities, and the other boy (in fourth grade) was aggressive and consistently picked fights with peers. Ms. Quincy received calls from the school almost daily, and as a result of this work interruption lost her job as a surgical technician at a local hospital. She felt that she was in constant conflict with the school and in fact complained that the school was out to target her children.

The MHP worked with Ms. Quincy to help her find ways to be proactive and volunteer at the school, rather than to continue being reactive. This work required several meetings and the support of the school counselor. Ms. Quincy was able to create some distance from the problems at school and to develop some strategies to approach the school when she needed to respond to situations concerning her children. She also worked out a way to reward the children for "good time" at school. She eventually became active in a program to increase parent awareness of bullying that was very successful.

An important technical aspect of reducing authority conflicts and teaching paradoxical skills to a family is avoiding triangles. This is a key concept borrowed from family therapy, especially Bowen (Kerr and Bowen 1988), who based his family therapy techniques on identifying and eliminating triangular behavior within systems. The idea that allies and enemies will always be forming in any large system (as posited by Volkan [1997]) extends this concept to the international arena, although Bowen originally described it in the context of the family system. Whether on a large or small scale, triangulation builds coercion within the system; the child is frequently caught between these power struggles. The dynamic of these struggles typically involves having authorities and children allied together against another adult or child. When a triangle forms, communication stops and actions are determined by an "us versus them" phenomenon that defeats the purpose of focusing on the child or ensuring that the best possible educational opportunities are available.

Another approach to clinical intervention involves helping the family understand the point of view of the professionals and agencies involved in the case.

This is a form of "knowing the other," or understanding how an adversary views a problem. Taking the other's viewpoint is typically difficult to do alone, and this is where the MHP can be quite helpful in assisting the family in developing and understanding their conflicts, discovering new ways to unravel them with the best interests of the child in mind. MHPs can help families to try not only to personalize the adversary but also to think the way the adversary is thinking. This allows for a humanizing process, as well as a strategic protocol that can help a family realign their authority, sending a single simple and consistent message to the child.

MHPs will also frequently appear alongside families, advocating for them in a variety of settings. It is important for the MHP not to simply be a "one way" antagonistic advocate, disregarding what others are saying, and simply defending and pushing the family's point of view. We have observed this frequently in school meetings where teachers and other school personnel may have one view of a situation, while the family has a completely different understanding. The MHP should listen and try to extract the critical elements. It is essential for the MHP to not allow the patient to be blamed or to be personally attacked in a meeting, but instead to model a more positive and information-seeking stance toward adults who may be seeing the child's problem in a more critical fashion.

Validating the child's problem and its impact on the school or community is an important first step in building trust and opening up dialogue. It is extremely important to "de-rail" blame when advocating for families. This strategy is meant to decrease the targeting of the victim, instead engaging in techniques and practices during meetings, as well as in sessions with families, that strive to understand the other's viewpoint of the problem. This is not possible without creating some way to generate the information without having it be a finger-pointing power struggle around who is responsible for not overcoming the problem.

MHPs are strongly urged to familiarize themselves with special education laws. There are certain standards that are generated on a federal level and interpreted by the state. The MHP is urged to know the standards that are being used in any special education protocol process. The MHP can be trained in this by attending workshops or by researching the criteria used in the special education decision-making process. The primary standard is "free appropriate public education" (FAPE). The government Web site on FAPE (U.S. Department of Education 2010) contains information to guide parents in understanding the rules of the special education process. Despite this unifying principle, each state has different measures and standards in place to qualify a student for special education, and also for developing a strategic plan to ensure that a child is receiving the best possible education.

MHPs will frequently enter a family that has been at war with the system for some time. Children from these families often are receiving very mixed signals and act this out at school by being aggressive, violent, or withdrawing into a submissive victim role. When an MHP enters a situation like this, it is critical to understand the need to rebuild burnt bridges. When a family is struggling to cope with a system without any support, they frequently will personally attack and alienate key people within the educational system. This will lead to a conscious or unconscious barricade against working together. Overcoming these obstacles is a function that can be incorporated into the MHP's work with the family, and the MHP can play a critical role in assisting the family to live in the present and look forward, rather than clinging to old resentments and angers toward the school.

Once these barricades have been eliminated, the MHP can then begin a process of teaching negotiation skills to the family. This is something that will require a mutual mind-set and will frequently involve the MHP having to take firm steps in order to teach the family to negotiate within the system. These negotiation skills are best modeled and practiced in therapy and then processed when the parent tries to interface with the school without the MHP's help. Teaching negotiation skills with the system can also include ways of dealing with the court system, police, community agencies, recreational programs, and other community supports.

The MHP is also tasked with discovering resources that can be used to assist the family in rebalancing itself within the home, school, and community. Every geographic area has a service landscape that needs to be understood by the MHP when working with school violence problems. It is no longer sufficient to understand symptoms and treatments in a vacuum. The solution to complex school violence problems requires that the MHP be consciously and continuously striving to identify resources within the community that can be unlocked and used as part of the re-stabilization of an emerging problem with violence. In all of the comprehensive treatment planning strategies outlined in this chapter, there is a need for some type of community support in order for there to be sustained success in developing an intervention that truly targets the problems that are creating difficulties in school.

Common Patterns of School Violence

In this section we outline five patterns of school violence that are commonly encountered in modern schools (Table 4–5). It should be emphasized that these problems can occur at all SES levels; they are not simply products of disadvantaged homes in poor neighborhoods. These problems are generic and apply to all levels of society, although specific elements will differ based on cultural realities and service landscape dimensions. How a problem is addressed or understood varies based on each individual school and community. Nevertheless,

TABLE 4–5. Patterns of school violence problems

Pattern I—Repetitive school disruption—illegal and aggressive behavior at
  school
Pattern II—Acute case of child aggressor or victim
Pattern III—Highly submissive victim or aggressive young student
Pattern IV—Child with self-injurious or self-defeating behavior
Pattern V—Truants and dropouts

**TABLE 4–6. Pattern I: repetitive school disruption—illegal and
aggressive behavior at school**

Student suspended from class or school
At-risk behaviors toward self and others at school
Possession of a weapon at school
Aggression toward a teacher
Drugs at school
Illegal behavior during school or at school activities
Early childhood aggression involving peers

there are certain patterns that emerge when dealing with school violence problems. An understanding of these five patterns of school violence can help the MHP to structure appropriate treatment strategies.

Pattern I: Repetitive School Disruption

School violence is not just fighting and dramatic eruptions of stabbings and shootings. There is a process that unfolds across the three arenas: home, school, and community. As with all school violence problems, there are victimizers and victims, both parts of the same process. When children or adolescents stop thinking, they behave mindlessly at school and reenact their conflicts, which typically take the form of repetitive disruptions within the classroom, in the school yard, and on the bus (see Table 4–6).

Case Example: John, the Identified Patient in a Very Disturbed Family

John was a 15-year-old white male attending a suburban high school. His parents owned their own home; his father was a businessman. John's mother had agoraphobia and was homebound, except for when she could be escorted out by her husband or by John. After fighting with a teacher, John was expelled from school. He had been asked to leave a classroom, but he had refused. The teacher approached John and demanded that he leave the room, so John pushed the desk against the teacher, injuring her knee; he was expelled, and criminal charges were filed.

John was referred to a local community mental health center for a threat assessment and treatment. A family stabilization team was dispatched by the clinic because of the acute nature of the stress that was being reported at home. After John's expulsion, his father became increasingly angry at his mother; John would begin to team up with his father, becoming aggressive toward the mother. John had been an excellent student up until the fifth grade, when his father's difficulties at work began. The family stabilization team quickly learned that there was a domestic violence situation between the mother and father, except that whereas his father used verbal aggression, John would frequently lash out physically at his mother when she tried to enforce a limit.

When the MHP began providing home-based family therapy with John, his parents, and younger sister, it became clear that John's behaviors did not begin in fourth or fifth grade. His mother reported that she'd had difficulty making him follow her rules since he had begun day care much earlier in his childhood. John's father quickly jumped to his defense and became aggressive, telling her that she did not remember anything correctly and that nobody would be able to respect her view since she could barely even leave the house. The father angrily blamed the mother for John's lack of success at school and felt burdened by the responsibility of having to cope with John's current problems given the fact that his business was almost bankrupt. The family was sinking quickly into a financial meltdown, and this was causing even more stress.

The MHPs also discovered that John had physically attacked his mother on a number of occasions, yet there were no official reports. John's sister was the first to communicate this in the family session and was quickly quieted by John's father who said that she was way too young to remember any of that. There were several incidents eventually discovered in which John had used a weapon to attack his mother; he had also at various times taken weapons to school when he had felt threatened by others who would bully him. The school was quite adamant about its disciplinary protocol. When the family stabilization team approached the school, they reported that the family was very difficult to engage and that the father was often hostile and defensive of his son's behavior, pointing a finger at the school instead and complaining that he paid plenty of taxes and expected better from a suburban school.

John was not active in any after-school activities. His primary interest was playing video games at home, and he had very few friends in the community. When he did have someone visit him, they frequently would smoke marijuana and then joyride. John presented as a rather arrogant and entitled young man who was socially quite inept with his peers and gravitated toward older kids. He frequently complained that people didn't understand him, that he was a misunderstood child who wasn't being given the proper resources. He felt constantly under attack and blamed, when in fact he frequently was provocative and would engage people in conversations that were bound to end with conflict.

In John's case, it was critical to understand the school's, family's, and student's perceptions of the problem; this began with home-based intensive family therapy. During this process, it was clear that the father's unconscious aggression toward the mother and the world at large was being acted out by the son, who was also allowed to act aggressively toward his mother.

This pattern transferred to school, where he acted out aggression toward an adult female teacher. The school aggression was not an isolated incident, and there had been ongoing mounting problems with John that were dismissed by the parents and dealt with by the school using a variety of disciplinary techniques. There was very little cooperation between the school and the family, since the family saw John's problems as being the school's problem, while the school saw John as being protected by the family. This resulted in having a probation officer assigned to the case; a petition was filed with the court by the school in addition to the criminal charges. A disciplinary hearing was arranged, but the family was unable to afford a high-priced criminal attorney. In fact, they qualified for a public defender and this was the beginning of a process that unraveled throughout the therapeutic intervention.

John flatly refused to participate in any psychiatric evaluation and so the therapy focused primarily on creating a simple set of rules that his father could enforce. Several meetings were arranged with the school counselor, and the family was shown how to negotiate a system of behavioral controls that included phone calls to the father so he could reinforce the message from the school. John was shifted out of classes where there were female teachers and was placed on a daily reporting system to the vice principal. This plan was overseen by his probation officer and became part of his conditional release.

John's case illustrates a common pattern that can occur in a variety of different settings. A number of the interventions outlined in Table 4–4 were used in this case. The treatment philosophy outlined in Table 4–1 was applied in this case and illustrates how an MHP enters a school violence problem from the community.

Pattern II: Acute Case of a Child Aggressor or a Victim

The second school violence pattern involves children who are living in homes that are recently reunited, are in the process of reuniting with homes, or are living temporarily in substitute care environments (see Table 4–7). These children attend community schools and are considered "extreme" behaviorally, or, in the clinical sense, as high-risk children in adolescence. This population of children may have a variety of family patterns that will reflect where they live. Each family will cope with problems in its own way, although there are commonalities in the problems experienced.

When these children come to school, they frequently will demonstrate either the aggression or the submission necessary for extreme acts of aggression to erupt. When children have some stability and are not suffering from serious impairments, they tend to exhibit their school disruption or violence in a progressive or less intense fashion. Children living under the circumstances described in Pattern II are extremely vulnerable with a tendency to reflect the intensity of their home and community worlds at school, resulting in acute and repetitive problem behaviors. These are not children who are easily engaged in school-based activities or counseling to resolve their issues at school. These children tend to be engaged in sustained activities of defiance or withdrawal that form a pathological process within a school system. Their problems are made more damaging when the school system ignores the need to create positive alternatives. There are secondary consequences of this pathological process in which the children may become alienated from their normal social peer groups and engage in highly self-destructive behaviors, such as suicide, substance abuse, promiscuity, truancy, and other social deviance.

Pattern II children are also likely to move from school to school on a frequent basis. It is possible, for instance, that a foster home from a particular neighborhood will often have high-risk children moving through the home and attempting to connect to a community school. In these cases, clinical interventions may already be in place, may be engaged by the state agency case management, or may be engaged by the school in response to problems that surely will begin at the school and continue if a proper treatment plan is not in place. These children are at risk for becoming either aggressive or submissive, sometimes directly in response to their involvement with the child protective service system. Many of these children have families that are required by the state to adhere to a service plan in order to begin or maintain the reunion process. This places already at-risk children in a situation where they are experiencing many strange and unsettling connections and disconnections. Supervised visitation is a process that many children are exposed to from a very early age; they are removed from school and then returned to school, often in the same day.

Case Example: Sonja, a Sexually Abused and Neglected Child

Sonja was a 9-year-old Hispanic female who was living in a foster home and was reported to have pulled a boy's pants down and engaged in a sexual act during recess. Sonja was in her fourth foster placement and had been moved from her biological family 2 years earlier as a result of sexual abuse at the hands of a male friend of her mother, who was at that time addicted to heroin and worked as an exotic dancer and part-time prostitute. Sonja was an only child and frequently was supervised by friends of her mother.

Sonja quickly became a behavior problem and the school indicated reports of child neglect. When Sonja did have difficulty at school, her grandmother would often be the only person the school could reach; eventually this resulted in a substantiation of the child neglect allegation and the removal of Sonja from her biological mother's care. Sonja entered foster care and was enrolled in a neighborhood school. There was very little communication, however, between

TABLE 4–7.   Pattern II: acute case of child aggressor or victim (e.g., child protection case with family at risk for placement of child, disrupted foster care, sudden homelessness)

High-risk circumstances

Child in custody of a child protective agency of the state investigating a report of abuse or neglect

Multiple prior child protective services placements (foster homes)

Caretaker compromised or overwhelmed (foster or biological)

Out-of-control child—aggressive or submissive child

Coercion in the family—supports failing

Limited social support

Exploitative male present or recently abandoned family

Acute windows of risk—presence of toxic adult or absence of supervision

Poverty, homelessness, domestic violence shelters

Parent addict during relapse

Therapy objectives with the family

Contact parents to provide support and technical information about clinical services crisis connection during the early phases.

Perform an intensive home-based family safety assessment.

Build an active relationship with the parent and child protective services to quickly identify resources needed to implement the service plan and determine how to access those resources.

Develop a family plan to cope with the absence of the child or continue to develop safety plans to keep the family functioning safely under stress. (Supervision of the therapist may be needed.)

Create open discussion with the family to review what individual roles each plays in the crisis behavior threatening the family.

Assist the family in making a 90-day plan to gain and improve stability. Help family set goals and assist in developing simple usable ways to measure their functioning.

Consult with child protective agencies concerning the progress being made and advocate for the desired family outcomes.

Assist parents in developing a plan to keep family safe from negative influences.

Review the economic supports that might be available, such as disability (short- or long-term); housing; or Women, Infants, and Children (WIC) nutrition program.

Maintain regular contact with school, state agency, family, and court if involved.

Offer backup psychiatry to assist in controlling aggressive outbursts or extreme withdrawal at school.

TABLE 4–7. **Pattern II: acute case of child aggressor or victim (e.g., child protection case with family at risk for placement of child, disrupted foster care, sudden homelessness)** *(continued)*

Therapy objectives with the family *(continued)*

Support school by increasing productive after-school programs.

Work with school on programs to prevent bullying and teach compassion and tolerance.

Community support

Provide in-home behavior management services to assist in decreasing aggression and increasing family harmony and productive use of time.

Offer transportation and support to visitations and model positive in-control behavior during high-stress and emotional circumstances.

Assist in accessing services required to get the family back together.

Develop an active relationship with a medical and dental provider so that all children under 21 in the family are current with their well-child care, including dental cleaning and diagnostic assessment and preventive dental interventions identified in the dental assessment.

Create a safety plan for whatever risk factors are identified by the family in therapy and make contact with accessible resources in the community.

Provide transportation and support in making applications to access resources to assist in the promotion of healthy economic functioning of the family.

Help develop a budget and a financial plan to save and obtain what the family needs. Provide help in learning to shop, store, and plan ahead for healthy living.

Provide in-home customized parental skill building.

the foster home and the school. Sonja entered the school and within several weeks was identified by her teacher, as well as by the school counselor as being a child with increasingly more aggressive problems. This pattern repeated itself over the course of 2 years and four schools. During one of the foster placements, Sonja was aggressively attacked by an older adolescent at the foster home. She was sexually assaulted over a period of 4 months while at the foster home until it was reported to a school counselor by another foster home.

At the time of her referral to a local psychiatrist, Sonja was beginning to decompensate at a rapid level. Sonja had a number of counselors over 2 years, none of whom were able to continue a course of treatment because every time Sonja moved, she needed another therapist; the foster parent would be marginally motivated to provide the transportation, and frequently Sonja would simply refuse to go to therapy altogether.

The psychiatrist quickly realized that this was not "simply" a case of medication; any long-term solution to Sonja's difficulties would require a much more extensive treatment plan. The first aspect of this was to make contact with the state agency case worker to consult about the extensive trauma history Sonja had experienced. The state agency case worker provided the psychiatrist with all of the background information and details about all of Sonja's placements as well as her difficulties at school. Sonja had undergone several educational assessments that indicated that she could function at grade level academically, but had serious social and emotional difficulties.

The psychiatrist also made a referral to a local clinic that offered a wide spectrum of services that could involve a variety of community supports, as well as ongoing home-based family therapy. He also continued to see Sonja on a weekly basis and worked to help her cope with the intense feelings of fear, hopelessness, and vulnerability she experienced during her time in foster care and during the latter part of her custody with her mother at the height of her addiction.

Sonja was extremely gifted athletically, especially with volleyball. The clinic's therapeutic mentor encouraged her to participate in an open volleyball league offered twice weekly by the local community center, and Sonja quickly became quite adept at the game and greatly enjoyed playing. She eventually was placed back into a community school and began having weekend visits with her mother. These visits proved to be extremely positive and highly motivating for Sonja. Her problems at the community school decreased greatly; psychiatrists continued to consult weekly with her, and the clinic consulted with Sonja's mother and Sonja at home processing visits.

This case illustrates treatment planning that began as a psychiatric referral and then evolved into a more complex system of care for Sonja. The psychiatrist immediately recognized the need for a more comprehensive approach and that Sonja represented a rare high-risk child who was experiencing multiple separations and placements. The psychiatrist also recognized the need for a more comprehensive involvement between home, school, and community and understood the difficulties of integrating children from foster care back into their biological homes. The psychiatrist became the care coordinator, using his office as a place to help the child process traumatic memories, as well as to direct the intervention through telephone and in-person consultations with the other professionals involved in the treatment plan. The efforts of a diverse group of natural and professional helpers in the community *can* be harnessed. The MHP is best advised to follow a comprehensive approach when attempting to consult with a child who presents with this pattern.

Pattern III: Highly Submissive Victim or Aggressive Younger Student

The third pattern forms an increasingly common part of daily practice in any clinical specialty that deals with child and family mental health (see Table 4–8). School violence is best known early in the educational cycle as bullying, and bullying is an accurate precursor of how children are likely to behave in school

TABLE 4–8. Pattern III: highly submissive victim or aggressive younger student

Circumstances with escalating risk for domestic violence

No state agency involvement

Family threatened by aggressive male

Battered woman syndrome

Child victims and bullies

History of violence

Woman and children held hostage

Jealous and controlling male influence

Therapy objectives with the family

Create a plan to protect the family by using a state agency, the court, and family to construct a boundary that reduces or eliminates contact with batterer.

Establish a family safety plan to identify any early warning signs of impending aggression.

Begin a psychoeducational process to help the family understand the cyclical nature of domestic violence and the battered woman syndrome.

Increase the assertive and protective skills of the family's caretaker and social support network.

Coordinate with child protective services agencies, if necessary, for child protection and services.

Ensure that child is functioning at school and that caretaker knows what to do, and if not, make a plan to access the needed resources.

Redirect the energy of the caretaking parent to pursuing self-improvement rather than being a participant in the cycle of domestic violence.

Provide daily support to reinforce new directions that are safe and healthy for victims in the domestic violence cycle.

Case management support: providing community support

Provide support for and transportation to appointments with law enforcement, court, district attorney, and/or state agency case worker.

Provide in-home parenting classes to develop positive discipline without aggression or loss of control and learn how to set appropriate boundaries within and around the family.

Offer transportation and educational support for new job training or education pursuits for parents.

Provide in-school support during the crisis and keep the school alerted to any spiking of risk; establish a strong link with school counselor.

throughout their educational life cycles. In creating treatment plans for school violence problems, it is essential to be alert to families that are beginning to show signs of erosion while one of the children is in early childhood education. This is an excellent point to begin a very intense and comprehensive intervention that can assist the family in coping with an isolated, yet highly dangerous intrusion into their family's safe living.

Pattern III problems commonly come to light when a young child behaves in a very unusual way. Many cases of sexual abuse are first noticed at this stage, since children often reenact the behaviors of the adults who are engaging them in sexual activity. Often, these children are the silent bystanders in families where there are protected aggressive and predatory adults. This is, unfortunately, a common pattern for young mothers who become victims of battered woman syndrome; the history of the victim begins with verbal transgressions and escalates to the physical. In these cases, there is typically not yet a child welfare intervention and there are frequently no indications outside of the school that there is a problem in the home. These children are frequently disconnected from community activities since most of the young mothers' attentions are directed toward gratifying the needs of the increasingly more possessive and disruptive males.

Case Example: Fred, an Abused Child With a Family Secret

Fred was a 5-year-old African American child whose mother was pregnant at age 14; Fred's father was incarcerated for drug distribution. Fred and his mother lived alone after his father's arrest, although there was some amount of extended family support offered. Over the course of the first 3 years of his life, Fred was exposed to many unstructured living arrangements. He was never enrolled in early childhood education and received no clinical services. Fred's mother was not a drug user, nor did she drink or "party." She was the youngest child in a large family who was been reluctant to assist her since she displayed a very independent and rebellious stance.

Fred first came to the notice of child protective services when he was in a Head Start program and his mother was in a battered women's shelter. Fred quickly became aggressive and the teachers noticed within the first several days that he was lacking in basic social skills necessary to participate in normal day care experiences. The school social worker intervened and asked Fred's mother to attend a consultation at the day care center.

Fred was referred to a child psychiatrist for an evaluation by the private-practice social worker. During this time, Fred's mother renewed her relationship with Fred's father, who had recently been released from prison. He was 24 years old and had been distributing drugs since he was initially recruited into a gang at age 14. Once Fred's father was living with them, he quickly returned to his previous street life. Fred's mother did not reveal any of this to the social worker or to the psychiatrist, and Fred continued in a diagnostic day care.

The social worker continued to receive reports from the psychiatrist and the

TABLE 4–9.   Risk areas for evaluation of student's level of home safety

Physical environment, fire risk, overcrowding

Sanitation

Adequacy of basic nutrition

Health and dental status of children under 21

Active addiction, crime, or uncontrolled mental illness

Domestic violence and battered woman

Exploitative males misusing power and control

Economic dependency on demeaning or overcontrolling males

Predation by adults, teens, or children

Sexually or aggressively reactive behavior

Adequacy of adult supervision for children

Violent community

Presence or absence of positive social networking

Housing and economic stability

Ongoing high-risk behavior in adults or children

Overt and covert aggression in family, school, or community

school and was convinced that there was some experience occurring that explained Fred's inability to function in the school setting. The school behavior remained consistent, and it appeared that it was not resonating with the messages from the social worker and Fred's mother. The social worker made a referral to a family stabilization team, who intervened and performed a risk assessment (see Table 4–9). In this risk assessment, it was clear that there were breaches of safety within the family. This was evidence that the home was not inhabited by just a mother and child, and there were extreme reactions when the family stabilization team met with Fred and his mother at home. Fred began to talk about the presence of the father and this again led to the filing of a child abuse/neglect report. Fred continued to act out at school and was at risk of losing his place in family day care. The situation became increasingly more complex and difficult to manage.

Although he was too young to participate in the organized team, Fred loved to run around the gym and displayed some gross motor flexibility that interested the community recreational department. Fred was allowed to participate as a ball boy in one of the athletic events for older children, and he quickly developed a close relationship with the soccer coach.

The family stabilization team discharged Fred, allowing him to remain in individual family therapy with the support of a child psychiatrist. This psychiatrist was able to manage Fred's medication by decreasing the daily dosage of stimulants, providing higher dosages and increased-frequency dosing during high-stress academic times only. He coordinated this through the clinical social worker who remained closely connected to the school counselor, beginning at the diagnostic day care and continuing through a community day care. Regular contacts were made between the community center and the social worker. Eventually, Fred was enrolled in a town athletic league by a therapeutic mentor who became involved at the request of the clinical social worker and the psychiatrist. This cemented the overall treatment plan and eventually the violence at school stopped before Fred entered the first grade.

Pattern IV: Self-Injurious or Self-Defeating Behavior

Karl Menninger (1938) wisely reminded us that aggression is a two-sided coin. There is a vital balance between the internalizing and externalizing forces that might force aggression in one direction or the other. In many instances, extreme aggressive behavior may stem from a variety of sources and may shift directions like the wind. In some conditions, such as pervasive developmental disorders (PDDs) or serious autism, the aggressive behavior is part of a communication breakdown complicated by difficulties with sensory integration and inability of the child to connect to normal social activities. In these cases, intensely aggressive tantrums can ensue when activities are suggested or shifted. Pattern IV violence—self-directed aggression (see Table 4–10)—is something that can reach an extreme level and may not always occur in the context of autism or PDD. There may be cases in which a student presents with an undiagnosed serious learning disability, a PDD with partially preserved social skills, Asperger's disorder, or a host of mental impairments that are sequelae of child abuse and neglect. The processes involved in a suicide at a school and a shooting at a school are very similar. The risk assessments, as well as the ways in which the suicidal or violent student becomes disconnected from normal social supports, are nearly identical, reinforcing the idea that school violence is not just an outward expression of aggression; it is the harmful misdirection of aggression that occurs within a social context controlled by adults.

Case Example: Luke, an Adolescent With a Pervasive Developmental Disorder

Luke was a tall (6 feet 5 inches) 15-year-old African American male who frequently engaged in high-risk behavior both in the community and at school. Luke had been diagnosed with a pervasive developmental disorder and had an IQ of approximately 54. Although he had the capability to participate in certain after-school activities (e.g., Boys and Girls Clubs), he regularly engaged in behaviors that resulted in his being at risk of attack by hostile forces in the community or aggressive youth at his community school.

Luke did not have any obvious mental deficiencies, yet he frequently would provoke an aggressive male into attacking him. He was not able to truly reflect on this behavior, which continued throughout his early education. Luke lived with his grandmother, and there was none of the social support at home necessary to control him if he had an aggressive outburst in response to some type of

TABLE 4–10. Pattern IV: student with self-injurious behavior

Risk areas in caretaker or child

Self-injurious behavior due to autism, pervasive developmental disorders, or communication disorders

Expressed suicidal ideation

Ongoing depression in parent or child

Ineffective medication or none tried

Parent gradually losing control of child

Caretaker giving up hope or overwhelmed

Few perceived options and resources

Therapy objectives with the family

Work with the family on a safety plan, 24-hour phone support, and follow-up psychiatry. Maintain daily contact to monitor self-destructive thinking or temptations to act.

Ensure that everybody impacted by the suicidal ideas or actions is involved in the behavioral health treatment needed to treat their problems. Identify barriers to treatment.

Organize the family to commit to a role in the close monitoring of self-destructive thinking and behavior within the family; identify roadblocks and emotions or fears expressed by the family about potential loss of life or serious injury.

Create a schedule with the family in which they identify productive and high-interest activities or services and develop a plan to increase the family's accessing of these protective resources and/or people in their social networks and community.

Refer the high-risk child or adolescent for a child psychiatric evaluation and psychological evaluation to determine the cause of the extreme behavior.

Use functional behavioral analysis to find a therapeutic intervention for self-injurious behavior.

Link school and home in understanding the "function" of the behavior.

Recognize the need to evaluate the role of the school climate in maintaining the self-injurious behavior.

Community support

Provide safety monitoring by phone and brief in-home support visits. Carry out the check-in plan designed in family therapy with the family.

Arrange for therapeutic recreation or parent respite offered during the day or weekend to reduce the overall pressure and sense of hopelessness in the family.

Plan, schedule, and transport to resources.

Offer a parenting class to help the family organize and plan for productive activities and maintain contact with resources.

Assist in the organizing of appointments, medications, prescriptions, and transportation to needed services.

Provide mentoring and social skill development.

verbal criticism or other disciplinary action from his grandmother. Luke did participate in an after-school Boys and Girls Club. Luke's mother was in early stages of recovery from a stimulant and opiate addiction.

The initial referral came from the child protective services that were called after Luke was in a fistfight in the school recreational area. He had taunted an older boy, who then struck him in the face; a rather vigorous fight ensued. The police were called, and both caretakers of the fighting children were assembled in the school. Luke's home-based MHP made a referral to an in-home behavioral management specialist who performed a functional behavioral analysis, a process in which the specific nature of Luke's behaviors could be identified and some alternative positive reward system established to encourage Luke to behave in a more socially appropriate fashion. Also, it was decided that a therapeutic mentor (who specialized in dealing with aggressive young men) would be dispatched to begin engaging Luke in some community activities where he could participate with his mentor and learn some expanded skills.

The school counselor was very active in welcoming the clinical team to coordinate with the special education team struggling to manage Luke's behavior, especially during transitional times and while waiting for transportation or in recreational activities outside. Once Luke was in a classroom, it was much easier for a teacher to individually direct him toward some type of activity that would hold his attention; he was less likely to act in a way that was provocative or aggressive. The functional behavioral analysis identified a series of five behaviors that appeared to be triggers for Luke's self-injurious behavior. The school agreed to identify the sources of these triggering behaviors and to include these in his educational plan. Luke's grandmother worked with the functional behavioral team to develop a way of rewarding prosocial behaviors, rather than the aggressive provocative behavior learned at the school.

In addition, Luke made a strong connection with the therapeutic mentor, who expanded his involvement with Luke and involved him in a local community center where he could participate in weightlifting. Luke had difficulties with an injured foot, and his size presented a barrier in his ability to participate in normal athletic activities. He was exposed by the mentor to a weightlifting program where he was able to quickly develop some remarkable body and leg strength. He seemed to enjoy the simple routines of free weights and they became his primary source of recreation, replacing video games and overeating. He continued in the after-school program, and his social awkwardness and tendency to provoke were reduced significantly.

Luke's school did not have any climate programs that would initially have been useful in redirecting Luke's difficulties. The school counselor was very aware of the problems in the school climate and the hopelessness expressed by the lack of care by the leadership within the school. The school clearly was a dumping ground, and Luke's grandmother—despite her good intentions—was in no position to add any kind of real support. In this situation, someone could have offered to work with the school to develop a climate intervention strategy (see Table 4–10).

Pattern V: Truants and Dropouts

In this pattern, the most common time at which problems begin to emerge is around 12–14 years of age. As a child approaches seventh grade, learning difficulties will clearly have done their damage, lack of support in the community will have eroded any solid foundations, and adolescents will be searching for ways to feel safe and secure in a world that may vary in providing them these basic survival needs. We have frequently observed a pattern in children between 14 and 18 years old in which these adolescents may have cycled through the substance abuse or mental health systems at one point in their earlier educational cycles. They are frequently engaged in school violence, starting early, and will frequently exhibit problems such as substance abuse, gang involvement, eating disorders, and suicidal behavior. Often, these young people are transitioning from caretaker to caretaker, and do not have strong family ties. There are frequently a number of service providers who have been active in the young person's life, although the young person is typically someone who is difficult to engage clinically or is unlikely to use any type of traditional human services.

Truancy is often the gateway to crime, aggression, and substance abuse. A Hawaiian study found that the highest early arrests for both boys and girls were due to truancy and running away (Pasko 2006). Hallfors et al. (2006) found that low grade point average and frequent school absence were predictors of later self-destructive activities such as suicidal behavior, drug abuse, and delinquency. Henry and Huizinga (2007) and Chou et al. (2006) used survey data to examine links between truancy and substance abuse. Both studies found a reciprocal relationship between truancy and drug abuse.

Truancy tends to follow a different pattern for older teens (Table 4–11) than for younger ones (Table 4–12). Treatment objectives for older and younger students differ somewhat because there are laws that compel younger children to go to school. It is critical to intercept truancy early, since it is the gateway to crime and aggression in school and in the community.

Case Example: Justin, an Older Adolescent in Need of Ongoing Assessment and Help

Justin was a 19-year-old white male who had graduated from high school and was beginning a 4-year college. Justin was removed from his biological mother's care at age 11 and lived in a series of specialized foster homes; he had participated in individual psychotherapy from the age of 11 to 17. He was eventually was adopted by a young couple who was extremely supportive of him as he began to increase his success at school athletically and academically. After 6 years of psychotherapy (1 hour per week), Justin's care was terminated. He was considered a success case and was going off to college. This outlook quickly changed within a year. Justin was placed in a psychiatric facility because of a drug-induced psychotic disorder, which resulted from his being immediately overwhelmed by his new independence, the college drug culture, and his own self-destructive tendencies.

TABLE 4–11.　Pattern V: truants and dropouts (older teens: ages 16–21 years)

Risk situations/circumstances

Early adult transitional disruption (dropouts, truancy, failed college), substance abuse, gang involvement, eating disorders, suicide

Truancy beginning at age 14 years

History of inpatient treatment for behavioral health:

• Substance abuse

• Mental illness

Transitioning from inpatient facility to community residence

Interruption of educational and vocational goals

In need of bridge work to community

Need for multiservice aftercare

At risk for readmission to inpatient care on multiple occasions in the course of 6 months

Therapy objectives for the family

Create "buy in" with the intervention team, the young adult, and the family; allow for the proper independence and confidentiality for the young adult as well as releases of information to facilitate resource development.

Set a stabilization timetable that highlights goals as well as roles and responsibilities for the accomplishment of these goals.

Work with the family to develop a weekly schedule that addresses vocational and recreational goals:

• Making all critical appointments

• Reengaging in vocational or educational pursuits

• Seeking short- or long-term disability

• Ensuring that all medical/dental care is current

• Providing vocational rehabilitation

• Arranging special accommodations for work, school, training, and driving

Establish a coordinated community team that offers support and guidance to any member of the family, connecting to needed supports.

Communicate with the family about their potential fears and any obstacles to successful community living.

Evaluate clinical usefulness of existing treatment resources and support those that are helping. Work with the family to access

• Psychotherapy or substance abuse treatment

• Psychiatric follow-up

• Recovery or support groups

TABLE 4–11.   **Pattern V: truants and dropouts (older teens: ages 16–21 years)** *(continued)*

Community support

Provide support and transportation to all critical meetings; organize appointments and monitor attendance.

Provide specialized support in exploring vocational or educational activities, including in-class support, work with special services to arrange accommodations, help with homework and study.

Provide in-home and one-to-one psychoeducation about the behavioral health problem that led to the inpatient referral.

Create a daily log to assist in the independent accomplishment of the needed activities of daily life.

Provide support and transportation for patient or family to support the social-recreational development of healthy community activities.

This is a case of school violence expressed as aggression turned toward the self, in which someone who had struggled through the system became trapped during the transition into adulthood. Young people who grow up as wards of the state in foster care and who try to set up independent living have a special set of needs in order to launch them into successful adult lives and careers. This is particularly true of young women trying to transition from lives of being victims into becoming empowered young women seeking educational opportunities. All too frequently, these young women become overburdened by the constant demands of parenting at a very young age. The males seem to lose contact with normal social supports and begin to use drugs, engage in repeated high-risk sexual behavior, and become involved in illegal activities.

Justin *(continued)*

When Justin was reengaged in psychotherapy, it was clear that he was disoriented and required inpatient care. After his release from the hospital, Justin was quickly engaged in employment by a landscaper friend of his adoptive parents. He was also reengaged with the same therapist who had treated him since he was a young boy. The therapist quickly ordered a therapeutic mentor to engage Justin in some social-recreational activities so that he would have options for filling his time after work with activities that did not include drinking or hanging with the same crowd that led to his earlier loss of control. He eventually became interested in martial arts and developed a positive relationship with a young woman; these factors greatly reduced his temptation and active participation in substance abuse. He now trains 5 nights a week with his new female companion, and his ongoing success is being supported in outpatient psychotherapy.

TABLE 4–12.   Truancy prior to age 16 years

Risk situations/circumstances

CHINS (Child in Need of Services) report made or family court involved;
  safety still compromised

Parent cannot enforce curfew or consequences

Persistent high-risk exposure during unsupervised community time

Defiance of authority

Failure to report for curfew

School refusal

Defiance at school

Running away

Common treatment goals and strategies

Referrals for services

Applications for resources

Consultations/family advocacy

Service accountability

Information sharing for treatment plans

Testimony

Written letters, phone calls

Stimulating the system

Conducting assessments

Advocacy in meetings

Repairing burnt bridges

Building new connections

Teaching negotiation skills in the system

Role modeling system management

System skills for parents

Finding resources

Designing an approach

Humanizing the system

Draining authority conflict

Paradoxical skills training

Use of silence

Value of respect

Assertiveness rather than aggression

Conflict management with collaterals

Building relationships with others before the trouble starts

Avoiding triangles

Understand collaterals problem with patient

Validating difficulties without blaming patient

TABLE 4–12.   Truancy prior to age 16 years *(continued)*

Common treatment goals and strategies *(continued)*
Derailing blame
Educational advocacy
Individualized Education Program (IEP) or Section 504 plan
Informal consultation/school meetings
Parent–school signal resonance

Justin's case illustrates that school violence is not something that stops at high school. School shootings such as those at Virginia Tech and the frequent reports of workplace violence are evidence that the process first experienced as school violence is expressed in many different social contexts. In the pattern of truancy and dropout, school violence is typically the way in which a child displays these tendencies earlier in the educational process, and this may cause the child to be disconnected from school or to be allowed to function in school as a sadistic bully, resulting in his increasing involvement with criminal activity when left unsupervised in the community. Again, this is the high-risk time for recruitment into gangs, which are an ongoing source of school violence whether the child is being recruited in school, being sold drugs, or being attacked and held up for money while trying to get to school.

Conclusion

Treatment planning in school violence is a complex task. MHPs are challenged to create powerful interventions that may combine traditional therapy strategies with social systems approaches involving the home, school, and community. Also, school climate is a key element in planning interventions. Why? The best individual and family therapy cannot undo a day of shaming at school. This model creates a framework to design flexible and comprehensive interventions into school violence problems.

KEY CLINICAL CONCEPTS

- Schools are becoming the most natural setting to intervene with children who display or are hurt by school violence.

- Understanding the child's interlocking social systems is a diagnostic necessity.

- The Internet has collapsed the boundaries between home, school, and the community. This causes increased pressure from shaming events in person or on the Internet.

- Treatment philosophy stresses the MHP's understanding of interlocking social systems and how they impact a child's behavior at school.

- Mentalization is a key process underlying the treatment philosophy. Enhancing a child's reflective capacity is used to increase self-control, decrease impulsivity, and improve his or her ability to accurately read social cues.

- Failure to launch into independent living is a common way in which students can become stuck and an easy target for involvement in destructive behaviors at school. This pattern may be more common among higher-SES families.

- Excessive pressure to perform is a destructive process observed in higher-SES homes with successful and competitive parents. These pressures will show in school and may result in suicide or extreme behaviors, truancy, substance use, or crime.

- When one of the child's interlocking systems is not mentalizing, there is disequilibrium that is often acted out at school.

- Diagnosis of school violence problems requires taking a very broad perspective in building an understanding of the impact of stressors on the various systems affecting the child's development in the home, school, and community.

- Treatment strategies aim to empower families to control their children at home, at school, and in the community.

- One essential treatment goal in school violence is containing aggression.

- The MHP is a quarterback or play caller for complex school violence interventions.

- There is one primary goal in treatment: a peaceful day at school.

- Psychopharmacology plays a core role in containing aggression at school, decreasing impulsivity, unlocking depression, and controlling anxiety.

- The MHP has an expandable role but remains anchored in traditional therapy ethics and values.

- Learning disabilities are frequent trigger points for school violence.

- It is critical in effective intervention in school violence problems to create common goals and synchronized signals for the containment of aggression at school.

- MHPs need to help humanize the system, including the school, for clients who are angry and distrusting of any authority.

- MHPs play a role in helping families empathize with others, especially those who may be perceived as adversaries (as is often the case with child welfare workers).

- There are five major patterns of school violence:

  — Repetitive school disruption in the form of illegal and aggressive behavior

  — Acute case of child aggressor or victim

  — Highly submissive victim or aggressive young student

  — Student with self-injurious behavior

  — Truants and dropouts: early and later school years

References

Blos P: The Young Adolescent. New York, Simon & Schuster, 1974

Chou L, Ho C, Chen C: Truancy and illicit drug use among adolescents surveyed via street outreach. Addict Behav 31:149–154, 2006

DeRosier ME, Cillessen AH, Coie JD, et al: Group social context and children's aggressive behavior. Child Dev 65:1068–1079, 1994

Erikson E: Childhood and Society. New York, WW Norton, 1963

Freud A: Normality and pathology in childhood: assessment of development (1965), in The Writings of Anna Freud, Vol 6. New York, International Universities Press, 1965, pp 3–273

Freud A: The ego and the mechanisms of defense (1936), in The Writings of Anna Freud, Vol 2. New York, International Universities Press, 1966, pp 1–191

Hallfors D, Cho H, Brodish PH: Identifying high school students "at risk" for substance use and other behavioral problems: implications for prevention. Subst Use Misuse 41:1–15, 2006

Henry KL, Huizinga DH: Truancy's effect on the onset of drug use among urban adolescents placed at risk. J Adolesc Health 40:9–17, 2007

Kerr ME, Bowen M: Family Evaluation. New York, WW Norton, 1988

Menninger K: Man Against Himself. Orlando, FL, Harcourt, Brace, and Jovanovich, 1938

Menninger K: A Manual for Psychiatric Case Study. Baltimore, MD, Waverly Press, 1952

Pasko LJ: The female juvenile offender in Hawaii: understanding gender differences in arrests, adjudications, and social characteristics of juvenile offenders. National Institute of Corrections, 2006. Available at: http://nicic.gov/Library/023426. Accessed December 4, 2010.

Perkins J: Medicaid EPSDT litigation. National Health Law Program, October 2, 2009. Available at: http://www.healthlaw.org/images/stories/epsdt/1-EPSDT-Docket.pdf. Accessed December 7, 2010.

Sacco F, Larsen R: Threat assessment: a critique of an ongoing assessment. Journal of Applied Psychoanalytic Studies 5:171–188, 2003

Sacco F, Twemlow S, Fonagy P: Secure attachment to family and community: a college proposal for cost containment within higher user populations of multiple problem families. Smith Coll Stud Soc Work 77:31–51, 2007

Twemlow SW, Sacco FC: The application of traditional martial arts in the treatment of violent adolescents. Adolescence 33:505–518, 1998

Twemlow SW, Sacco FC, Fonagy P: Embodying the mind: movement as a container for destructive aggression. Am J Psychother 62:1–33, 2008

U.S. Department of Education: Free Appropriate Public Education for Students With Disabilities: Requirements Under Section 504 of The Rehabilitation Act of 1973, August 2010. Available at: http://www2.ed.gov/about/offices/list/ocr/docs/edlite-FAPE504.html. Accessed December 4, 2010.

Volkan V: Bloodlines: From Ethnic Pride to Ethnic Terrorism. New York, Farrar, Straus, & Giroux, 1997

5

Bullying Is a Process, Not a Person

Inviting the Community Into the School

"Power does not corrupt people, people corrupt power."

Andre Gide

"We can easily forgive a child who is afraid of the dark, the real tragedy of life is when men are afraid of the light."

Plato

THIS chapter defines bullying and its related facets, focusing on what a mental health professional (MHP) can do to help schools manage bullying from a clinical and systems perspective. In other words, we view destructive bullying as a process and as a social dynamic that grips a child's entire world, not simply when the child is at school. There is a difference between a child who is "at risk" and one who is also victimizing others at school and has evolved into a true bully. Thus, when a child or adolescent is "at risk," an MHP needs to conduct a very thorough assessment of the risk and protective factors, and should be careful of using the pejorative label "bully." It not only badly stigmatizes the child, but can be reacted to angrily by parents and may even obstruct a potentially seamless process of risk and protective factor assessment, preventing useful early and quick preventive care from occurring.

As an interconnected process within many schools, "the bullying process" can become the way both at-risk victimizers and true bullies attack their victims. We argue that most bullying is generated from unmonitored pathological power dynamics with the collapse of mentalization, and that is what allows coercion within a school. We posited in 2008 that any antibullying program will work if the process of implementing change at the school stresses teacher buy-in and the creation of a reflective process that spans school years (Twemlow and Sacco 2008). Conversely, even the best program will not work if it is forced, short-lived, and not embraced by the school.

The essence of this systems approach is that a bully is an individual caught up in a complex social systems network (one that we will attempt to define in this chapter) that makes the bully part of a group process, not simply a sick individual driven by his or her own psychopathology. We view bullies as generally unwilling scapegoats in a dysfunctional social system. The MHP needs to not just "know" this, but also know how to use this information. Simply put, the bully–victim–bystander equation creates the basic framework of the power dynamics in question. Bullying is the use of power and position to create public humiliation for a submissive target. A victim or target is submissive and becomes the antagonist with the bully as protagonist. The rest of the school is the bystanding audience for this power theater but is inextricably involved with it, as we will demonstrate.

Etymologically, the word *bully* (according to the *Oxford English Dictionary*) is quite obscure, having evolved from the "bully boy" of medieval times, a swashbuckling figure who was a protector of the weak, to later definitions describing a hurtful ruffian (rather than protective) who overwhelms people for no good reason. What is most interesting is that the victim has no role in either of these definitions. We do agree with most of the authorities in the school bullying literature that the "true bully" is primarily a child with psychopathic tendencies who may end up in serious trouble with the law before becoming a fully grown adult. Later we will describe the group dynamics of a very pathological social system in which all individuals are eventually sucked into submissive victim roles with a bully tyrant leader protected by special "henchmen," as often occurs in cults (Twemlow and Hough 2005).

The impact of bullying essentially depends on how the bully's social context accommodates the activation of bullying behavior at school. In a narrow psychiatric analysis, we can view the bully as a defective psychopath. The community, as an abdicating social system, tends to treat such young people as being unsuitable for the school. When the child ceases to contain and express the aggression of the community in a socially acceptable fashion, that community ejects the child. This process of community abdication of responsibility for that child inevitably may lead the child to a life of criminality, forcing the community then into the role of victim of the criminal's activity. Our collective observation is that less than 2% of the population in most schools consists of children of this nature. They may have been brought up in environments where they have seen a great deal of parental aggression, and they may be genetically oriented toward a callous disregard for human feelings. The MHP can assist in intervening in these special circumstances as well. Children living in this type of home tend to use aggression to manage their peers as part of their identity. Such children, if they get into serious trouble at school, do require special management and psychiatric care, and often should be removed from school for their own sakes.

Redefining Bullying From a Social Systems/Bystander Perspective

Destructive bullying is more than "simply" fighting; it is an interpersonal and large-group process that creates humiliation for a victim in front of a bystanding audience. In order to be considered true bullying, the humiliation needs to be sustained, not just an isolated occurrence. Bullying tends to be a compulsively repeated psychological process that begins between individuals or groups of unequal power, and then often evolves into a peer group phenomenon. Cliques grow quickly; social war zones are formed within the school environment. True bullying is not the periodic stupidity of young people hurting one another's feelings; it is a sustained process of a peer group or adults consciously using humiliating strategies in public toward a targeted individual. True bullying is clearly coercive and is not just an occasional misplaced comment or broken allegiance to a friend; it is by definition a mean-spirited and sadistic sequence of activities targeting an individual. True bullying involves a clear intention to humiliate a victim, but this also functions as a stepping-stone toward overall social dominance. As children move into puberty, they shift from physical intimidation—pushing, shoving, and threatening—to more socially based bullying: exclusion, name calling, humiliating photos, Internet bullying, and other forms of more subtle nonphysical coercion.

In comparison, the at-risk victimizer can do all of these things as part of a prematurely foreclosed identity: Erikson (1963) described the young person as "…fallen prey to overidentifications which isolate the small individual from his budding identity and his milieu" (pp. 239–241), as part of a group-influenced peer mind-set whose standards are both demanding and often pathological and irresistible. Such victimizers are often troubled by their reluctant compliance, which they describe as not what they would normally do outside the school setting.

Dr. James Gilligan (1996) eloquently described the role of shame in the evolution of violence, drawing on firsthand experiences from decades of working as a prison psychiatrist in various Massachusetts state prisons. Gilligan noted the powerful role that shame plays in the causal factors in the evolution of violence, citing numerous examples of how young people may be incarcerated for long periods of time as punishment for seemingly petty crimes. When interviewed, many of these young prisoners explained that they were not fighting over material goods, but rather to gain respect of others or to create better images for themselves. Shame is a causal factor in many of the destructive decisions made by adolescents who may be caught up in a group dynamic that insists on respect (obedience to the bully leader), and in creating a macho self-image in that way. Such children may look like true bullies but are instead at-risk victims of the dynamics of the social group.

Figure 5–1 summarizes the group relationships that are part of normal everyday human interactions (Twemlow and Harvey 2010). As illustrated in the figure, the co-created roles of victimizer, victim, and bystander cannot exist without each other and are occupied by all of us at different times in our lives. We may perform as all three during the course of a single day, although certainly not to the extent defined by extreme instances of bullying. In other words, power issues are a part of what goes on in normal human relationships every day. All of us at some time or another are in a submissive relationship to somebody else. This can be perfectly comfortable if an individual makes the choice to be there and is not coerced into it. A simple situation can quickly become a power struggle as coercion, and finally humiliation, are added to the equation.

It is important to differentiate group relations involving normal power issues from the pathological roles of sick victimizer and victim, in which power issues have devolved into power struggles. Apart from being confused with psychiatric diagnoses, these fixed unequal power roles can lead to the repetition of pathological behaviors, and thus are frequently evident in situations where power dynamics form an intrinsic part of an illness or are triggers for unhealthy behavior. For example, the pattern of choosing an abusive spouse is commonly seen in borderline personality disorder (self-destructiveness).

The "Stuck in Role" Victim as Fuel for Bullying and Victimization

The MHP must consider the perennial "stuck in role" victim within this power dynamic regardless of whether there is a bullying process obvious. The stuck-

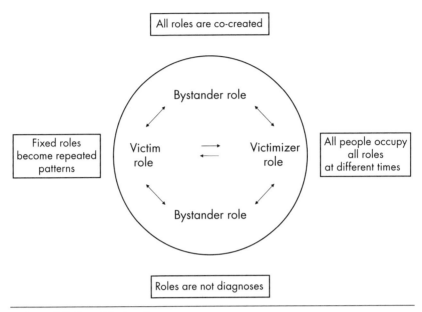

FIGURE 5–1.   Circle of power.

victim role is characterized by submission, which activates both the attention of the bystanding audience and the sadistic wishes of the bully. These observable victim–victimizer interactions are played out in school corridors, at bus stops and playgrounds, on athletic fields, and in gymnasiums, and they continue after hours at student's homes, enhanced by the Internet and cell phones. Certain victim roles can become fixed early in life, and the life for that victim becomes burdened by constant public humiliation. True bullies tend to seek out easy targets to ensure that their public displays of humiliation are seen by the audience. They are sucked into that role by both the stuck victim and their own proclivities to hurt. People picked out as problems will be the ones who make the loudest noise, and these tend always to be the bullies and their victims.

This is the pattern tragically illustrated by the suicide of Phoebe Prince in South Hadley, Massachusetts (Oliver 2010). In this case, a vulnerable victim (recently emigrated to the United States from Ireland) became trapped in a vicious peer onslaught of hurtful communications. There were no victimizers stalking the corridors. This victim was pulled into a bullying process with multiple students in bullying roles devolving into a form of school psychosis.

Victims seem to attract the bully, just as the bully pursues the victim. The result of this dynamic is, again, a public show of humiliation. However, the most commonly forgotten element in this equation is the audience of bystanders. Essentially, this audience fuels the process of bullying. There would be little reinforcement for the bully and victim without the presence and involvement of the bystanders. This group of audience members identifies with different roles in the coercive process from a number of different positions within the larger group. For instance, some bystanders identify with the victim, while others may instead live vicariously through the bully, all but forgetting how their own engagement can be fueling a destructive and harmful process (as indicated in Table 5–4 ["Bystanding roles"], later in this chapter).

Victims of the drama of bullying are typically easily targeted by the school and the MHP for help. They tend to withdraw and act in self-defeating ways. The school will notice the withdrawn and miserable states of mind victims display. Counselors can diagnose a victim's condition and begin to try to help him or her deal with the residual effects of the bullying process. However, it is often very difficult for school administrators to know what happens to these students when they are not at school. They may, for instance, be bullied at home by parents or older siblings, or they may be experiencing problems that play a role in their victimization at school as well. Some children may have dysfunctional parents who neglect them and sent them to school unprepared and dressed for ridicule. These children can become targets very early in their school lives.

While studying a large group of Jamaican schoolchildren, all of whom wore uniforms, we were surprised to learn that the children still honed in on the differences in each other's appearance. The uniforms may have been the same color, but their conditions varied greatly, as did the children's footwear, belts, and accessories, or lack thereof. Children will always find differences to pick on (Twemlow et al., in press); Freud (1918/1957, 1930/1957) defined this human process as "the narcissism of minor differences." In other words, to establish who is the best (most dominant), people will notice differences in each other through a narcissistic exaggeration of minor differences between them, something as insignificant as shoe type, for instance. Caring and involved parents take the time to make sure their children look their best, and students show the result of that parental investment. Many of the very poor children from rural Jamaica had uniforms, pressed and ironed to perfection. The children's teeth sparkled; they had clearly benefited from what Jamaicans call "good broughtupsy," or concerned caretaking, from their families, whether extended or immediate. Distracted and dysfunctional upper-income parents may heap material goods on their children yet fail to invest the time and quality of involvement needed to teach positive values.

We must be mindful of the damaging effects being bullied can have on individuals and find ways to prevent bullying from escalating. In Alaska, a middle school student attempted to hang himself, and although he survived his suicide attempt, he remains severely mentally and physically impaired as a result. Where was the school while this was happening to one of its students? Where were his friends? How could a child become so desperate and miserable that he would take his own life without anyone noticing and intervening? In this case, as in others we have studied, the social context became a causal ingredient in the escalation of violence. The school dismissed the significance of the bullying, and parents are often the last to know. It is up to schools to penetrate this often-undiscussable underground "peer conspiracy" of silence. Without information from the peer network, it is virtually impossible to predict and stop violence within a school. No system of therapy designed to help at-risk students can be successfully implemented unless students have an adult they can talk to and whom they trust. Devine (1996) approached this problem in his social anthropological work in New York City schools, concluding that schools have distanced teachers from students by adopting procedures and policies that stress mechanical safety over teachers' relationships with students. Teachers are forced into roles by institutional policies that promote fear of the student and encourage abdicating "hands-off" approaches because of the fear of lawsuits.

Group Dynamics and the School Social System

At either socioeconomic class extreme, bullies become part of a pathological social group capable of usurping the leadership of the designated leaders (principal, teachers, and administrative staff) of the school. A bully is traditionally surrounded by a number of bully (aggressive) bystanders and "identification with the aggressor"–style bystanders who become part of the social clique that coerces and induces fear in the school. Following the group dynamics theories of both Bion (1959) and Volkan (2004), this bully group dynamic, if not clearly recognized and dealt with, will induce and ensure a constant state of fear, affecting the school as a whole.

Teachers will become upset by the need to punish more and will often unintentionally and unconsciously adopt methods that are pathological, knowing these approaches are not what they would normally take. One teacher caught in such a setting slapped a child across the face in a classroom. This act led to her suspension from the school, and in counseling she realized that she had been trying to manage an impossible situation in the school, as the therapist helped her modify the projected aggression she embodied. This state of mind—defined in psychoanalysis as "projective identification"—allowed this teacher to be trapped into embodying the aggression the group projected onto her (that is, not her aggression), and she was subsequently controlled by it through interpersonal pressure of the group. The teacher reported experiencing this aggression as a foreign body in herself which made her "act crazily," as she put it. After appropriate psychotherapy and a university course in child development, she moved to another school and was able to see the contrast in group processes. Projective identification is a defense that can occur very painfully in intense group settings where people's normal boundaries and common sense are overwhelmed. The reaction of the teacher is a submission to the controlling force of the bullying student group, due to her own unconscious problems and boundary issues (countertransferences).

Freud spoke of group power and its effect on individuals in *Group Psychology and the Analysis of the Ego* (1921/1955). He said, in his consideration of large groups like the church and military,

> In order to make a correct judgment upon the morals of groups, one must take into consideration the fact that when individuals come together in a group all their individual inhibitions fall away and all the cruel, brutal and destructive instincts, which lie dormant in individuals as relics of a primitive epoch, are stirred up to find free gratification. But under the influence of suggestion groups are also capable of high achievements in the shape of abnegation, unselfishness, and devotion to an ideal. While with isolated individuals personal interest is almost the only motive force, with groups it is very rarely prominent. It is possible to speak of an individual having his moral standards raised by a group. (p. 79)

One might add to this that moral standards can also be lowered, as in the case of the teacher. The power and example of the leader is critical to the moral (peaceful school), or immoral (cult) outcome of the group social process. The power of the large group is remarkable to behold as in the cases of people's submission to pathological dictators like Stalin and Hitler. Can this occur in a school? It can indeed.

Such an incident occurred in a school dominated by serious "gangstas" (children in gangs created by adult criminals to distribute drugs). The school principal decided, with the support of the staff, to give over discipline in the school to the gangstas to see if responsibility and accountability would reshape their attitudes. The school was peaceful for about a month; the gangstas immediately established a discipline code that operated through hidden threat. They were also using their newfound power to distribute drugs which, as you can imagine, eventually led to the collapse and closure of the school, as well as hundreds of out-of-school suspensions.

The principal who made this decision was not mentally ill; he was simply overwhelmed by the unconscious dynamics of the large group. Bion (1970) would say that a "Negative K" situation exists in a school whose designated leadership is usurped in this way. Knowledge (K), in this context, is not an intellectual value, but refers instead to what the school community knows about itself that makes that place desirable and worth maintaining. The goal of "Positive K" is to build the school's climate into a place children value and want to belong to. Thus, in "Negative K" schools, the principal operates under a fright–flight unconscious basic assumption, responding to threats with short-term Band-Aid solutions. In such schools, the environment often seems frayed at the edges: children may fight over games and the use of equipment, the grounds tend to be unkempt, and the classrooms themselves are cluttered and often dirty. Teachers escape from these schools as quickly as they can and resent any extra time they have to spend preparing lessons or working after hours.

Teachers are not the only ones who contribute to the group dynamic, however. Coaches are often bullies and view failure of any kind as humiliating. Intervening in such large-group dynamics requires a psychological approach to the school as a large dysfunctional group. The MHP has a major role in understanding these group dynamics at school and in showing how protective factors can be realistically created. Much of what goes on in a devolved school is unconscious and cannot be modified by merely trying to adapt the conscious mind to healthier ways of thinking. These efforts, however well-intentioned, are simply drowned out by the pathology of the unconscious.

We are not suggesting that all schools need full-blown psychoanalytic consultation, but they may benefit immensely from simple interventions that recognize these unconscious dynamics at work. As an example, during a school-wide assembly to discuss problems within a school, the school bully and his henchmen grouped together at the back of the room, talking and laughing among themselves. The leaders of the assembly recognized them and, during the large-group interaction, brought them into the group process by designating them as leaders, asking them to create a play that would illustrate the problem of bullying within the school. This play was performed for the whole community, was very successful, and led to a paradoxical shift in the school's environment immediately afterward.

Since the play had been so successful—both with the children involved in it and within the community around the school—it became very well known and discussed, but many students were identifying with the bullies, especially in wanting to become stronger like them. This obviously alarmed the school leaders. However, after several brief school meetings with an MHP who specialized in dealing with group regressions, the children realized that what they wanted was not to control others, but to live together peacefully with the common purpose of being friendly, happy, and having fun. One student said, "I am now friendly with kids I don't even like." The leader of the bullies even refocused himself and became the captain of the soccer team. The value of encouraging friendship through shared goals (rather than pathological personal intimacy and idiosyncratic regressions) helped to unite the school community. The school became an effective symbol with which children could connect with pride and with respect for each other—that is, a "Positive K" school again.

As we will continue to emphasize, the group dynamics of a successful intervention must view bullying as a process, not a person. The collapse of mentalization is induced by complex social factors, such as active power struggles,

crime, or poor leadership in the surrounding communities, subsequently creating a dynamic within the school in which the principal emerges as a flight–
fight leader. The flight–fight leader typically responds to school violence problems by implementing action-oriented short-term solutions that put out fires
but fail to establish a long-term policy for the school. Such schools can end up
feeling like prisons.

In one such school system, the elementary school was surrounded by walls
topped with coiled barbed wire, not unlike a POW camp. When the school no-
tified the police of any disturbance, children and teachers were instructed to lie
motionless on the floor, and a squad of heavily armed detectives were brought in
to manage the disturbance like a prison uprising. If any children moved, they
were punished. The police once released a picture on local television of a fifth-
grade child handcuffed to a chair because he had moved when he should have
been lying still on the floor. The community had created this pathological dynamic in a school already dominated by bullies. Although this was an extreme
example, schools like this are not uncommon in the United States. In such examples, the school students lose respect for teachers and tend to band together
in small groups to protect themselves.

Frequently, the bullying may be more subtle, especially in affluent schools
where competition for grades becomes a focal point. The victims in those conditions are the children who "only" achieve placement in state universities
rather than the Ivy League schools, and who might attempt suicide over state
university placement. (This issue is discussed in more detail in the section "The
Problem of Excellence: Achievement Pressure in Affluent Families and Schools"
[see Chapter 1, "School Violence: Range and Complexity of the Problem"].) In
one such school that we observed, the top academic group angrily viewed themselves as victims of a school system that made them hate studying. The school
staff refused to evaluate the problem, instead utilizing questionnaires that
showed notably few problems; they would not allow the word *bully* to be part of
the school vocabulary or be discussed further. The principal focused on new
building projects (avoidant bystanding). This school adopted a watered-down
character-building antibullying program and continues to be dominated and
controlled by avoidant, controlling bully parents and frightened, abdicating,
and victim–bystander staff. The number of suicidal crises and completed suicides in the school is increasing.

The so-called normal child—that is, a child without a predisposition either
to bullying or to being a victim—is caught in the devolution and might act this
dilemma out in troubling ways, thanks to the pathological sadomasochism and
aggression of the group. Such a child can become envious of the bully group's
power and triumph, entertaining an unconscious wish to identify with the aggressor, and will be disturbed by the envious arousal and triumph he or she experiences vicariously. Thus, for reasons that are entirely psychological, such

---

TABLE 5–1. Bullying myths

Bullying is a normal part of growing up.
Bullying involves children only.
Bullying is always physical.
Bullying is worse in boys than in girls.
Interventions must target the bully.
Victims are best treated as sick.
Bullying only happens in poor schools.

TABLE 5–2. New thinking about bullying

Bullying is most destructive as social aggression.
High-achieving schools are at the highest risk for social aggression.
Bullying is a process, not a person.
Bystanders are the causal agents in bullying and prime targets for intervention.
The process of change is the key, not the antibullying program.

---

children will not be able to learn very well, nor will they wish to go to school, and they are much more likely to act out this behavior at home and in the community.

Tables 5–1 and 5–2 summarize some of the myths about bullying current in our society and also some of the new thinking about bullying.

Revisiting Social Dynamics From a Bystander Perspective

One hypothesis of this chapter is that the social context—rooted in the Latin word *contextus,* meaning "a joining together"—situates the bystander in an unavoidably active role created, in the case of school violence, by the victim–victimizer interaction; being passive is not possible from this perspective. The victim, victimizer, and bystander roles are co-created and dialectically defined (Twemlow et al. 1996). In these roles, mentalizing (i.e., self-awareness, self-agency, reflectiveness, and accurate assessment of the mental states of oneself and other people) is impaired (Fonagy 2001). Fonagy's concept of mentalizing takes a Hegelian perspective in that the individual is defined through social feedback from interactions with others. Over time, the individual's "theory of mind" regarding self and others is continuously modified by feedback from this interaction with others. In the case of the infant, for example, if the caretaker gives feedback in an empathic, constructive, and accurate manner, the child develops a theory of mind of others that can process reality in a healthy and adaptive fashion. If, however, pathological feedback is received, the child's mind may develop in distorted ways, manifested in overt and covert psychopathology in later adult life.

The pathological bystander plays an active role with a variety of manifestations, in which an individual or group indirectly and repeatedly participates in the victimization process. Bystanding may either facilitate or ameliorate victimization. The community bystander role could be described as an abdicating one. *Abdication* then is avoidance of acknowledgment of the role in the bullying process by the abdicating bystander, who projects the blame onto others. The bystander is propelled into the role through interactions with the victim and victimizer, and the ongoing interaction can be activated in a helpful or harmful direction.

The roles of bully, victim, and bystander represent a dissociation process; the victim is dissociated from the school community as "not us" by the bully on behalf of the bystanding community. From this vantage point, interventions in a school setting must focus on the transformation of the bystander into a committed community member and witness. Interventions from this perspective should promote recognition within the large school group of the dissociated element (represented by the victim), as a part of themselves about which they are anxious. The recognition of the dissociation process (represented by the bully) should occur as a defensive action for which the bystanders are, in part, responsible.

A peaceful learning environment is then restored when the fragmenting effect of the dissociation process is interrupted by first understanding that it is a largely unconscious effort to deal with anxiety in response to a dysfunctional, coercive, and disconnected social system. Dissociation is a violent process, and the goal of any intervention is the transformation of brute power into constructive and respectful communication. This requires a clear conceptualization of the group's task from a perspective that does not permit scapegoating, empowers bystanders into a helpful altruistic role, and does not overemphasize therapeutic efforts with the victim or victimizer. This triadic approach is summarized in Table 5–3.

Symptomatic behavior, such as violence and bullying within such a system, is, from this perspective, a consultation-in-action to the authority structure of the administrative system. That is, the symptom is not merely a problem to solve, but a dysfunctional solution or adaptation, which keeps a larger more painful and more meaningful problem unseen. The abdicating bystander projects blame onto the victim and victimizer. We summarize several other bystander roles in Table 5–4.

Approaches to school and community violence that focus solely on correcting pathological bystanding roles and/or bully and victim roles ignore what we believe is an important part of the solution: to activate the helpful and often altruistic bystander role.

TABLE 5–3.   Redefining bullying: from a dyadic to a triadic approach

Dyadic
Bully and victim are primary focus
Individual roles of bully or victim are seen as fixed
Bystander audience is passive observer
Purely external definition
Bully and victim are behavioral roles
Focus is on behavioral change
Interventions targets individuals

Triadic
Social context of bully and victim is primary focus
Co-created bully–victim–bystander roles are in flux
Bystander initiates the stress
Bully–victim–bystander interactions have complex internal meanings
Focus is on mentalizing
Interventions aimed at climate

Dyadic definition of bullying
The repeated harmful exposure of a person to interactions that produce social
  reward for the bully, are hard to defend against, and involve an imbalance of
  power with the bully stronger and the victim weaker

Triadic definition of bullying
The repeated harmful exposure of an individual or group perceived as weaker
  than the bully to negative interactions inflicted by one or more dominant
  persons and caused mainly by the active or passive role of the bystander
  audience linked with the bully and victim in complex, ever-changing
  dynamic roles and social rewards. **Note:** The helpful bystander can play a
  major role in reversing these negative interactions.

Who are helpful bystanders? Any individual in the school environment can be
one: teachers, students, support staff, volunteers, parents, and others. Such people are not really bystanders any longer, but move from passive to active and altruistic roles. Such people are often natural leaders who enjoy being helpful in a
way that is not self-centered; they do not seek the limelight, but instead gain pleasure simply from the act of being helpful. In schools and communities, they rarely
occupy traditional elected leadership roles, such as class president or committee
chairman; they may doubt their own leadership skills, and need encouragement
to emerge. Such individuals often are turned to by others with their problems. Instead of directing and advising, they tend to listen and mentalize (Patterson et al.
1992). To our knowledge, there are no evidence-based methods by which such altruistic bystanders can be identified, but in a school setting, staff members (espe-

TABLE 5–4.   Bystanding roles

Type	Mentalization	Subjective state	Role in the system
Bully (aggressive)	Collapse of mentalization	Excitement, often sadomasochistic	Establishes a way to set up victimization within the school community
Puppetmaster variant* of bully	Authentic empathy and reflectiveness collapses. Capable of logical planning and nonfeeling empathy	Arrogant, grandiose sense of powerfulness	Committed to violent outcomes, achieved by conscious manipulation
Victim (passive)	Collapse of mentalization	Fearful, apathetic, helpless	Passively and fearfully drawn into the victimization process
Identification with aggressor	Mentalization collapses	Desperately wants to be part of popular and powerful groups; willing to do anything to achieve social dominance	No euphoria. Often assumes the "bouncer" role or servant for the popular group, thereby enhancing victimization
Avoidant	Mentalization preserved by denial	Defensive euphoria—an individual action	A staff reaction facilitating victimization by denial of personal responsibility
Abdicating	Mentalization preserved by projection and projective identification	Outraged at the "poor" performance of others—an agency or group action	Abdicates responsibility by scapegoating; seen in community members
Sham	Mentalization preserved	Uses conscious, largely verbal manipulation; deliberate and calm	Neither victim nor victimizer; role is adopted for personal or (often) political reasons

TABLE 5–4.   Bystanding roles *(continued)*

Type	Mentalization	Subjective state	Role in the system
Helpful (altruistic bystanders have been called "Upstanders")	Mentalization enhanced	Compassionate, outraged at harm to others, but not a "do-gooder"	Mature and effective use of individual and group psychology to promote self-awareness and develop skills to resist victimization

*In a recent school shooting, a boy set up a shooting to occur at a school dance, taking few pains to hide the plan and recruiting a resentful victim bystander into the role of killer. The puppetmaster bystander did not attend the dance, but came later to observe the murders at the prearranged time, as the dance was ending.

Source.   Adapted from Twemlow S, Fonagy P, Sacco F: "The Role of the Bystander in the Social Architecture of Bullying and Violence in Schools and Communities." *Annals of the New York Academy of Sciences* 1036:218, 2004. Used with permission.

cially counselors and social workers) can use their clinical skills to help, and will often intuitively know such natural leaders. Dr. Peter Olsson (personal communication, 2005) created a clinical characterization of self- and other-focused leaders, which we have modified to assess altruistic helpfulness (Table 5–5).

Although we will not focus extensively at this time on the research literature on altruism, there is convincing evidence that altruism is a fundamental drive or impulse in humans and several other species (Shapiro and Gabbard 1994) that can be harnessed in the service of ameliorating violence. Such pragmatic forms of altruism, although lacking the mysticism and selflessness of well-known forms of it in spiritual leaders, focus on benefit for the community as a whole. This quality of commitment to the community as a whole often serves as inspiration for others, often catalyzing unexpected and dramatic change in the system (Gladwell 2000).

In our experience in a violent secondary school in Jamaica (Twemlow and Sacco 1996), a remarkable systemwide restoration of order began as a sort of epidemic of helpful bystanding seemingly created by a playful chant, the brainchild of a police officer in the altruistic bystander role. In an effort to get boys to be more tidy, a chant of "tuck your shirt in" (set to reggae music) was employed, which rapidly inspired songs and jokes and even created a minicraze to be tidy among boys seeking the police officer's positive attention. In the space of a few days there was hardly an untidy child in the school, and notably fewer incidents of violence too!

TABLE 5–5. Comparison of natural leaders and narcissistic leaders

Natural leaders	Narcissistic leaders
Noncutting sense of humor that connects and empathizes with peers to encourage their autonomy and participation	Cutting, sarcastic, cold, aloof humor that puts down or victimizes peers
Sanguine ability to empathize with peers in a way that helps self and others	Empathy that largely promotes the self above others, eventually at their expense or harm
Creativity and leadership promote creativity in group projects and in individual members	Creativity promotes destructive subgroups that cause isolation or alienation from the larger group
Personal needs met by benevolent reaching out to challenge the peer group to connect with their community via helpful projects and activities	Personal needs met or psychopathology deepened by efforts to dominate the peer group
Often do not see themselves as leaders and prefer to characterize themselves as helpers	See themselves as the only ones capable of leading, often in a martyring way
Reaches out to foster and mentor positive leaders in younger grade-level children modeling future leaders	Bullies or puts down younger aspiring leaders so as to maintain his or her fiefdom

Source. Peter A. Olsson, M.D., personal communication, 2005.

In this case, the helpful bystander was part of a highly corrupt police force in Jamaica, where an unusual group of senior police officers (more than 10 years in the force) had volunteered for training as an add-on to their usual police work. These police officers worked at poverty-level wages under conditions that few American police officers would tolerate. Personal qualities of these altruistic peacemakers are listed in Table 5–6.

Viewed from the perspective of the bystander, contemporary definitions of bullying may need revision. Leading researchers in the field of school bullying, like Peter Smith in England (Smith and Ananiadou 2003), Dan Olweus in Norway (Olweus 1999), and Ken Rigby in Australia (Rigby and Slee 2008), define bullying as repetitive, harmful, and producing gain for the bully, involving an imbalance of strength in which bullies are dominant, while victims struggle to defend themselves. Physical harm is usually of less concern than the insults, ostracizing, teasing, social isolation, and humiliation, which cause much of the harm.

We believe, however, that bullying should be redefined in triadic terms, as an interaction effect between bully, victim, and bystander, one in which the re-

TABLE 5–6. Personal qualities of altruistic peacemakers

Being more altruistic than egoistic
Awareness of, and takes responsibility for, community problems
Willingness to take physical risks for peace and not easily frightened
Relationship oriented and humanistic
Self-motivated and a motivator of others
Alert, strong, and positive
Self-rewarding with low need for praise
Personally well organized
Advocate for and protector of the vulnerable and disempowered
Able to see potential in all people
Low in sadism
An enthusiastic advocate, committed and understanding of "the cause"

sponses of each directly affect the severity of the outcome. The bully does not act as an individual, as for example in a private vendetta, but becomes, in part, an agent of the bystanding audience, which fuels the fire, so to speak, and perhaps even intensifies the harm done. In our clinical experience, we have found that bullies usually fantasize about the impact their actions will have on the bystander even if the bystanding audience is not physically present, suggesting prominent grandiose, sadomasochistic, and voyeuristic elements. To recontextualize traditional definitions in triadic terms, bullying is the repeated exposure of an individual to negative interactions directly or indirectly inflicted by one or more dominant persons. The harm may be caused through direct physical or psychological means and/or indirectly through encouragement of the process or avoidance by the bystander. This abdicating bystander group dynamic, with replacement of designated leaders (the school staff) by bystanders in active roles allowing severe bullying to occur, is illustrated in the following case example.

Case Example: Defeated Teachers and Administrators Replaced by In-Control Bystanders, Bullies, and Victims

We were invited to visit a large K–8 school serving a very poor minority neighborhood in an East Coast city, to assess the school's need for a violence prevention program. Its problems included criminal activity in and around the school; trash on school property, often in the form of discarded needles; and pedophiles cruising its perimeter. The school principal had assured us that the school had few bullying problems. Moments after entering the lunchroom, however, one boy knocked another out as the culmination of a long process of verbal abuse of the first boy's mother. After the principal hastily settled this matter, a school counselor rushed up in rage after a student had pelted her in the chest with full milk cartons.

The principal was an outstanding individual with idealistic concepts for her school and worked very hard and under very difficult conditions, including a school policy that penalized school administrators for poor student academic performance and disciplinary problems. The avoidant bystander role of the principal is not always based on denial in the strict sense, but rather on self-preservation, accompanied by the hope that nothing terrible will happen if one takes a positive attitude.

In the incident that followed several days later, during the first outside recess of the spring, two sixth-grade students faced off in front of 125 peers, who interlocked arms and cheered on the fight. When one of the fighters was knocked to the ground, 10 students continued punching the downed victim. The victim suffered serious facial damage from a ring worn by one of the students bullying him, a "dirty trick" similar to the ones seen on the World Wrestling Federation television show, as proudly announced later by one of the bullies.

Teachers were unable to intervene in the fight for more than 90 seconds because of the audience of bystander children, their interlocked arms surrounding the combatants. Although students had been talking about the upcoming fight throughout the day, teachers were not aware of the brewing problem. The whole peer grade became invested in one side or the another, and excitement built up throughout the day.

Bystanders were active in fanning the flames of the violent act, beginning with the ride in the school bus earlier that day. The two kids were matched up by rumor and innuendo, not actual personal conflict; this fight was staged by the bystanders through a peer group fantasy enacted in the fight.

Selected Literature Review: The School Bully–Victim–Bystander Problem

Smith et al. (2002), in an interesting survey of the use of the word *bully* and related terms around the world, found that the words are subject to substantial variation in the 14 countries surveyed. Clinical and research findings suggest that these are descriptions of temporary states of mind and will vary enormously, depending on the current dynamics of the social system.

With rare exceptions (for example, the genetically established psychopath [true bully]), bullying may not simply be one person repeatedly bullying another, but one individual being repeatedly victimized by many often at-risk individuals who, not through conscious malice or psychopathy but through failure to understand the impact of unpleasant behavior on others, follow a peer-set pattern of behavior; these at-risk victimizers would not even consider themselves bullies, nor would their parents or (for that matter) teachers. From this very broad social systems perspective, we are speaking here of essentially the manifestation of aggression in the social system and the violence it causes, violence being defined of course as harmful aggression.

Pontzer (2010) has found that a bully tends to be male, to be impulsive, to have been bullied as a child, and to be harassed and stigmatized by his parents. A study in Finland (Sigfusdottir et al. 2010) of 15- and 16-year-old bullies found that anger was a strong emotional component of being both a bully and a victim. Quality of life was very much affected in both bullies and victims and more so in older bullies and victims than in younger ones (Frisen et al. 2010).

Walden and Beran (2010) suggest that the quality of the attachment of the child and empathy in connection with the school are associated with variations in the way aggression is manifest. For example, they suggest that children with poorer-quality attachment are most likely to bully others and/or be victims. Eiden et al. (2010), in a study of parental alcoholism in 160 families, carefully evaluated the attachment patterns. Children were evaluated at age 18 months and in the fourth grade, showing that a father's alcoholism predicted bullying for boys, but not girls.

A cross-national study showed few differences by country in sex of the children and responses to bullying (Hussein 2010). In this study, an Egyptian, a Saudi Arabian, and a U.S. sample were compared using gender as the constant variable. Boys had higher levels of bullying than girls in all three cultures, but boys and girls were similar in their levels of peer victimization. Bush (2010) found that dangerousness at school was highest in youth who believe that their parents endorse fighting and who lack adult mentorship.

The complexity of how psychopathology manifests in bully, victim, and bystander behavior is illustrated in a wide range of studies. Both rural and urban studies show that victimization produces depressive symptoms, which are enormously influenced by parental support. A study of almost 1,000 children and adolescents (grades 5–11) in a rural southern U.S. community (Conners-Burrow et al. 2009) found that symptoms were fewer when parental support was high, and also supported the value of the teacher for the student's health. When parental support was low, the teacher could substitute for home support.

There are all sorts of variations in teacher attitudes and how that relates to the incidence of bullying in schools. Copeland (2010), in a study in Missouri, showed that more experienced superintendents believed that little or no problems existed with bullying in their schools, whereas the least-experienced superintendents saw bullying as a tremendous problem. One study conducted to measure the ability of teachers and counselors to differentiate between bullying and other forms of conflict (Hazler et al. 2001) noted that both had a rather poor understanding of bullying. Teachers often rated all physical conflict as bullying and underrated verbal, social, and emotional abuse. Kupersmidt (1999) looked at whether teachers could identify bullies and victims and found that elementary school teachers were more likely than middle school teachers to accurately do so. Kasen et al. (1990), in research over many years, showed that well-organized schools have less bullying and that if there is more adult supervision and a better climate between teachers and students, students will perform better academically. Research studies of bullying are beginning to look at ethnic groups in the United States. Nansel et al. (2001), in a survey of students in grades 6 through 10, found that black students reported less victimization than did white or Hispanic youth; Juvonen et al. (2003), in a study of sixth graders, found that black students were more likely than white students to be called bullies and victims. Sexual orientation has been found to be very important (see Swearer et al. 2010), with more victimization and physical assault of homosexual individuals.

Studies of Bystanding Behavior

Until recently, bystander behavior has largely been overlooked as a major variable in the literature on victimization. Henry et al. (2000) showed that students of teachers who openly discouraged the use of aggression were less likely to show the usual developmental increases in aggressive behavior over time. Slee (1993) showed that students of teachers who did not intervene in bullying often would also not help victims. In an earlier book Twemlow and Sacco (2008) we summarized the helpful impact on school interventions of retraining the bystander/natural leader.

A study of 10,000 Canadian children in grades 4–11 (Trach et al. 2010) found that younger females were more likely than boys and older females to intervene in bullying; percentages of children who did nothing at all increased with grade level and showed no gender bias. A number of high-profile school shootings over the last several years have placed bystanders squarely in the public eye (Twemlow 2008; Twemlow et al. 2002), with articles highlighting the inaction or aborted actions of students, teachers, and parents who were aware of threats by fellow students but did not act, either out of denial (avoidant bystanding) or because of fears that they would be targeted for tattling on peers (the conspiracy of silence). In some California schools, bystanders who did not report a shooter's previous threats were considered to be in need of protection from retaliative violence by members of the public (CNN 2001).

On a more positive note, several high schools encourage bystanders to help prevent or stop violence by providing confidential or anonymous online and phone-line reporting (Cromwell 2000, Sarkar 2000). In a Finnish study (Salmivalli et al. 1996) of several hundred children, participant roles were categorized into several groups: victim, bully, reinforcer of the bully, assistant of the bully, defender of the victim (i.e., helpful bystander from our perspective), and outsider. Boys were found to be more closely associated with the role of bully, reinforcer, and assistant; girls were more likely to identify with defender and outsider. Cowie

(2000), studying gender differences, suggested that part of the difficulty in targeting boys to take on helpful roles results from the fact that they are more likely to drop out of such interventions because of "macho" values, especially as the socially modeled concept of masculinity develops. In other studies, passive bystanders were found to reinforce the bully by providing a consenting audience, which sent the implicit message that aggression is acceptable (O'Connell et al. 1999). Craig and Pepler (1997) reported that child bystanders are often effective in trying to stop bullying. They also found that in 85% of bullying episodes observed by videotaping children in the playground, other children joined in either with the aggression or against the aggression. It is a well-known fact that children, especially during their adolescent years, tend to look to their peers for clues about how to respond to everything in their social environment. Studies have shown that watching or laughing can encourage and prolong bullying (Craig and Pepler 1995, 1997) and peers may see powerful aggressive and harmful behavior as valuable.

There is yet another piece of this complicated puzzle: in a study of teachers' perceptions of other teachers who bully students (Twemlow et al. 2006), 116 teachers from seven elementary schools completed an anonymous questionnaire reflecting their feelings and perceptions about their own experiences of bullying and how they perceived their colleagues. Forty-five percent of the teachers in the study admitted to having bullied a student; many recognized that the roles of bully, victim, and bystander are roles, not moral indictments or diagnoses and usually become damaging only if repeated frequently and if the roles become fixed. In our study, teachers' openness to seeing and admitting bullying suggests that efforts to prevent bullying by training teachers to recognize and deal with it in themselves, students, and colleagues can be quite helpful.

Our study also showed that few if any teachers perceived a current school policy or training experience that might help them handle this particular problem. Teachers who self-reported a tendency to bully students also reported having been bullied when they were students in school, and they were far more likely to report seeing other students bullied by teachers. They also reported having been bullied by students inside and outside the classroom. Lack of administrative support, lack of training in discipline techniques, overcrowded classrooms, and being envious of smarter students were found to be elements that were part of the pattern of these bullying teachers. Statistical analysis found two main types of bullying teachers. Sadistic teachers tended to humiliate students, appeared to act spitefully, and seemed to enjoy hurting students' feelings. By contrast, bully-victim teachers were frequently absent, failed to set limits, let other people handle their problems, and tended to see lack of training in discipline techniques as the primary cause of their behavior, acting in many ways as an abdicating bystander by blaming others for their problems. Such teachers often explode in a rage and react in a bullying fashion when they have "reached their limits."

The Peaceful Schools Project: A Social Systems–Psychodynamic Antibullying Intervention

The Peaceful Schools Project (Fonagy et al. 2009) began as an attempt to test a social systems–psychodynamic approach to bullying and violence in an elementary school setting. The theory driving the intervention was an evolving one, focused on trying a variety of ideas and approaches. During the pilot phase, the intervention was modified as various ideas worked or did not work. Between 1993 and 1996, a pilot study was launched in three elementary schools in a midwestern city (Twemlow et al. 2001). The intervention was largely implemented by the teachers, who were also closely involved in coauthoring articles and creating the actual interventions and were not reluctant bystander participants forced into the research by the administration.

The pilot study involved two intervention schools—one affluent and one poor—and one control school demographically matched to the nonaffluent intervention school. The nonaffluent intervention school had a very high out-of-school suspension rate, a high rate of violent incidents (including the attempted rape of a second-grade girl by a group of elementary-age boys), and a record of very poor academic achievement. The demographically matched control school was built in an almost identical way as the nonaffluent intervention school and was in the same socioeconomically deprived area. This control school received only weekly psychiatric consultations, as has been the convention in school psychiatry for many decades. A dedicated group was organized for children who had experienced a murder in the family or seen a murdered body. The cost of the overall project was minimal, and interested teachers collected and scored the data, illustrating very high buy-in to a project they conceived.

The project did not pathologize psychiatric groups or at-risk children and did not call for expensive referrals to medical care and other experts. Since the project addressed a current need that was considered urgent and was designed by those who experienced the need, the buy-in problem was minimal, and schools were willing to tolerate longer-term, more difficult solutions rather than pushing for quick fixes designed to placate a possibly impatient school board. We found that instead of overloading teachers and students with massive initial training, ongoing supervision based on a psychoanalytic/psychodynamic model was a more practical way to problem solve.

When considering all three schools in this pilot phase, it is interesting to note that the poor intervention school maintained its progress and continued through numerous changes, becoming a very quiet school with low suspension rates, clean and attractive classrooms, and drastically fewer incidents of racial discrimination.

We had initially tried doing some therapeutic work with teachers and found very quickly, as other have, that teachers do not like that sort of work at all, and are not responsive to it. We also learned that teachers are likely to speak positively but often hide their negative reactions. It took a while as MHPs for us to realize these factors. After we did so, and began listening more carefully to the children's and teachers' interactions, we steered ourselves toward management of the bystanding audience, rather than the bully and the victim. We had started by trying to manage bullying children alone, which exhausted the instructors as well as the teachers.

Elements of Mentalization Particularly Relevant to the Social Intervention

The randomized school intervention focused on reducing pathological bystanding through the use of two mechanisms: enhancing mentalization and fostering healthier power dynamics (observations derived from the pilot phase). The concept of mentalization has been mainly applied in psychotherapeutic settings. We believe this program may be the first formal application of mentalization as part of a social systems intervention.

The intervention applied the following elements of mentalization:

- The capacity to reflect upon interpersonal events and experience in terms of the protagonist's mental states
- The capacity to modulate one's own affect in relation to these experiences so that reflective thinking (mentalizing) is maintained
- A sense of agency and intentionality—that is, one is acting in line with one's intentional states of feelings, wishes, beliefs, and desires rather than being controlled by the actions of others
- The capacity for interpersonal relating (emerging from the prior three elements), in which one is able to generate a balance between individuation, establishment of boundaries that protect the individual self, and relatedness
- The capacity to closely cooperate with, rely on, and even become attached to others

We noticed that mentalization in violent schools was significantly lower. In violent schools, the power dynamics featured control over others, using coercion and humiliation. We also observed that efforts to address this type of power dynamic by identifying and attempting to deal with the bully did little to change the school climate. A system characterized by ignoring the mental states of self and others creates systems of social influence, with coercion and humiliation playing key roles. High levels of emotional arousal could be expected to make both bully and victim inaccessible to a mentalization-based intervention. The key to solving a problem of pathological power dynamics could be the facilitation of thinking about the bystanding group, since in our view parents, school administrators, schoolteachers, and students are the participating audience in this power play.

Because bystanders' involvement is not direct, the intervention focused on enhancing mentalization to create a social environment in which ignoring the feelings and thoughts of others was no longer seen as acceptable or experienced as necessary. Thus, the project was focused more on the role of the bystander than on the bully or victim role. Its immediate aim was to provide a mentalizing alternative that begins with perceiving and accepting bystanders' own unthinking role in maintaining the bully–victim relationship through abdicating responsibility and making an unconscious decision not to think about what either the bully or the victim is experiencing in any but the most superficial or schematic ways.

Understanding the psychological backdrop of the pathological power dynamic in which one person uses physical or psychological coercion to change the behavior of another was a starting point for the intervention. The intervention aimed to change the way the entire school social system viewed bullying, to promote acceptance of universal "blame" for the problem, and to encourage helpful bystanders to see themselves as an organic and essential part of the power dynamic.

The program used five main devices:

1. A positive climate campaign highlighting the subjective experiences of bully–victim and of bystander.
2. A classroom management plan requiring teachers to elaborate the thoughts and feelings associated with aggressive acts in the classroom
3. A defensive martial arts program based on principles of mindfulness
4. Peer or adult mentorship to create additional opportunities for reflective interpersonal interaction and a healthier acceptance of power issues as part of everyday life
5. Reflection time to allow the class to consider immediate past experience as a group. The last 10 minutes of each day was spent reflecting on how students had performed over the course of the day in managing power dynamics and focusing on the thoughts and feelings of others. Teachers felt that children were often a lot harder on themselves than they, the teachers, would have been, but after the reflection period the class would decide whether or not to hang a banner outside the classroom indicating that the class had had a good day of reflectiveness, mentalization, and helpfulness to others.

Study Method

Over a 3-year period, beginning in 1999, the theoretical ideas derived from the pilot study and from clinical observations of schools were formally tested in a cluster randomized controlled trial in which nine schools (involving a total of 1,345 students in grades 3–5) were randomly assigned to one of three conditions: 1) Creating a Peaceful School Learning Environment (CAPSLE), which was designed to encourage mentalization and reduce pathological power dynamics, as already described; 2) traditional school psychiatric consultation involving assessment of children through classroom observation referrals but no direct contact with children; or 3) treatment as usual (these schools, although they received no intervention, were promised the most effective of the other two interventions after a 2-year period if they desired it; this was an attempt to provide a motivated control group). The program was implemented intensively in the first 2 years, and the intervention was reduced in the third year to see whether the effects could be maintained.

Training in defensive martial arts with role-playing helped the children to think about how they responded to victimization and how the victimization affected their capacity to think clearly and creatively. These bully–victim–bystander role-plays involved the entire group, so that children gradually began to see themselves as more powerful.

It became obvious that daily reinforcement was necessary to help community members keep the importance of empathic awareness of self and others in mind. Poster campaign stickers and badges were used to create a climate where feelings were (quite literally) labeled and distress was acknowledged as legitimate. The emphasis was on the need to reflect on the importance of understanding, rather than reacting to others and avoiding the problems created by regression into the victim, victimizer, and bystander roles in a system controlled by the bully.

A further major component was the helpful bystanders. While these individuals may be thought of as natural leaders, they do not naturally emerge, but need to be chosen. They were very powerful in their capacity to motivate large groups of other children and appeared able to understand the needs of many, if not of the entire group, but were not interested in using their abilities to achieve social status by becoming high-mentalizing bullies themselves. There was no attempt to focus on helping individually disturbed children or, for that matter, to pathologize them by singling them out. Over time, bullies came to be disempowered, initially complaining that the work done on the program was "boring," but gradually the social system tended to recruit them into more helpful roles, ones that made use of their leadership skills.

Results

As might be imagined, teacher buy-in to the program was closely related to its overall effectiveness. Biggs et al. (2008) suggested that students whose teachers reported greater fidelity to the intervention protocol had greater empathy (defined as a student's awareness of the negative effects of victimization on other students) over time than students whose teachers reported less fidelity. The results also suggested that students whose teachers reported greater fidelity were viewed by peers to show less aggressive (bully) bystanding than did students whose teachers reported less fidelity. Over the second and third years of the program, helpful bystanding behavior was significantly related to the adherence of teachers to the elements of the program and awareness of its usefulness. Students whose teachers reported greater fidelity were viewed by peers as showing more helpful bystanding over time than did students whose teachers reported less fidelity.

As part of this study, 254 children in grades 3, 4, and 5 participated in the Gentle Warrior Program, the martial arts intervention (Twemlow et al. 2008). Boys who had participated more frequently in Gentle Warrior training reported a lower frequency of aggression and a greater frequency of helpful bystanding over time, relative to boys with less frequent participation. The effect of participation on aggression was partially mediated by empathy. The effect of participation on helpful bystanding was fully mediated by changes in students' empathy levels. There was no significant statistical effect for girls, but the trainers and teachers felt that the quiet "wallflower" girls (especially in third grade) became much more comfortable with their aggression and thus were more easily able to participate in social and emotional learning.

Fonagy et al. (2009) provided a detailed analysis of overall outcomes of the study over the 3-year period. CAPSLE moderated the developmental trend of increasing peer-reported victimization ($P<0.01$), peer-reported aggression ($P<0.05$), self-reported aggression ($P<0.05$), and aggressive (bully) bystanding ($P<0.05$), as compared with treatment-as-usual schools. CAPSLE also moderated a decline in empathy and an increase in the percentage of children victimized compared with school psychiatric consultation ($P<0.01$) and treatment as usual ($P<0.01$). Instances of self-reported victimization and helpful bystanding, and beliefs in the legitimacy of aggression, did not suggest significantly different changes among the study conditions over time. CAPSLE produced a significant decrease in off-task ($P<0.001$) and disruptive classroom behaviors ($P<0.001$), while behavioral changes were not observed in the school psychiatric consultation and treatment-as-usual schools. The intervention's superiority with respect to treatment as usual for victimization ($P<0.05$) and aggression ($P<0.01$), as well as for both helpful bystanding ($P<0.05$) and aggressive bystanding ($P<0.01$), was maintained in the follow-up year.

We concluded from these results that a teacher-implemented and -invested, schoolwide intervention that does not focus on disturbed children substantially reduced aggression and improved classroom behavior. One educator cogently noted that education is the cure to the extent that ignorance is the disease. We wish to note that overemphasizing intellectual approaches to problems in the learning environment causes teachers and curriculum or policy planners inadvertently to occupy avoidant and abdicating bystander roles.

To examine the effect of CAPSLE on educational performance, a total of 1,106 students were monitored before and after the program across the school district for academic attainment, as measured by standardized Metropolitan Achievement Test scores (Fonagy et al. 2005). An equivalent control sample of 1,100 children who attended schools in school districts that did not join the program was compared. CAPSLE was associated with pronounced improvement in the children's achievement tests scores. We were able to track children moving to schools without the CAPSLE program and who were not in any of the clusters of schools being studied. In general, the notable improvements in reading, math, and overall scale percentile test scores were maintained. If children had spent 2 or more years in the program, transferring to a less peaceful school brought no change in their academic performance, which actually continued to improve. If children had been there less than 2 years, there appeared to be a decrease in their academic achievement, as if they were still unsure of what to do in a less peaceful school environment.

After the randomized study was concluded, one of the school administrators called us; he noticed that children who went on to middle school from the CAPSLE schools appeared to perform better academically and also had fewer out-of-school suspensions. We obtained the data from the school district and were able to show that the trend for children to be able to carry what they had learned and use it to improve their quality of life continued into middle school. Table 5–7 illustrates how changing the power dynamics in the bully, victim, and bystander roles results in mentalization.

Relationship Between Community Health and School Violence

In a study of a developing country, Jamaica, we saw how a community could devolve as the country became a way station for cocaine trafficking (Twemlow and Sacco 1996). Table 5–8 summarizes the psychological and structural attributes we observed as the situation deteriorated over a number of years. This type of deterioration has also occurred in certain areas of developed countries, including the United States.

Studies of school violence in Jamaica provide a potentially useful microcosm for understanding school violence in the context of violence in the surrounding community. Schools have often failed to realize that education also depends on the social and emotional climate surrounding learning, as seen by the largely behavioral training of schoolteachers in educational psychology with

TABLE 5-7. Changing the power dynamics in Creating a Peaceful School Learning Environment (CAPSLE) schools

Role	Type	Changing the power dynamics	Resulting in mentalizing
Bully	Sadistic bully	If you stop forcing people to do things your way	you will have more friends
	Bully victim	If you stop bullying and complaining about people bullying you	then you may be seen as more stable and more self-reliant
Bystander	Avoidant	If you acknowledge a problem with bully–victim–bystander relationships	then you have the chance to be more honest with yourself in other situations
	Bully	If you stop looking like you are enjoying other people's pain	you may be seen as more gentle and considerate of others
	Helpful	In making a decision to help others	you will show people your courage and kindness
	Victim	In saying no to the bully	you will show self-respect and your assertiveness to others
Victim	Submissive	If you stop giving in and giving up	others will respect you and you will respect yourself more
	Martyr	If you stop showing self-pity	you will have more friends
	Rescuer	If you stop letting others take advantage of you	you will show others your assertiveness and self-control

IF YOU DON'T, YOU WILL →   IF YOU DO, YOU WILL →

BE an angry, whiny, often complaining, threatening student with very few friends   BECOME a respectful, reliable, honest, kind, assertive student with lots of friends

AND   AND
You will hate school   You will like school

Source. Adapted from Twemlow S, Fonagy P, Sacco F: "Feeling Safe in School." *Smith College Studies in Social Work* 72:303–326, 2002. Used with permission.

TABLE 5–8. Psychological and structural attributes of violent communities

Anti-intellectualism	Reflection is seen as antithetical to the need for urgent responses in the struggle for survival
Altruism is weak; power comes from violence	Powerful narcissistic subgroups protect themselves
Unstable political and family systems	Lack of respect for the leader; collapse of the nuclear family
Powerlessness, despair, and anomie	Individuals do not feel connected to each other or the system
Escapism	Drug and alcohol addiction is inversely proportional to hope and stability of community
Increase in school bullying	Results in truancy, dropout, and possible homicide and suicide
Community denial of violence	Direct denial, oversimplification, overgeneralization, and stereotyped response patterns

↓

RESULTING IN

Disconnection of police from community members, who are seen as nonhuman (animals, pigs)

Population redistribution: squatters seize land or are "homeless"

Buildings are poorly or cheaply designed; trash and overgrown lots abound

Lack of functioning social welfare programs

Increase in criminal enterprises

Abuse and rejection of the vulnerable (elderly and children)

little emphasis on normal and pathological development, unless the teacher personally pursues specialized training. Given this narrow focus on intellectual training, it is not surprising that coercive power dynamics and mentalizing are paid insufficient attention. One result of this limited focus is that community leaders can scapegoat agencies, particularly those that have been delegated the responsibility to educate children and to provide a safe learning environment, such as teachers and law enforcement officers. Without sophisticated awareness of pathological bystanding roles, problem children can be labeled as aberrant or sick and unnecessarily "evacuated" into the medical or criminal justice system and special classrooms and schools. Such an action causes considerable expense for the community and does not address the universal responsibility of everyone in the community for how schools function.

Education is not just a right or a service; it is a defining necessity for a healthy society, and addressing the social and emotional needs of children is an imperative of even greater importance than attention to structural issues in the school climate, such as the use of increasing security surveillance and increased presence of law enforcement. The work of Sampson and others (Sampson and Ramedenbush 1997) on the collective efficacy of communities in the Chicago area provides a helpful model. *Collective efficacy* refers to social cohesion among neighbors combined with a willingness to intervene on behalf of the common good. These researchers' large-scale studies in more than 300 Chicago neighborhoods showed very strong evidence of a link between collective efficacy and reduced violence.

Figure 5–2 represents a summary model for the social and psychological factors in a dialectical, co-created relationship with each other. Helpful (altruistic) bystanding will promote mentalization, and vice versa. In such a community, social affiliation and the needs of the group as a whole are the dominant concern. The Peaceful Schools Project described in this chapter addresses these two elements in a primary (universal) prevention approach to school violence. Coercive and humiliating power dynamics (defined as the conscious and unconscious use of force and humiliation by individuals and groups against other individuals and groups) and social disconnection (the feeling of being actively separated from a social group in the community) are two other factors that research has linked to violence and other forms of community disruption. Such factors create a social crucible of at-risk groups and individuals who may be violence prone. When coercive power dynamics and social disconnection, with the collapse of mentalization, become a fixed modus operandi of a social group, outbreaks of lethal violence occur, as in the adolescent homicide perpetrators in the spate of murders in schools beginning in the 1990s. Treating such children and their victims is a tertiary prevention action to address a collapsing and fragmented community.

This research suggests a testable model for fostering social harmony in our communities and for improving the learning environment in schools by connecting all stakeholders as passionate and committed members of the community, rather than as bystanders in fragmented, self-centered subgroups. From this perspective, then, connected and mentalizing people make safer communities and schools. Bullying as a process is best impacted by activating positive bystanders in the school to aid in this process.

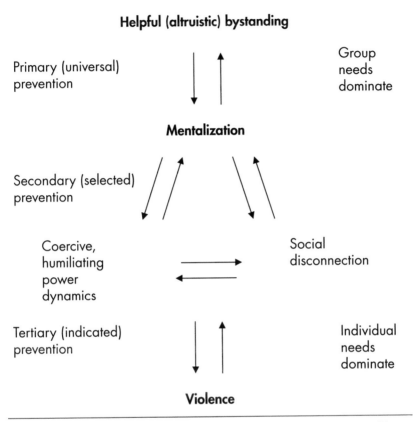

FIGURE 5–2. Clinical–social systems model of community health.

Source. Adapted from Twemlow S, Fonagy P, Sacco F: "The Role of the Bystander in the Social Architecture of Bullying and Violence in Schools and Communities." *Annals of the New York Academy of Sciences* 1036:230, 2004. Used with permission.

KEY CLINICAL CONCEPTS

- Examining the underlying theory of what renders a school environment coercive and humiliating introduces a way to understand the power dynamics of the family and community and the role this social drama plays in the creation of a peaceful school learning environment.

- Bullying is a group power dynamic.

- Bullying is the result of shame in a public setting.

- Bullies will only do what bystanders allow.

- Bullying is a coercive action that spreads through a school.

- Changing a school climate demands that the underlying power dynamics be understood, whatever program is used.

- Bullying is a social process with three main roles: 1) bully or victimizer, 2) victim or target, and 3) bystanding audience.

- Denial of bullying fosters a group sense of powerlessness, leading to resignation and eventually to physical and emotional disturbances.

- Bullying can take many forms and exists all over the world.

- Bullying differs depending on the type of school. In schools in affluent communities, the main type of bullying is based on social inclusion/exclusion, while in schools in poorer communities, bullying is more survival oriented and based on intimidation.

- Adults play a huge role in shaping how children manage social power. When adults in elementary schools allow bullying to occur, children's mean-spirited social aggression is reinforced. This is further complicated by the role of the parent, who may come into conflict or agree with the school and might be the cause of the oft-reported decrease in empathy for victims of bullying as the student grows up.

- True (psychopathic) bullying is NOT NORMAL. It involves

  — Intention to shame and cause discomfort

  — Sustained humiliation

  — Predatory stalking of victims

  — Lack of empathy

  — Sadomasochism

- Bystanders are a causal link in the evolution of coercion in a social environment. School systems can become abdicating bystanders and spark violence through their dismissiveness.

- The bully–victim–bystander relationship involves co-created roles. There cannot be a bully without a victim, and the bully will not be reinforced without the audience of bystanders. People change roles throughout the day. Students who are victims of domestic violence may bully other students at school. There are, of course, many variations in the co-creation of all of these power roles.

- Within schools, it is essential to keep the door open for peer communication about bullying and victimization. Social cliques evolve as hiding places within the war zone that can develop in socially aggressive schools. Peer communication to adults is a key pressure valve and primary prevention tool.

References

Biggs BK, Vernberg EM, Twemlow SW, et al: Teacher adherence and its relation to teacher attitudes and student outcomes in an elementary school-based violence prevention program. School Psych Rev 37:533–549, 2008

Bion W: Experiences in Groups. Basic Books, New York, 1959

Bion W: Attention and Interpretation. London, Heinemann, 1970

Bush MD: A quantitative investigation of teachers' responses to bullies. Dissertation Abstracts International Section A: Humanities and Social Sciences 70, 2010

CNN: District Bars Students Who Allegedly Heard of Shooter's Plans. March 8, 2001. Available at: http://archives.cnn.com/2001/US/03/08/shooting.students.knew/index.html. Accessed December 5, 2010.

Conners-Burrow NA, Johnson DL, Whiteside-Mansell L, et al: Adults matter: protecting children from the negative impacts of bullying. Psychology in the Schools 46:593–604, 2009

Copeland DA: Bullying in public schools in Missouri. Dissertation Abstracts International Section A: Humanities and Social Sciences 70:3284, 2010

Cowie H: Bystander or standing by: gender issues in coping with bullying in English schools. Aggress Behav 26:85–97, 2000

Craig W, Pepler D: Peer processes in bullying and victimization: an observational study. Exceptionality Education Canada 5:81–95, 1995

Craig W, Pepler D: Observations of bullying and victimization in the school yard. Canadian Journal of School Psychology 13:41–59, 1997

Cromwell S: Anonymity spurs students to report potential violence. Education World, November 29, 2000. Available at: http://www.educationworld.com/a_admin/admin/admin202.shtml. Accessed December 5, 2010.

Devine J: Maximum Security: The Culture of Violence in Inner-City Schools. Chicago, IL, University of Chicago Press, 1996

Eiden RD, Ostrov JM, Colder CR, et al: Parent alcohol problems and peer bullying and victimization: child gender and toddler attachment security as moderators. J Clin Child Adolesc Psychol 39:341–350, 2010

Erikson E: Childhood and Society. New York, WW Norton, 1963, pp 239–241

Fonagy P: Attachment Theory and Psychoanalysis. New York, Other Press, 2001

Fonagy P, Twemlow SW, Vernberg E, et al: Creating a peaceful school learning environment: impact of an antibullying program on educational attainment in elementary schools. Med Sci Monit 11:317–325, 2005

Fonagy P, Twemlow S, Vernberg E, et al: A cluster randomized controlled trial of a child-focused psychiatric consultation and a school systems-focused intervention to reduce aggression. J Child Psychol Psychiatry 50:607–616, 2009

Freud S: The taboo of virginity (1918[1917]), in Standard Edition of the Complete Psychological Works of Sigmund Freud, Vol 11. Translated and edited by Strachey J. London, Hogarth Press, 1957, pp 191–208

Freud S: Group psychology and the analysis of the ego (1921), in Standard Edition of the Complete Psychological Works of Sigmund Freud, Vol 18. Translated and edited by Strachey J. London, Hogarth Press, 1955, pp 65–143

Freud S: Civilization and its discontents (1930), in Standard Edition of the Complete Psychological Works of Sigmund Freud, Vol 21. Translated and edited by Strachey J. London, Hogarth Press, 1957, pp 57–145

Frisen A, Bjarnelind S, Frisen A: Health-related quality of life and bullying in adolescence. Acta Paediatr 99:597–603, 2010

Gilligan J: Violence: Our Deadly Epidemic and Its Causes. New York, Grosset/Putnam Books, 1996

Gladwell M: The Tipping Point. New York, Little, Brown, 2000

Hazler JR, Miller DL, Carney JV, et al: Adult recognition of school bullying situations. Educational Research 43:133–147, 2001

Henry D, Guerra N, Huesmann R, et al: Normative influences on aggression in urban elementary school classrooms. Am J Community Psychol 28:59–81, 2000

Hussein MH: The peer interaction in primary school questionnaire: testing for measurement equivalence and latent mean differences in bullying between gender in Egypt, Saudi Arabia, and the USA. Social Psychology of Education 13:57–67, 2010

Juvonen J, Graham S, Schuster M: Bullying among young adolescents: the strong, the weak and the troubled. Pediatrics 112:1231–1237, 2003

Kasen S, Johnson J, Cohen P: The impact of school emotional climate on student psychopathology. J Abnorm Child Psychol 18:165–177, 1990

Kupersmidt SS: Factors influencing teacher identification of peer bullies and victims. School Psych Rev 28:505–518, 1999

Nansel T, Overpeck M, Pilla R, et al: Bullying behaviors among US youth: prevalence and association with psychosocial adjustment. JAMA 285:2094–3100, 2001

O'Connell P, Pepler D, Craig W: Peer involvement in bullying: insights and challenges for intervention. J Adolesc 22:437–452, 1999

Oliver K: Phoebe Prince "Suicide by bullying": teen's death angers town asking why bullies roam the halls. CBS News, February 5, 2010. Available at: http://www.cbsnews.com/8301-504083_162-6173960-504083.html?tag=mncol;lst;10. Accessed December 5, 2010.

Smith PK, Morita Y, Junger-Tas J, et al (eds): The Nature of School Bullying: A Cross-National Perspective. New York, Routledge, 1999, pp 7–27

Olweus D: Norway, in The Nature of School Bullying: A Cross-National Perspective. Edited by Smith PK, Morita Y, Junger-Tas J, et al. New York, Routledge, 1999, pp 28–48

Patterson S, Memmott J, Brennan E, et al: Patterns of natural helping in rural areas: implications for social work research. Soc Work Res Abstr 28:22–28, 1992

Pontzer D: A theoretical test of bullying behavior: parenting. Personality, and the bully/victim relationship. J Fam Violence 25:1573–2851, 2010

Rigby K, Slee PT: Interventions to reduce bullying. Int J Adolesc Med Health 20:165–183, 2008

Salmivalli C, Lagerspetz K, Bjorkqvist K, et al: Bullying as a group process: participant roles in their relations to social status within the group. Aggress Behav 22:1–15, 1996

Sampson R, Ramedenbush S: Neighborhoods and violent crime: a multilevel study of collective efficacy. Science 277:918–925, 1997

Sarkar D: Georgia taps web for school safety. Federal Computer Week, August 23, 2000. Available at: www.fcw.com/civic/articles/2000/0821/web-georgia-08–23–00.asp. Accessed December 5, 2010.

Shapiro Y, Gabbard G: A reconsideration of altruism from an evolutionary and psychodynamic perspective. Ethics Behav 4:23–42, 1994

Sigfusdottir ID, Gudjonsson GH, Sigurdsson JF, et al: Bullying and delinquency: the mediating role of anger. Pers Individ Dif 48:391–396, 2010

Slee P: Bullying: a preliminary investigation of its nature and the effects of social cognition. Early Child Dev Care 87:47–57, 1993

Smith P, Ananiadou K: The nature of school bullying and the effectiveness of school-based interventions. Journal of Applied Psychoanalytic Studies 5:189–209, 2003

Smith PK, Cowie H, Olafsson RF, et al: Definitions of bullying: a comparison of terms used, and age and gender differences, in a fourteen-country international comparison. Child Dev 73:1119–1133, 2002

Swearer S, Espelage D, Vaillancourt T, et al: What can be done about school bullying? Linking research to educational practice. Educational Researcher 39:38–47, 2010

Trach J, Hymel S, Waterhouse T, et al: Bystander responses to bullying: a cross-sectional investigation of grade and sex differences. Canadian Journal of School Psychology 25:114–130, 2010

Twemlow SW: Modifying violent communities by enhancing altruism: a vision of possibilities. Journal of Applied Psychoanalytic Studies 3:431–462, 2001

Twemlow SW: Assessing adolescents who threaten homicide in schools: a recent update. Clin Soc Work J 36:127–129, 2008

Twemlow SW, Harvey E: Power issues and power struggles in mental illness and everyday life. International Journal of Applied Psychoanalytic Studies 7:307–328, 2010

Twemlow SW, Hough G: The cult leader as an agent of a psychotic fantasy of masochistic "group death" in the Revolutionary Suicide in Jonestown. Emory Across Academe 5:24–32, 2005

Twemlow SW, Sacco F: Peacekeeping and peacemaking: the conceptual foundations of a plan to reduce violence and improve the quality of life in a midsized community in Jamaica. Psychiatry 59:156–174, 1996

Twemlow SW, Sacco F: The prejudices of everyday life with observations from field trials, in The Future of Prejudice: Psychoanalysis and the Prevention of Prejudice. Edited by Parens H, Mafhouz A, Twemlow SW, et al. Lanham, MD, Rowman & Littlefield, MD, 2007, pp 237–254

Twemlow SW, Sacco F: Why School Antibullying Programs Don't Work. New York, Jason Aronson, 2008

Twemlow SW, Sacco F, Williams P: A clinical and interactionist perspective on the bully-victim-bystander relationship. Bull Menninger Clin 60:296–313, 1996

Twemlow SW, Fonagy P, Sacco F, et al: Creating a peaceful school learning environment: a controlled study of an elementary school intervention to reduce violence. Am J Psychiatry 158:808–810, 2001

Twemlow SW, Fonagy P, Sacco FC: Assessing adolescents who threaten homicide in schools. Am J Psychoanal 62:213–235, 2002

Twemlow SW, Fonagy P, Sacco FC, et al: Teachers who bully students: a hidden trauma. Int J Soc Psychiatry 52:187–198, 2006

Twemlow SW, Nelson T, Vernberg E, et al: Effects of participation in a martial arts anti-bullying program on children's aggression in elementary schools. Psychol Sch 45:947–959, 2008

Twemlow SW, Fonagy P, Sacco FC, et al: Reducing violence and prejudice in a Jamaican all-age school using attachment and mentalization approaches. Psychoanal Psychol (in press)

Volkan V: Blind Trust: Large Groups and Their Leaders in Times of Crisis and Terror. Charlottesville, VA, Pitchstone Publishing, 2004

Walden TN, Beran TN: Attachment quality and bullying behavior in school-aged youth. Canadian Journal of School Psychology 25:5–18, 2010

6

Children Need to Feel Safe to Learn

"People are disturbed not by things, but by their perception of things...."

Epictetus

IT is a well-recognized fact that safe children learn more easily (for a review, see Office of Safe and Drug-Free Schools 2010). The more difficult fact is that we cannot seem to make our schools safe havens for our children. Driven by the search for the quick fix, our culture has an insatiable appetite for programs that promise such a "fix," and there are plenty of them. These programs often deceive people into thinking that the task of psychological change is easy; just follow the formula. The equivalent in schools is simple curriculum add-ons that imply that the key to change is just a matter of teaching nonviolent attitudes.

We have gone a step further, suggesting that the community be invited into the school (see Chapter 5, "Bullying Is a Process, Not a Person"). How to deal with underlying resistance to making antiviolence programs work is an underrepresented area in the literature of our field. We believe that it is crucial to

147

address resistance to community involvement and to provide the skills for addressing the psychological needs that interfere with the way all people in the school relate to each other, including children, teachers, school administrators, custodians, secretaries, lunchroom staff, paraprofessionals, teachers' aides, substitute teachers, and anyone else who comes in contact with students. Parents functioning as teachers offer potentially useful contributions for mental health professionals (MHPs) with psychodynamic background and experience. Learning can be a mutual process. A deepened understanding promotes respect and healthy interrelatedness in the community as a whole.

A study of 26 industrialized nations (Bleich et al. 2000) reported that 73% of all child homicides occur in the United States. Our homicide rate is 10 times higher than the rates in Western Europe and Japan and 5 times higher than the rates in Canada, New Zealand, and Australia. The homicide rate for 15- to 17-year-olds in the United States is 22 times higher than that in any other industrialized nation. Our work with the Federal Bureau of Investigation (FBI) and study of school shooters has shown that the most terrified children are the ones who feel the most unsafe, often the shooters themselves (Twemlow et al. 2002). How can we create safe schools?

Literature About Feeling Safe

What makes children feel safe is an elusive and complex topic in existing literature. Feeling "attached and contained" (Haigh 1996) has been observed to be related to a person's experience of belonging and feeling safe. The quality of the child's early attachment relationship with the primary caregiver plays a vital role in personality development (Bowlby 1988) by influencing the capacity of a person to modulate affect (Fonagy et al. 2000) and to rely on the internal representations of the caregiver (object constancy) to feel safe and soothed (Main 1995; Sroufe 1996).

People do not feel safe when they see violence on a regular basis. Overstreet and Braun (2000) surveyed 70 African American children between the ages of 10 and 15 years about neighborhood safety and learned that (as common sense might suggest) children feel less safe in their neighborhoods when they have ongoing exposure to violence. Feeling safe is clearly related to the effectiveness of public safety in keeping overt instances of violence in a community low. Espelage et al. (2000), in studying the social context of bullying, found that feeling safe in a community was related to the presence of adult supervisors and the absence of negative influences. Children feel safer when they can see and feel their protectors and when those protectors are effective in combating the negative influences leading to bullying. In a large British study of the impact of neighborhood trustworthiness and safety on psychopathology among more than 3,000 11- to 16-

year-olds, it was noteworthy that children who identified trustworthy and honest people in their lives showed far less psychopathology (Meltzer et. al 2007).

Does ethnicity or gender affect one's feelings of safety? There are few studies available. A study of more than 400 children, spanning a variety of ethnic groups, found that African American children felt safest and had the best relationships with adults and also the most evolved social skills, whereas Asian, Pacific Islander, white, and Hispanic children all showed weaker internal feelings of safety (Lee et al. 2009). A study of nearly 10,000 secondary school students ages 9–13 years in New Zealand found that females had the highest rates of attempted suicide, but rates of self-injury were lowest in children who reported caring homes and fair, safe school environments (Fleming et al. 2007).

In Israel, a country under constant threat of terrorism and/or war, an intervention to foster resilience was found to be significantly effective in promoting an internal feeling of safety in three major aspects: the mobilization of social support, the capacity to solve problems, and the attribution of meaning to the experience. All three of these are part of what a resilient child may have genetically, but this particular program demonstrated that in chronically violent countries (like Israel), much can be done to foster resilience in young people but not without the attention of adults in the school settings (Slone and Shoshani 2006).

Children are children throughout the world, and as such, they need adult and older peer support to feel safe. This type of support can be expressed as a physical presence for younger children, but all young people must have others to talk to about their insecurities, and these other people need to be attuned to the young person's developmental level. Reeves et al. (2010) was able to show that to feel safe, children must not only know that their school is secure but also have someone to talk to about safety concerns. Vaillancourt et al. (2010), in a study of 12,000 Canadian schoolchildren in grades 4–12, found that students reported that they felt least safe in areas of the school that tended not to be well supervised by adults. One lesson we learned from this research is that the younger the child, the more the presence of adults is needed. A child with secure attachment patterns is likely to respond better to adult mentorship.

Children's exposure to television violence has been studied quite extensively. Federman (1996, 1997, 1998) found that television violence contributes to children learning aggressive behavior, desensitizes children toward violence, and increases their fear of victimization. Joshi and Kaschak (1998), in a study of high school students, showed that exposure to media violence promoted posttraumatic stress disorder (PTSD)–like symptoms, including fear of being alone, nightmares, and withdrawal from friends. The influence of violence from other media, such as video games, the Internet, and popular music, has been less extensively researched. Clearly, unsafe feelings can be generated through exposure to repeated violence on television, causing effects that are much greater in preschoolers and that are no doubt aggravated when family members are similarly feeling unsafe.

TABLE 6–1.   Risk and protective factors for vulnerability to media violence: a summary

Factor	Risk/protection weight
Maleness/testosterone	R2
Low cerebrospinal fluid serotonin	R2
Smoking/substance abuse problems	R3
Callousness/antisocial personality disorder	R3
Conduct disorder in childhood	R3
Affective lability	R1
Thoughts of self-harm	R1
Shame and humiliation experiences	R3
Being a loner	R1
"Black and white" perceptions of others/self	R1
Poor school performance	R1
Head trauma and organic brain disease/injury	R2
Poor social skills	R1
Pertinent exposure to stress	R2
Poor prenatal care, maternal stress	R1
Attachment pattern: security of parent–child interaction	R3
Parental modeling of aggressive behavior	R2
Authoritarian parental discipline style	R2
Parental substance abuse	R3
Maternal depression	R2
Child abuse: painful sexual and/or physical abuse	R3
Recent loss/individual and social rejection	R2
Bullying (perpetrator/victim or involved bystander)	R2
Lack of feeling attached to family/school/community	R2
Community violence/gangs	R1
Access to weapon	R2
Underemployment	R1
Overcrowding	R1
Overwhelming arousal with average stimuli: heat, fear, noise, aggressive sports	R1
Dismissive families (parental lack of caring and involvement with children)	R2
Available support during time of loss	P2
Resilience	P3
Age and developmental stage of child	P/R3

TABLE 6–1. Risk and protective factors for vulnerability to media violence: a summary *(continued)*

Factor	Risk/protection weight
Youth: the younger the child, the more media vulnerability	R3
Capacity to symbolize and abstract: flexible operational skills	P2
Security and stability of adults (parents, schoolteachers, etc.)	P3
Amount of exposure to media violence	R2
Media depiction of weapons and use of humor to minimize violent media images; realistic violence, video games/MTV	R2
School and community resilience programs	P2
Promoting mentalization and awareness of power struggles and power dynamics with coping skills	P3

Note. No single factor will invariably cause psychological harm in all children. R=risk; P=protection; 1=small risk/protection weight; 2=moderate risk/protection weight; 3=high risk/protection weight.

Source. Adapted from Twemlow SW, Bennett T: "Psychic Plasticity, Resilience, and Reactions to Media Violence: What Is the Right Question?" *The American Behavioral Scientist* 51:1155–1183, 2008. Used with permission.

Identifying factors that increase or reduce a child's vulnerability to the effects of media violence may well be a fruitless task, given the vast range of contributing variables (see Table 6–1). The pivotal feature in this complex equation is the state of mind and experience of the individual child (Twemlow and Bennett 2008).

Feeling safe is also related to the social climate. Caprara et al. (2000), in a 5-year study of 294 third graders, found that when students engaged in altruistic behaviors such as cooperating, helping, and consoling, academic achievement improved. Having friends and being helpful contributed to a sense of safety and success. Gilgun (1996) examined a variety of factors protective against violence and identified the role of close personal friendships and the presence of older prosocial role models in the experience of feeling safe in a community.

There are a number of other useful studies of the concept of feeling unconnected in a school environment. One such study (Bonny et al. 2000) of nearly 4,000 children in grades 7–12 demonstrated that early signs of disconnection and alienation from the school environment (creating a child who feels unsafe) are indicated by the child's withdrawal from the peer group and by the adoption of habits that may negatively distinguish the child from his or her peers, such as cigarette smoking and alcohol consumption. The "Small Schools" movement among North American educationists (Wasley et al. 2000) represents a reaction to the same phenomenon of alienation and lack of safety by assuming that smaller schools might make children feel safer, all other factors being favorable. Table 6–2 summarizes factors that might affect a young person's feeling of safety and well-being in a school setting.

Feeling Safe Is an Internal Decision

As discussed in Chapter 5 ("Bullying Is a Process, Not a Person"), Bion (1970) has pointed out that a healthy group is one in which the knowledge (K) of the group as a whole, defined as what the group has found out about itself that is of essential value for its continued existence as a cohesive group, becomes a critical part of what binds it together and makes people feel safe and creative within it ("Positive K"). As communities become more fragmented, this knowledge becomes spoiled and destroyed, as evidenced by traditions being lost and families becoming transient. The stories that unite people and make them proud of their community become garbled and forgotten ("Negative K"). In such violent communities (Twemlow and Sacco 1999), individuals break away and form small subgroups, often of a highly pathological, self-centered nature. These pathological subgroups frequently have as their central concern the need for individuals to feel safe through coercive power using violence and money.

Unfortunately, pathologically cohesive communities (like urban street gangs) offer little forgiveness, little freedom of choice, and no permeability to the outside. You're either in or you're out. It is not only children's gangs that form these structures; many dictatorships share similar characteristics. A colleague from Paraguay pointed out that under a dictatorship between 1954 and 1989, the country's overall climate was quite peaceful, but there was no freedom. Singapore is another example of how a nonpermeable and unforgiving community can be peaceful and safe, but without the freedom of choice that our democracy demands. In the countries of the former Soviet bloc, safety was hardly an issue through the 1960s and 1970s. With the awakening of democracy and personal freedom came a massive increase in violent crime, particularly mafia/gang-related criminal activity. The dilemma for Americans is how to achieve safety without overwhelming bureaucratic or tyrannical control.

It is interesting to note here that one etymological root of the word *safe* means "whole." The Latin *salvus* also implies healthiness. These dimensions of feeling safe are often forgotten. In other words, a whole and healthy person feels safe both inside and outside. That feeling of safety derived from feeling whole then pervades the individual and the community. Commonly, intactness is a quality of the social system within which the individual finds him- or herself.

TABLE 6–2.   Factors contributing to a feeling of safety and well-being in schoolchildren

Negative factors

Exposure to constant family and community violence

Presence of drugs and alcohol

Exposure to media reports concerning community's lack of safety

Exposure to media depictions of violence

Being rejected by peers

Positive factors

Good quality of caregiver–child relationship in early life

Presence of protective adults whom the child trusts and who are seen to be effective in providing protection (i.e., feel safe themselves)

Presence of a safe haven or retreat

Training in personal safety techniques and social skills, which can mobilize social resources, problem solve, and provide children with a feeling that the situation is understandable

Having good relationships with peers and friends

Having predictable routines

Feeling valued and respected at school

Engaging in altruistic behaviors

Having a sense of belonging to the school

A colleague recently visited Israel with his wife. I asked her if she felt safe there, and she said, "Of course." When I asked her why, she replied, with a look of some surprise, "Because I'm with my husband." Secure human relationships create a feeling of safety. Behaviorists of the 1960s and 1970s tried to explain this phenomenon by suggesting that the attachment figure who could make a "dangerous" environment "safe" for the phobic patient represented a "learned safety signal" (Rachman 1984). Attachment theory offers insight into the almost magical decrease of anxiety that occurs in children in the presence of primary attachment figures (Ainsworth 1989).

Defenses Against Fear and Threats to Personal Safety

No one wants to think of themselves as being constantly vulnerable to the threat of violent attack. No woman walking home from work wants to picture an attacker looming, ready to force himself on her violently. No man relishes the thought of being caught in a situation where a desperate and violent attacker might destroy his ability to continue to provide for his family with one slash of a knife or a single gunshot. No parent welcomes the nightmarish image of his or her child's abduction, rape, mutilation, or murder. Pondering the possibility of death, torture, or attack of oneself or one's family is clearly not a comfortable state of mind. It is not surprising that people choose not to spend all their waking hours dwelling on potential dangers.

People use many internal strategies to keep themselves from thinking about the threat of violence and to make themselves feel safe. Some of these ways are normal and adaptive, but others are not. For example, certain psychopathological conditions, including mania and other grandiose psychotic states, may allow an individual to feel omnipotent and to deny potential danger. Dependent and avoidant character pathology may create a spurious feeling of safety for different reasons. Obviously, *feeling* safe is not synonymous with *being* safe. Thus, some of the things that people do to make themselves feel safe are actually quite detrimental to their safety, weakening their ability to react to and defend themselves from an attack.

What, then, is a healthy way to feel safe? Survival depends on having a fully conscious and integrated mind-set dedicated to monitoring inner arousal and maintaining alertness to escape options (Twemlow 1995a, 1995b). Feeling safe obviously also requires an awareness of danger, including adequate self-defense and negotiation skills.

In the following subsections, we describe a number of strategies that people—and, by extension, schools and communities—use to distract themselves from fear, worry, and awareness of threat: denial, false hope, avoidance, role immersion, and dissociation.

The Denial Mind-Set

Animals don't think; they use their instincts to survive and respond to danger in a world filled with predators. Denying violence is a uniquely human trait and represents a clear disconnection from our evolutionary ancestors, whose primary instinct was survival in a violent world. Becoming aware of violence may be painful, but it is a necessary first step in preparing for any eventual violent attack that may occur as a result of one's personal or professional pursuits.

It is easy to understand the allure of denial. Awareness is frightening. Preparation is tough and demands discipline and commitment. It is simpler in a modern world to use a handy defense to deny and avoid the anxiety associated with awareness of violence. Stories about gang violence, carjacking, mass murders, serial killings, rapes, and domestic violence dominate all forms of the media. When a particularly brutal murder or rape occurs, most communities react with shock and confusion. Task forces are formed to seek answers to decrease the fear. Community members look to their leaders for protection and guidance. After the meetings and speeches, the most effective solutions begin and end with us all facing the ugly realities of this increasingly violent world. Personal safety is your responsibility, not your community's full obligation.

Further, maintaining mindless defenses against fear requires a great deal of energy that is chronically questioned as a resource for coping with the demands of living in a violent world. Using defenses to deny violence is a natural and common method of human behavior in modern society. The demand for daily survival awareness has decreased as society and human beings have evolved into a more industrialized culture. Centuries ago, it was second nature for nearly every human to be armed and ready for an attack from man or beast. Today, the basic instincts that have kept us alive for millennia have been softened by the relative ease of modern life, thus making us more vulnerable to predators.

Thinking about violence causes a biochemical change that prepares you for action by stimulating the secretion of hormones that you experience as fear. Thinking about danger and violence causes ongoing anxiety. This anxious feeling is a survival signal that prepares you to freeze, flee, or fight in the face of danger. Watching the news or reading about violent attacks causes you to feel vulnerable and nervous. Fear begins to shape the way you live your life. Eliminating the discomfort of the signal has replaced responding to the warning. In the United States, some studies (American Institute of Stress 2010) suggests that we are in fearful denial 24 hours a day, and the recommendation to relax creates more anxiety because it is seen as a fear-increasing challenge! We do not compare well with other countries, including China, where the average person can relax.

Denying violence is a quick way to reduce the constant anxiety and fear of living in a violent world. Denying violence is comparable to ingesting an anti-anxiety medication that quickly numbs your senses. The threat of violence becomes remote during the exhilaration of the numbing of anxiety through denial. Closing your eyes to danger opens your mind to a magically clean and clear reality without the discomfort of fear. You can guarantee yourself invincibility by simply closing your eyes. The tighter your eyes close, the more you can feel safe. But remember: if it sounds too good to be true, it usually *is* too good to be true.

It is simple to recognize why this is an attractive option. Most people don't have the necessary tools and equipment to prepare correctly for a violent attack. In the face of being ill-equipped, the simplest solution to mounting fear and anxiety is quick and easy denial. Shutting out reality is uplifting. Illusions of survival can be easily spun from the web of denial. Unfortunately, reducing the awareness of anxiety also greatly diminishes your alertness toward danger signals. Denying violence coats your brain's danger-receptor sites, effectively wrapping a blindfold around your natural biochemical alarm system. In addition, the denial of anxiety confuses your ability to monitor your own self-arousal. You will not be able to look into yourself and become aware, as danger approaches, of your own internal cues. Being able to tune into one's own inner reactivity to fear is the first step in preparing for a defensive or offensive response in a dangerous situation.

Reducing anxiety and awareness of fear also minimizes the available biochemical and mental resources necessary to take evasive action. While numbed by denial, your escape options are greatly reduced at the outset of a violent attack. Your use of denial cuts off your available energy for counterattack or running away. Also, a great deal of mental and physical energy is used to erect and maintain the defense of denial. The net result is a late and tired personal response during a violent attack. The bottom line is that you render yourself unable to respond in the face a violent attack.

Denial removes your motivation and ability to prepare yourself realistically for a violent attack. Safe escapes must be learned and practiced under simulated attacks. You do not have to become a dedicated martial arts student to be safe. In fact, training in martial arts does not guarantee safety. Many a trained martial artist has frozen in real-life situations. Knowing several simple techniques for physically releasing oneself from an attacker's grasp is rarely sufficient to safely escape an attack. Surviving an attack requires a clear and alert mind, combined with a few good "natural self-defense" techniques like poking, pinching, stomping, biting, and hair-pulling. As obvious as this may sound, it is hard to do. Model Mugging (http://modelmugging.org/), a popular and useful self-defense training, was developed by a karate master after he had been humiliatingly beaten to a pulp by a street person.

> A young and bright female college student, and a senior brown belt in martial arts, was in her apartment studying one day when a knock on the door revealed a man who said he had political material to show her. Through her chained door, she looked at his pamphlet and saw that it wasn't political. He then asked to use her phone. She let him in and remembers noticing that he wasn't going toward the phone, in spite of her instructions, and that he was taking off his coat. She got the message at this point and luckily was skilled enough to disable him; she then ran to get help.

When you are immersed in a denial mind-set, your ability to survive a violent attack is greatly reduced. Instead of preparing your body to defend itself, this mind-set spawns a complex progression of regressive physiological and psychological responses characterized by helplessness and hopelessness, which we call the *giving-up/given-up-on syndrome* (see Figure 6–1).

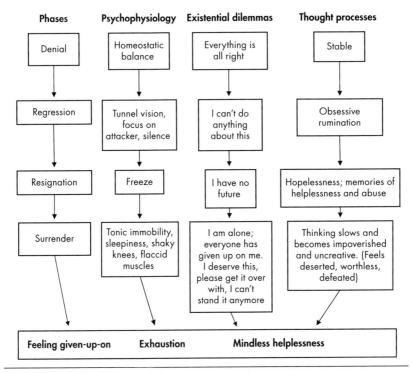

Phases	Psychophysiology	Existential dilemmas	Thought processes
Denial	Homeostatic balance	Everything is all right	Stable
Regression	Tunnel vision, focus on attacker, silence	I can't do anything about this	Obsessive rumination
Resignation	Freeze	I have no future	Hopelessness; memories of helplessness and abuse
Surrender	Tonic immobility, sleepiness, shaky knees, flaccid muscles	I am alone; everyone has given up on me. I deserve this, please get it over with, I can't stand it anymore	Thinking slows and becomes impoverished and uncreative. (Feels deserted, worthless, defeated)
Feeling given-up-on	**Exhaustion**	**Mindless helplessness**	

FIGURE 6–1. Giving-up/given-up-on syndrome.

Source. Adapted from Twemlow SW: "Traumatic Object Relations Configurations Seen in Victim/Victimizer Relationships." *Journal of the American Academy of Psychoanalysis* 23:563–580, 1995. Used with permission.

The Pollyanna Defense

The "Pollyanna" approach to dealing with fear is a reaction that simply denies the negative aspects of violence and inserts an overly friendly and often exaggerated sense of goodness in the world around. This all-powerful illusion of safety is used in order to create a sense of predictability and safety in the world. The world is made safe because it is only seen as having good intentions. It is a pretend world, though. Pseudo-safety illusions are key elements to denying violence. It is very easy to convince yourself that you are invincible and will be safe in almost every situation. This is a very calming, numbing fantasy that is easily spun personally and interpersonally; it commonly is contagious in groups of friends and relatives, who repeatedly reassure each other that everyone is safe from all danger.

Adopting this sweet attitude toward the world is also often socially expected in certain groups. Women, for instance, may be forced into socialization patterns that demand this attitude and that teach women that they must be submissive to men in order to survive. Many feminists believe that violence toward women is bred into cultural institutions in many obvious and some not-so-obvious ways. The Pollyanna defense may result from women's socialization patterns and may be the essential ingredient that leads tragically to many women being battered, raped, and murdered.

Pollyanna illusions clearly cloud your ability to sense danger. So much energy is expended in developing positive images that realistic cues in dangerous situations quickly become converted to the sweetened Pollyanna version. Arousal monitoring becomes impaired and loses its ability to guide and direct proper survival maneuvers. Prevention consciousness is eliminated since the fantasy is that no real danger exists. Thus, any violent situation is guaranteed to freeze you when clear, fast thinking is critical to survival.

Your ability to take evasive action becomes greatly delayed if danger cannot be seen until it is too late to escape. Your escapes become limited, since you consider that all potential enemies are friends until proven otherwise. The net result of this strategy is that you turn yourself into a submissive target for aggression.

It is easy to understand why feeling good and believing that people are good is comfortable and reassuring. It is not healthy to always think that someone is out to hurt you at every turn. It is, however, an excellent survival maneuver to plan and prepare yourself for a personal attack. Realistic orientation to safety precautions needs to be inserted into everyday personal and professional life. Pretending that everything is okay may make it easier to continue to perform tasks on a day-to-day level; however, staying alive in a violent world demands a realistic approach to preparation and alertness to signs of threat.

Risk Taking as Denial

Another common form of denying violence is to flood yourself with stimulation associated with self-created risk taking. You deny violence by constantly challenging violence to hurt you. Taking risks can be a numbing, almost aphrodisiac-like experience that leaves you with the impression that violence is under control. Thrill seeking and high sensation cravings overwhelm your nervous system, tricking you into believing that violence can never touch you. You feel reassured by surviving a high dive or a deep-sea scuba exploration. You indulge the illusion that you have conquered death and physical harm by attending a cage fighting match or professional wrestling event. Simply overwhelming ourselves with artificial pseudo-high-risk challenges allows us to believe that we are prepared for violent attack. This high level of stimulation mimics the high level of intensity and focus required in responding to violence. Unfortunately, this mirroring of stimulation only pumps up your arousal without training you to focus and harness your arousal state under violent attack.

By compulsively taking risks, people are denying the real risks in life by creating a false sense of well-being through conquering artificial, self-made risks.

This counterphobic approach is similar in its defense functions to being phobically afraid. Thus, those fascinated with danger are at heart really scared of it and try to desensitize themselves through frequent exposure. The real focus on imminent risk of violent attack is shifted and compartmentalized into happy activities as well as cavalier states of mind when confronting potentially violent situations that may unfold at home, on the way to work, or as part of work. Constant risk taking confuses people's abilities to sense danger. The planned re-creation of high-risk activities oversensitizes you to the high-arousal states often found in violent situations. Thus, danger becomes a false ally and does not spark the necessary first blast of preparatory energy needed for people to safely escape a violent attack. The heightened sense of arousal associated with risk taking confuses your ability to truly monitor internal arousal states efficiently during an attack. High-risk numbing and desensitization create confusing internal signals and falsify the accuracy of your internal emotional reactions to fear and danger.

High-risk activities reduce your motivation to realistically prepare for violent attack. Thus, the rush experienced from high-risk activities (e.g., skydiving, scuba, bungee jumping) is mistakenly confused with the arousal caused by actual life-threatening violent attacks. Someone participating in high-risk activities may believe that the thrill of a violent attack is the same as skydiving. Generating focused energy becomes difficult when people become preoccupied with increasing levels of stimulation rather than learning to balance and focus their attention and energy in the face of high stress or danger.

It is essential that we begin learning the difference between fun and reality. A healthy balance between the two is a simple prevention device that will allow people to enjoy taking risks without confusing the high-risk stimulation with insulation from possible danger associated with violence.

False Hope

The threat of violence often stirs up an impulse to manufacture false hope in order to gain an immediate sense of relief from the inescapable hopelessness of violence. Most people inherit their false hopes from their parents and mirror those behaviors long after separating from them. False hopes are soothing stories you fabricate to reassure yourself against the fear that accompanies thoughts of violence. "There's a little good in everyone," "Just treat others as you want to be treated," and "Nobody will bother you if you mind your own business" are only a few of the reassurances we all heard growing up. Your insight into potential danger is blocked by the growing number of stories you told to yourself.

It is understandable that the notion that "everything will be okay" is very appealing, especially in an increasingly visible violent world. As a modern individual, you are bombarded with violent images through every form of media available. The "anti-media" consists of these self-created false hopes that combat the information from media sources. The false hope spawns a belief that violence can be staved off indefinitely.

> Sometimes whole communities and cities engage in false hopes, as we observed when we consulted with a city school that had a bullying problem with a tiny minority of Asians, the children of wealthy business executives. These children were shunted into special eating areas in the school canteen, where the school had hired Korean chefs to help the children acclimate. It had the opposite effect, since many of the children were born in the United States and were accustomed to eating American food!
>
> In researching the city, we found low rates of violence, high rates of property crimes, and very high average real estate prices. The schools had no classes or provisions available for behaviorally and mentally ill children; such children went to schools in surrounding cities. Poor people regularly robbed the wealthy, and the police department was charged with maintaining safety. The unspoken philosophy was to purify the community by eliminating the poor and the needy, which included racial and intellectual minorities. Our suggestions to open the community to diversity were not well received, except by the city manager, with whom we became friendly. Three years later, he remembered a prediction we had made when the school became a disgrace for its abusive bullying of girls.

False hopes can be exchanged and reinforced socially over long periods of time. Parents and spouses can spin a web of false hopes to calm themselves and their offspring. Moving to seemingly quiet or "safe" neighborhoods is an example of creating false hopes through physical moves. Removing yourself and your family from known violent environments and populations is a classic example of striving for the false hope of safety through economic distancing from violent communities. False hopes create relief through the generation of competing information. The more intense the outside signals of danger become, the harder the mind works to create competing mythologies of safety.

False hopes distort reality and prevent proper planning and realistic preparation for potentially violent situations. This artificially created sense of hope decreases people's motivation to seek training that might have prepared them for an attack. During an attack, the calming preattack stories cloud one's ability to clearly read danger signals and deliver an effective escape or de-escalation tactic. The escape response requires a realistic perception of both internal and external stimuli. Proper execution of an attack avoidance maneuver or a counterattack demands clear thinking and decisive action. False beliefs distort the clarity of your mind and the readiness of your body to respond to threatening situations.

Withdrawal and Avoidance

"Shying away" from discomfort and fear is not abnormal. Avoiding and withdrawing from danger is a sensible move, since being aware of violence can cause great discomfort. Naturally, avoiding violence is everybody's goal. When you withdraw, you pull your awareness away from the outer world, directing your energy inward. However, looking exclusively inside cuts off your ability to accurately scan your environment, impacting how your sensory receptors perceive the outside world. For example, activities in the outer world may seem as if they are happening very far away.

As an interpersonal strategy, avoidance is based on phobic logic. This strategy involves creating endless mental lists of potentially fearful places, people, and actions and then using this list as a safety check for life's everyday activities. Withdrawal and avoidance can be accomplished using the following mechanisms:

1. *Internalization of stress into the body* is a common method of avoiding awareness of violence. The withdrawal is accomplished by cutting off your active awareness and attention from the real danger cues in the world and redirecting the mounting stress back into your body. In this scenario, anxiety about violence is swapped for physical body pain such as headache, lower back pain, and ulcers. Coping with pain daily creates a wall against a violent world.
2. *Task immersion* essentially involves bypassing the anxiety and stress associated with violence awareness by keeping very busy with daily tasks. The individual relying on this strategy resembles a busy worker with blinders on, avoiding distress by focusing on concrete tasks. Violence is viewed as an encumbrance on the efficiency of task-completion rituals. The sense of control and success experienced by completing tasks creates an antidote for the sense of impending doom associated with violence awareness.
3. *Mind numbing* is a redirection of mental energy into a circular defensive maneuver designed to keep the focus off danger and the fear that accompanies violence awareness. Today's media surround us with continual blasts of graphic violence with strong impacts on our arousal systems. Numbing allows you to experience information without internal or external arousal.
4. *Escapism* is a form of avoidance that often takes a very self-destructive path. Addictions are one of the most glaring examples. Living in a violent world can be tolerated by numbing the senses and decreasing inhibitions through intoxicants. Running away from the painful realities of a violent world becomes easy under the influence of mind-altering chemicals. Not all escapism is self-destructive; however, this defense becomes dangerous when violence is denied through the excessive use of chemicals that create the illusion of personal safety or toughness in a pretend world.

The principal problem with avoidance as a reaction to threat is that it weakens you by allowing fear to be the central power that governs your every move in life. Avoidance behaviors can be extreme and thus become very successful at reinforcing themselves. For example, a person afraid of being robbed may stay at home for years and is, consequently, not robbed. It can be tough to argue with the power of this formula, although, unfortunately, most rapes and murders occur at home. However, unless one can truly create a secure and protected bubble, the avoidance tactic leaves a person vulnerable to rare and unsuspected attack. Fear is instinctively perceived by predatory attackers.

Withdrawal and escapist strategies are often self-destructive and add to the burden of vulnerability to violent attack by being unhealthy and clouding your judgment. Alcohol intoxication is one prime example. The act of defensive avoidance carries with it a health risk that adds exponentially to the risk formula. Not facing facts in the violent world requires a high level of escape and withdrawal.

Role Immersion

In an earlier time in America, community professionals such as teachers and police officers were universally respected. Parents were very involved in their children's lives, whether it was in the city or on a farm. Children were connected to extended families, which in turn were connected through churches and civic groups as members of a community. A parent was likely to be angry at the child if a teacher had been forced to discipline him or her at school, so the child could expect a double punishment. The police were known neighborhood protectors, not high-tech and anonymous in their police cars. Respect for authority was a key value shared by the vast majority of people in the community. Dysfunctional children and adolescents were quickly separated and punished. The mentally ill and developmentally disabled were institutionalized away from the mainstream of the community.

The sad reality today is that those days of close family and community ties are gone. School discipline problems have become much more serious. In America, the role of teacher or police officer no longer engenders the same unqualified respect it used to. Teachers are assaulted every day. Police officers are killed or disabled on the job with alarming regularity. In a violent world, there are no safe professions. Even librarians have to walk to their cars in dark parking lots.

There are many examples of how professionals are harmed because they have not adjusted to the realities of a violent world. Jumping into arguments is second nature to many teachers, but this behavior can be fatal in a violent world. In a recent FBI survey of the murders of police officers (Pinizzotto et al. 2006), findings suggested that the victims were mostly veteran officers who let down their guard during seemingly routine tasks. In other words, it is not the rookie who is most at risk. The experienced officer of 10 or more years is the most vulnerable because of a false sense of security.

Role immersion is a defense that creates a sense of being protected and a decreased motivation to prepare for possible attack. The idea that what you do every day as a professional protects you soothes the growing fear of working in a violent world. As you get immersed in the role of police officer ("You wouldn't dare") or affluent child ("My father will get you fired"), you become unconsciously exposed to harm. This "they wouldn't dare" attitude is further buttressed by a false sense of invincibility that rests on the belief that the threat of consequences would be sufficient to scare off potential harm; thus, for example, a teacher might think, "They wouldn't want to stay after school or, even worse, have me call their parents."

Police officers and teachers are not alone in this fantasy. Nurses, doctors, social workers, and probation officers (just to name a few) often believe that they are safe because they are neutral authorities that people respect and leave alone. Case workers who intervene in child abuse allegations are at extremely high levels of risk for an unexpected violent attack, but they often approach their job with a cavalier attitude of false security fostered by the authority nature of their job. Role immersion as a defense against violence is often reinforced by the larger organization. Teachers are reinforced for downplaying violence in school systems. Often, the teacher is faced with the choice of physically intervening—at great personal risk—in a student fight or just walking away and knowing a student may be seriously hurt by their lack of action. Thus, the teacher and the school system cooperate in a mutual denial that violence is a job-related issue.

Role immersion also has a characteristic pressure-release valve to reduce the pressure built up by denying the fear of violence. Blaming the victim allows the professional the chance to safely distance and devalue the potential attacker. A sense of power and control is developed by putting down the student, client, patient, or suspect and morally disengaging themselves from the problem (Bandura 1999). Distancing oneself from the source of threat is accomplished through construction of a false image of accepted power and dominance. The expected protection stems from the presumed fear of authority in the potential attacker. The aforementioned "they wouldn't dare" attitude creates a sense of distance and protection while a person is at work.

Routine can help facilitate role immersion. Completing daily tasks helps distract from the growing realities facing everyone in a violent world. The threat of not performing at work or school dominates your attention, rather than a broader perspective that includes violence awareness. Every day brings a new chance to make a long list of tasks and run around thinking there is no time left for anything but the routine chores on the list. Somehow, the task of preparing your mind and body to live in a violent world never quite makes it onto the list.

Immersion in one's job or schoolwork as a denial of violence is made much more dangerous when the mounting stresses of life are added into the formula. Everybody accumulates their own stress; many people lack effective ways to cope with stress and live lives crippled by addiction, depression, abuse, and emotional pain. Stress and lack of realistic preparation for an attack combine to create weakness, increasing the risk of personal injury. Thinking that your safety is guaranteed by your job title or professional role is a dangerous move in a violent and competitive world. Survival requires a prevention consciousness and mental alertness. Hiding behind these roles prevents a person from acquiring the necessary knowledge to survive. The individual and his or her school or organization need to work together to make violence prevention and training a priority. School systems must develop policies that prepare and protect teachers and students.

Abdicating Bystander Defense

The abdicating bystander defense essentially says, "Violence (and preventing it) is someone else's job." Personal safety is unconsciously subcontracted to society, the police, schoolteachers, other co-workers, and spouses. The urge to "stay out of it" may seem to make sense, but abdicating personal responsibility for safety requires that you trust your life and personal security to strangers. No ordinary person has a bodyguard 24 hours a day, and even that is not a perfect guarantee of personal safety. This defense demands the development of a series of safety "subcontractors" that you feel compelled to use as a means of gaining safety and security.

Many teachers believe that discipline is the principal's job. School administrations and school committees don't protect teachers with clear protocols on how to act in violent situations. Again, the higher-ups think it is someone else's job. Teachers are then forced to make decisions "in the heat of the moment." When nurses walk to and from their cars in the hospital parking lot, their awareness of danger may be reduced because they believe that it is "Security's" job to keep them safe. Fear and anxiety are lessened when we project responsibility for our own safety onto others. Projection allows people to divest themselves of the heavy responsibility of taking charge of their own personal survival.

Although the President of the United States is required to subcontract his own and his family's personal security to another group, few ordinary citizens have the burden or luxury of needing Secret Service security. Short of this style of coverage, projection of responsibility to another always places us at some measure of risk, especially when we are alone. Not taking charge of our personal security weakens our chances for long-term survival. Skills can't be learned if people believe there is no need for the knowledge. Projection can block knowledge acquisition and might establish weakness through allowing us to place false confidence in others. In addition, projection indirectly implies that we view ourselves as weak and needy. This creates an increased probability for people to act submissively during an attack. When subcontracted personal safety leaves, the moment of truth can be very painful. Dependence on others creates vulnerability and frailty in the face of attack, as schools and communities have found. Fears and weaknesses are easily sensed by predators, and the net result is that we send out signals inviting an attack.

Predators and attackers look for weakness in potential victims. Why struggle? Common sense dictates that skilled predators know what easy prey looks like and how it behaves. Muggers sense when people are lost, fearful, and confused in a strange neighborhood. When you are accustomed to being protected by someone else, you will be likely to exude signals of fear when you are by yourself in an unfamiliar environment. In order to learn to protect ourselves, we must acknowledge and face the threat of danger to our own survival.

Identification With the Aggressor

Identification with the aggressor is another type of defense against fear; for example, a frightened young man may join the Marines to cope with his fear. Anxiety is often managed by tempting fate. The feared person or event becomes the target of a strange friendship. Fear becomes neutralized by creating a secret "deal with the devil." The victim becomes the attacker or bully, in other words, by becoming part of a violence franchise. Thus, the discomfort of feeling overwhelmed by fear is decreased by making friends with or imitating that which is feared. Identification with the aggressor is a weak and misguided attempt to cover one's own vulnerability.

In the classroom, a teacher sometimes becomes a bully and picks on a student. A nurse may push around an aggravating patient, or a police officer may become brutal or corrupt. The identity of the feared aggressor becomes incorporated into the person's own identity. This is an empty form of puffing up and provoking danger, rather than serious preparation. The person engages in chest-beating and self-aggrandizement in the face of nameless evil and danger. Nothing scares people while they are identifying with a potential fear. Thus, they lose the ability to accurately gauge their own inner arousal, as well as external cues during any real violent attack. The normal signaling power of fear and anxiety becomes neutralized by the maneuver of identifying with an imagined foe.

Identification with an aggressor creates an empty and boastful person living a lie. Toughness is advertised; weakness is never acknowledged. Trouble becomes a game of truth or dare, and violence becomes bearable because of the minimization of exposure to risk. Since danger is sought in the identification process, the approach of real violence will be masked. The "boy who cried wolf" fable teaches us not to overuse the danger alarm signal. Fear and anxiety should become a danger alarm system for the alert and prepared individual. Identifying with aggression and becoming a bully both attempt to cheat violence by becoming related to it, or marrying the enemy.

The denial of violence through identification with the aggressor relies on provocation as a sign of strength. Bravado is used to inoculate people against feeling overwhelmed by the fear of violence. Chest-beating is used to signal strength, while privately people may be praying that nothing actually happens. An example of this type of behavior might a series of stupid, empty challenges issued by a teacher to a potentially violent student. Other examples of this defense include the following:

> A middle-aged male teacher publicly confronts and tries to grab the jacket of a young man from a street gang. Risk of violence is denied by identification with the aggressor. The confronted youth waits until after school, when together with a small group of his fellow gang members he attacks the teacher as he is trying to get in his car.

> A female middle school principal witnesses an argument between two 13-year-old female students. She grabs one of the students by the back of the jacket and marches the girl to her office roughly, speaking harshly about how nobody will act as she did in her school. She then escorts the student to her locker and forces her to open it. The student opens the locker, grabs an ice pick from inside, and stabs the principal.

> A police officer is walking the beat in a high-risk neighborhood with racial tensions that are high. He tries to break up a group of young men on a corner by shoving, pushing, and flinging insults. The group surrounds the officer, grabs his gun, and shoots him with it.

These examples illustrate how professionals can fail to maintain alertness to how violence might be avoided. In all three examples, the opening moves of the professional involved an out-of-control escalator or provocation of violence. De-escalating techniques were not even considered. In each case there were many points where the professional could have used a prevention intervention to accomplish the desired goals. The fear and anxiety did not trigger more "heads up" or alert behavior, but the danger signals prompted an act of toughness and empty, needless bravado that quickly made the situation worse.

Dissociation

If you are in extreme pain and your pain levels cross a particular threshold, you will faint as a survival response to excruciating pain. The mental counterpart of fainting is dissociation. When fear becomes overwhelming, dissociation takes you mentally away from the discomfort and threat, as though the danger were about to happen to somebody else. In fact, dissociation is often described as an experience of hovering above oneself and looking at the action, or even forgetting it. This defense is a dangerous option in the face of violence. Pulling away mentally from danger is like wearing a blindfold during a fencing match. Dissociation can occur as an acute response to danger, or it can be adopted as a lifestyle. In either case, this defense pulls you away from fear by pushing awareness out to a distant point. People with a dissociative identity disorder cope with early life abuse by creating different personalities. The host personality is protected from the awareness of the torture by tricking the mind into believing it is happening to someone else. In extreme examples of dissociation, the humiliation and degradation of the trauma is passed on to somebody else, an alter personality.

As a lifestyle, dissociation can be very helpful in decreasing fear. Violence can be managed by simply convincing yourself that violence will only happen to "someone else." Realistic threats are minimized by "spacing out"—choosing to be mentally remote from the danger signals. Personal safety cannot be achieved when you believe you are above the possibility of attack. The classic movie *Looking for Mr. Goodbar* (1977) provides an excellent example of this defense. The heroine was a special education teacher by day and a seeker of sexually aggressive men by night, representing a splitting of her personality into two realities. Danger exists only in one half of the equation. A person begins to believe that his or her "other self" will take care of personal safety. During the day, a teacher may be cautious and exercise excellent control, but somehow dissociates at night and invites danger. This could easily apply to a nurse, teacher, or police officer.

The need to dissociate is motivated by the intensity of the fear and the extent of the perceived lack of control during threatening situations. Dissociation quickly turns to submission during an attack. As your worst fears become real, dissociation quickly takes over and virtually paralyzes your ability to think and act under attack. As a lifestyle, dissociation gives rise to split existences: a teacher may be a skydiver; a librarian, a bungee jumper. A police officer may believe that danger alertness is only needed on the job, and thus may be injured by an attacker while out walking the dog. Dissociation as a lifestyle creates compartments for fear and anxiety and develops alternative mind-sets and roles in life to further those mind-sets. Survival depends on a fully conscious and integrated mind-set dedicated to monitoring inner arousal and maintaining alertness to escape options.

Being Safe Requires a Healthy Mind-Set

All of the defenses described in the preceding section share the unrealistic hope that violence can be avoided or denied. What lessons can we learn from examining these ineffective mental defenses against fear, and counterproductive internal responses to threats to personal safety? How can we prepare ourselves mentally to withstand an attack? What is the best state of mind for survival? (The topic of mental preparedness is discussed further in the section "Clinician Safety: Assessment of Personal Risk" in Chapter 10, "Risk and Threat Assessment of Violent Children," which explains how MHPs might organize themselves when examining a potentially violent referral from a school setting.)

A healthy mind-set can be described as one of clear-eyed awareness and relaxed intensity. Safety mindedness does not mean worrying constantly about safety; rather, it is an automatic thinking process—an acquired habit, like brushing your teeth—that involves a realistic orientation to safety precautions throughout one's daily life. Denial is an active defense; the opposite is a calm and open consciousness that can be learned and is best reinforced by people talking about risk and danger rather than attempting to deny its existence.

A positive attitude is also created through measured practice and preparation. Like a vaccination, preparation for protecting yourself against violence requires exposure to a small bit of it. Relaxation, poise, and comfort stem from readiness to respond decisively and strategically if attacked. Preparation requires a sustained awareness of both inner arousal cues and external danger signals.

The School as a Securely Attached Family

A rather quaint early definition of the school (Chessick 1999, p. 77) was that it was "a theatre for self-improvement of the young." As old-fashioned as this eighteenth-century concept seems, it was in many ways ahead of its time, if psychology is an integral part of the process. In many ways, pathologically unsafe school environments mimic poor-quality parenting. Attachment researchers over recent years have highlighted the importance of affect modulation as the primary task of the caregiver–infant relationship (Ainsworth et al. 1978; Fonagy 2001; Sroufe 1996). The child's signals are understood and responded to by the caregiver; the signals gradually acquire meaning and, through internalization, become part of a process of self-regulation. Ultimately, the expectation is acquired that arousal no longer leads to disorganization; security is an expectation of safety.

In the context of the dyadic affect regulatory system of child and caregiver, it is the child's expectation of being comforted, soothed, and made to feel safe, in the context of fear generated by internal or external conditions (Bowlby 1988), that creates an internal feeling of safety and security. The securely attached child explores a strange environment readily in the presence of the attachment figure, becomes anxious in the presence of novelty in the absence of that figure, and actively seeks contact with the caregiver upon the reunion that follows a brief separation.

The burgeoning field of attachment research has described a variety of problematic attachment patterns that lead to pathological outcomes later in life (Dozier et al. 1999; Lyons-Ruth and Jacobovitz 1999; Main 1995; Main and Morgan 1996). Schools clearly have a role in continuing the process of internalization leading to affect regulation. The school plays a role in modulating the affect of children to create the expectation of control by its staff, which is a central factor in children feeling safe. Schools, as systems, may be characterized in terms of the manner in which they deal with fear. The attachment system has as its primary function the regulation of fear in the presence of conditions that biologically provoke it. A secure system accurately recognizes the emotional state of those within its confines and creates the well-founded expectation that distress will reliably be met by comforting. Confidence in this belief leads to a system that may be characterized as secure, where the systemic strategies for regulating affect would enable the school and any or all of its subsystems to restore homeostatic emotional balance relatively rapidly once emotion has been aroused.

The characteristics of this system will only be revealed when dysregulation has occurred, such as when the school has been challenged by some external or internal event (e.g., lack of discipline, community violence). A secure school will adopt a tolerant, open strategy, dealing with dysregulation through well-structured interactions, a flexibly applied range of communication patterns that permit individual expression, and meaningful responses. Signs of dysregulation are neither exaggerated nor minimized; language is respectful and participatory. Communications are clearly acknowledged, and individual contributions are expanded by other participants rather than ignored, denied, or dramatized. Evaluative comments are taken seriously, and there is a sense of coherence in communication patterns that implies collaborativeness.

How do such systems contrast with insecure systems? Insecure schools may carry the appearance of well-regulated organizations, but this appearance collapses under the pressure of a dysregulating event. Behind the apparently harmonious picture presented to a visitor are significant imbalances in communication and limited self-expression for the members of the group with the aim of avoiding tensions. A dismissive attachment pattern can develop in a school environment where there is little interest in children and where parents and teachers are preoccupied with their own problems and overwhelmed by feeling unsafe, by dealing with an unresponsive administration, by conditions of employment, by low salaries, and so on.

As these schools fail to provide a sense of safety in relation to threat both in children and adults, there is no sense of belonging on the part of those who participate in these systems. Truancy rates on the part of the students and absenteeism rates on the part of the staff are expected to be high. The emotional character of relationships is avoided in communications between students and teachers and between teachers themselves. There may be a false bravado and denial of all problems ("There is no bullying in our school"), as well as an idealization of the school environment. Just as the anxious-avoidant insecurely attached infant in the strange situation does not seek the caregiver upon reunion, children in avoidant or dismissive schools deny the importance of interpersonal relationships; they neither feel known by others nor wish to know others in the school. The school thus divides itself; small subsystems within the school exist without reference to or concern for the others. Children feel unknown and therefore are able to perform violent acts that they might not perform in a school that provides a sense of safety, where a feeling of belonging might be expected to serve a powerful inhibitory function.

In other schools, the anxious-resistant attachment pattern applies. Like the infant who fails to be comforted by the parent following separation, these schools, at a systemic level, tend to be "anxious" systems that upregulate problems, readily panic in the face of challenges, and are likely to call in consultants to assist with the difficulties they face, yet are unlikely to successfully implement any recommendations that such consultants might make. There are no clear lines of communications in these schools. The school is likely to have a well-studied and often-considered history of problems. There is likely to be an absence of a clear hierarchical structure, or if such structure exists, the participants mostly undermine it. There is confusion about most relationship issues, and domains of discipline are often confused with other domains, such as relationships or safety. The absence of clarity creates an environment where high levels of affect are often evident and where teachers frequently express anger to students and to each other.

A number of school systems have even further eroded feelings of safety by the ways in which they group grades. For example, it is not uncommon for middle schools to have only two grades, such as grades 6 and 7 or grades 7 and 8, with the inevitable 50%-plus turnover every year. In such settings, it becomes virtually impossible to develop a cohesive connectedness between children.

Modern theories of school functioning reserve an important place for the helpful involvement of parents. Such involvement is an almost impossible task in most inner-city schools and, ironically, in many affluent schools as well, where there is often too much parental involvement. Overly involved parents tend to be more interested in their own children getting a fair deal than in helping the school and viewing it as a community. Thus, parental involvement can be very much a double-edged sword. Lack of parental involvement should, however, not discourage the MHP, who even without parental participation can influence staff to become sensitive to the child as an independent sentient being with a unique mind, thoughts, and feelings.

In summary, in order for a school environment to be safe, the egos of all of its participants must engage and enable the development of a background of safety by helping the ego perceive a cohesive, understandable whole. At first, this atmosphere is provided by the parent or teacher, who must be sensitive to the developmental tasks of the child, allowing for a gradual weaning process as the child grows into the adoption of a peer-related, more externalized focus in high school. Group dynamics, power dynamics, competitive schools, and verbal and symbolic capacities can enhance or inhibit the child's ability to crystallize, identify, and deal with the frightening aspects of separation from that home environment. It is inevitable that the school will function as an important piece of the child's psychological matrix. The structure of the school (both physically and psychologically) can create a connection between children that is healthy or pathological. Attachment research suggests that schools that do not cultivate a feeling of involvement with the teaching staff (dismissive patterns) may be setting the scene for violence (Twemlow et al. 2002).

How a school functions is greatly influenced by social factors such as media pressures toward violence; abusive and neglectful child-rearing practices; the destruction of the nuclear family, including the climbing divorce rate; and the increasing mobility of families. All of these factors militate against the possibility of a safe, stable school and community.

Social Aggression in Schools

The complex social context of the school and its group and power dynamics have a potent influence on the individual's feeling of being safe. A concept from the Tavistock model of group relations is helpful in understanding this phenomenon. *Authorization*—that is, being able to act within a role determined by the task that one has—is one example of such a power dynamic. A well-functioning social system authorizes tasks that create a feeling of safety and connectedness. In pathologically authorized systems, there are internal pressures created by administration, politics, power struggles, media, pathological child-rearing fads, and other cultural factors that can yield what the writer Saul Bellow called a "moronic inferno" (Chessick 1999, p. 76). Anyone connected with the functioning of the school must feel authorized to act in a role, according to a defined healthy task.

The way schools are created, funded, and administered are also important parts of this feeling of safety. Alan Bloom (1988), in *The Closing of the American Mind,* indicted higher education for the degradation of a quality educational environment by teaching an oversimplified "democratic" concept of equality that encourages conformity. The punishment/surveillance philosophy of our culture encourages paranoia, exemplified by the highly visible presence of metal detectors and video surveillance equipment. In some inner-city schools (Devine 1996), the first one or two periods of the day are spent shuffling children through metal detectors, rather than through any academic learning process.

In our research (Twemlow and Sacco 1996), we have documented that a pervasive and untrammeled attitude of competitiveness at all costs can lead to an individual violent mind-set reflected later in community philosophies that breed an unforgiving attitude, materialism, and envy. Such mind-sets can lead to a downgrading of the quality of life in communities, which we have described as violent communities (Twemlow and Sacco 1999). Such communities harbor unforgiving attitudes toward the poor and the weak, valuing economic success far more highly than compassion. Since, to paraphrase an African proverb, "It takes a whole village to educate a child," it is no surprise that such socially aggressive attitudes are reflected in the children in schools and the atmosphere within schools. We have hypothesized that there is a social power dynamic operating between the victimizer, the victim, and the bystander audience to this sick drama. These co-created roles are, by definition, dependent for their viciousness on the intensity and sadism of the power struggles; we have formulated an explanatory model of lethal violence in schools based on an understanding of this dynamic (Twemlow 2000).

A helpful addition to these speculations is the chronic failure of mentalization in violent environments. A partial failure of mentalization creates ideal conditions for a witness to the power struggle (the bystander) and an avenue to the pleasure of sadism. In order for the child to be able to enjoy being witness to the suffering of another, he or she must be able to create distance from the internal world of the other, at the same time benefiting from using the other as a vehicle for the projection of unwanted (usually frightened and disavowed) parts of the individual's own inner self. Bystanders do not lack empathy, because it is precisely through projective identification with the victim (and/or the bully) that children are able to experience themselves as more coherent and complete. Thus, affect inconsistent with a coherent sense of self is seen as belonging to the victim of the vicious power dynamic. The child's mentalizing, however, is limited by the environment; the suffering and pain of the victim need never be represented as mental states in their consciousness. We must remember also that the fault does not lie with the child. Mentalizing is a fragile developmental function that is not acquired fully until early adulthood, if then and at all. In most social contexts, mentalization requires environmental support and a social system to scaffold it, ensuring that reflection on the mental states of self and other can be relatively comprehensive, covering painful as well as neutral mental states.

How pervasive is this social aggression we are describing? We examined 10,131 children and adolescents in grades 3–11 in a West Coast city as part of a violence audit of the school system. In this midsized community of public schools, the children were predominately lower income, with 73% of the school community being nonwhite. Four broad areas were measured: victimization of self, aggression toward others, perceived responses to victimization, and attitudes toward aggression. The findings (Eric Vernberg, personal communication, 2008) showed that somewhere between 10% and 20% of all children in all grades received a vicarious thrill and were not hesitant to express pleasure at seeing other children bullied. The middle grades (7, 8, and 9) scored lowest in empathy for the victim and highest in aggression toward others. The entire sample showed disturbing evidence of a slow social conditioning toward seeing violence as positive, feeling less distress for victims, and increasingly avoiding any involvement with victims of aggression. In some schools in that system where this tendency was not present, however, clearly some other quality present had created a climate of safety.

The school is a unique culture and is the main stage for the development of a social identity in children. Adolescents are especially sensitive to peer pressures and are psychologically more responsive to their peers than to adults, especially when immersed in an "identity diffusion," including conflicts around authority that appear to be part of normal adolescent development (Erikson 1974). Adolescents are secretive about emerging new roles and identities that often collide with the ideals of their parents. Consequently, a child may experiment with many faces, a number of which come into direct conflict with the important social attitudes of parents.

Erik Erikson described "negative identity" as a reaction formation identity for a child. Extreme examples would be the minister's daughter who becomes a prostitute and the marine officer's son who becomes a hippie. Complex role shifts like these are sometimes a part of the normal extremes of adolescence and require considerable understanding and tolerance from teachers, school staff, and parents.

Adults play a critical role in constructing a sense of safety for children. Every child is unique, and every school, teacher, and parent is also unique. Children can begin to feel safe only when the adults are all on the same page. However, it is clear that parents often hold incorrect assumptions about children and what happens in school. Some of the most common assumptions are as follows:

1. Teachers always know what is going on at school.
2. Children instinctively know how to relate to each other.
3. Children grow out of their problems quite quickly.
4. Power struggles between children are not the parents' business, and children should be left to solve their own problems.
5. The popularity of children is a passing phase and is harmless.
6. All or most problems at school are caused by mentally disturbed or learning-disabled children.

These assumptions are often wish-fulfilling and enable parents to avoid responsibility for what might be happening, both with their children and in the climate of the school. In addition, parents and teachers frequently overemphasize or overvalue the following traits or accomplishments:

- Academic success
- Attendance at school
- Prowess at sport
- Self-disciplined activities, including homework
- Participation in school activities and clubs
- Popularity with peers
- Children causing no problems and asking few questions ("no problem" children)
- Obedience

In other words, parents and teachers value the aspirations that they had for themselves when they were in school, but that (most likely, if they were honest with themselves) they rarely achieved, at least consistently. Such perfectionistic standards ignore the fact that obedient, high-performing children are not necessarily healthy.

One factor that sets up a climate for social aggression is when parents and teachers are not good examples or models for children by virtue of their own behavior. For example, adults often participate in dominant social groups that humiliate others (Twemlow 2000). We have pointed to institutionalized social rituals such as

- Hazing in colleges
- Excommunication in churches
- Blacklistings in unions
- Racial discrimination in country clubs

These bullying exclusion rituals are practiced by the very adults who expect their children to be nonviolent and affiliated with each other without power struggles. Social aggression in schools is not likely to abate until the aggressiveness of both teachers and parents is also admitted and dealt with. Such highly valued social aggressiveness involves

- Being relentlessly goal focused
- Active upward social positioning
- Destroying obstacles to success
- Performing for approval
- Intense competitiveness
- An us-versus-them mentality

In children, social aggression can be and often is physical, especially with children in middle schools, but later becomes less physical and more focused on rumors, scapegoating, exclusionary games, loyalty battles, teasing, public humiliation, nasty tricks, feuds, and numerous forms of backbiting. Parents and teachers often confront children caught in the cycle of social aggression with an impossible task: children who have been beaten down by this aggression or grandiosely enhanced by it do not have the mind-set to achieve the type of assertiveness that adults, including teachers, wish for them.

As we discuss throughout this book, there needs to be a parent–school–community team where parents, even if not present at school, support schools in a program to develop a collaborative attitude toward social aggression, including the following beliefs:

- Social aggression must be viewed as a school–home–community problem. (No member of the team expects another member to solve the problem alone.)
- Social aggression needs to be dealt with immediately when it appears.
- Aggressive behavior needs to be handled in a nonblaming, collaborative way, with a group rather than an individual focus.
- An ongoing assessment of the climate of the school must be established, with the enhancement of prevention programming.

Feeling Safe: Challenges for the Future

Ethological research, especially into complex primates like chimpanzees as models of human behavior (DeWaal 1989), suggests that chimpanzees are capable of terminating serious and violent conflict for the greater good of the social structure. Chimpanzees, for instance, embrace and kiss after fights; other nonhuman primates engage in similar reconciliation behavior. It is as if primates know that because survival depends on mutual assistance, the expression of aggression must be constrained by the need to maintain beneficial relationships. DeWaal commented that it is only when social relationships are valued that one can expect the full complement of natural checks and balances. Herein lies the main problem and paradox. With the size and complexity of the human brain, we seem to be able to override survival-related checks and balances, displaying instead narcissistic cruelty and sadism of untrammeled viciousness and horror, without a single survival benefit.

The school is a community of families engaged in educating the younger generation. When that community is connected, members respect one another. They communicate openly, and they value creativity and altruism. Change is a natural part of responding to new challenges. The modern world bombards children's minds with violent images through the media, Internet, and family life.

Schools are pressured to demonstrate increased academic achievement as an indication of success. The focus shifts from the child as a sentient and feeling individual to the child as a responder to questions. "Time on learning" is the modern anthem of educational reform. Oddly, there is a reverse logic to this focus on numbers rather than human children. When children and teachers feel safe, they learn and teach better. Numbers should go up and children should be better able to answer questions. Creating safe schools begins with developing an understanding of what makes people feel safe in schools and in the communities that schools mirror. Over time, creativity and achievement can thrive only in open, compassionate, connected, and noncoercive large groups (Twemlow 2001).

KEY CLINICAL CONCEPTS

- Feeling safe is an internal decision influenced by many factors.

- Feeling safe is a necessary ingredient for children to learn effectively in school.

- Safety can be marginalized when people deny violence and adopt mind-sets that hide out of fear, such as

  — A denial mind-set

  — Reducing fear through denial

  — Pollyanna defense

  — Risk taking as denial

  — False hope

  — Withdrawal and avoidance

  — Role immersion

  — Abdicating bystander defense

  — Identification with the aggressor

  — Dissociation

- Attachment theory provides a useful way to conceptualize safety as being related to the physical presence of an attachment figure.

- A positive school climate free of coercion contributes to a child feeling safe at school.

References

Ainsworth M: Attachments beyond infancy. American Psychologist 44:709–716, 1989

Ainsworth M, Blehar M, Waters E, et al: Patterns of Attachment: A Psychological Study of the Strange Situation. Hillsdale, NJ, Lawrence Erlbaum, 1978

American Institute of Stress: Job stress. 2010. Available at: http://www.stress.org/job.htm. Accessed December 6, 2010.

Bandura A: Moral disengagement in the perpetration of inhumanities. Personal and Social Psychology Review 3:193–209, 1999

Bion W: Attention and Interpretation. London, Heinemann, 1970

Bleich J, Ingersoll S, Devine J: National Campaign Against Youth Violence Academic Advisory Council Report. Boston, MA, John F. Kennedy School of Government, Harvard University, 2000

Bloom A: The Closing of the American Mind. New York, Touchstone Books, 1988

Bonny A, Britto M, Klosterman B, et al: School disconnectedness: identifying adolescents at risk. Pediatrics 106:1017–1021, 2000

Bowlby J: A Secure Base: Parent-Child Attachment and Healthy Human Development. London, Routledge, 1988

Caprara G, Barbanelli C, Pastorelli C, et al: Prosocial foundations of children's academic achievement. Psychol Sci 11:302–306, 2000

Chessick R: Emotional Illness and Creativity: A Psychoanalytic and Phenomenological Study. Madison, CT, International Universities Press, 1999

Devine J: Maximum Security: The Culture of Violence in Inner-City Schools. Chicago, IL, University of Chicago Press, 1996

DeWaal F: Peacemaking Among Primates. Cambridge, MA, Harvard University Press, 1989

Dozier M, Stovall K, Albus K: Attachment and psychopathology in adulthood, in Handbook of Attachment: Theory, Research, and Clinical Applications. Edited by Cassidy J, Shaver PR. New York, Guilford, 1999, pp 497–519

Erikson E: Dimensions of a New Identity. New York, WW Norton, 1974

Espelage D, Bosworth K, Simon T: Examining the social context of bullying behaviors in early adolescence. J Couns Dev 78:326–333, 2000

Federman J: National Television Violence Study, Vol 1. Thousand Oaks, CA, Sage, 1996

Federman J: National Television Violence Study, Vol 2. Thousand Oaks, CA, Sage, 1997

Federman J: National Television Violence Study, Vol 3. Thousand Oaks, CA, Sage, 1998

Fleming TM, Merry SN, Robinson EM, et al: Self-reported suicide attempts and associated risk and protective factors among secondary school students in New Zealand. Aust NZJ Psychiatry 41:213–221, 2007

Fonagy P: Attachment Theory and Psychoanalysis. New York, Other Press, 2001

Fonagy P, Gergely G, Jurist EL, et al: Affect Regulation and Mentalization: Developmental, Clinical, and Theoretical Perspectives. New York, Other Press, 2000

Gilgun J: Human development and adversity in ecological perspective, part 2: three patterns. Fam Soc 77:459–476, 1996

Haigh R: The matrix in milieu: the ghost in the machine, in Contemporary Psychology in Europe: Theory, Research, and Applications. Edited by Georgas J, Manthouli M, Kokkevi AE, et al. Kirkland, WA, Hogrefe & Huber, 1996, pp 288–302

Joshi PT, Kaschak DG: Exposure to violence and trauma: questionnaire for adolescents. Int Rev Psychiatry 10: 28–215, 1998

Lee S-A, Borden LM, Serido J, et al: Ethnic minority youth in youth programs: feelings of safety, relationships with adult staff, and perceptions of learning social skills. Youth and Society 41:234–255, 2009

Lyons-Ruth K, Jacobovitz D: Attachment disorganization: unresolved loss, relational violence and lapses in behavioral and attentional strategies, in Handbook of Attachment: Theory, Research, and Clinical Applications. Edited by Cassidy J, Shaver PR. New York, Guilford, 1999, pp 520–554

Main M: Recent studies in attachment: overview with selected implications for clinical work, in Attachment Theory: Social, Developmental, and Clinical Perspectives. Edited by Goldberg S, Muir R, Kerr J. Hillsdale, NJ, Analytic Press, 1995, pp 407–474

Main M, Morgan H: Disorganization and disorientation in infant strange situation behavior: phenotypic resemblance to dissociative states, in Handbook of Dissociation: Theoretical, Empirical, and Clinical Perspectives. Edited by Michelson L, Ray W. New York, Plenum, 1996, pp 107–138

Meltzer H, Vostanis P, Goodman R, et al: Children's perceptions of neighborhood trustworthiness and safety and their mental health. J Child Psychol Psychiatry 48:1208–1213, 2007

Office of Safe and Drug-Free Schools: Safe Schools: Academic Success Depends on It. The Challenge, 2010. Available at: http://www.thechallenge.org/vol14_2/safe.html. Accessed December 6, 2010.

Overstreet S, Braun S: Exposure to community violence and post-traumatic stress symptoms: mediating factors. Am J Orthopsychiatry 70:263–271, 2000

Pinizzotto AJ, Davis EF, Miller CE: Violent Encounters: A Study of Felonious Assaults on Our Nation's Law Enforcement Officers. Washington, DC, U.S. Department of Justice, Federal Bureau of Investigation, August 2006

Rachman S: Agoraphobia—a safety-signal perspective. Behav Res Ther 22:59–70, 1984

Reeves MA, Kanan LM, Plog AE: Comprehensive Planning for Safe Learning Environments: A School Professional's Guide to Integrating Physical and Psychological Safety-Prevention Through Recovery. New York, Routledge/Taylor & Francis, 2010

Slone M, Shoshani A: Feeling safe: an Israeli intervention program for helping children cope with exposure to political violence and terrorism, in Terror in the Holy Land: Inside the Anguish of the Israeli-Palestinian Conflict. Edited by Kuriansky J. Westport, CT, Greenwood Publishers, 2006, pp 173–182

Sroufe L: Emotional Development: The Organization of Emotional Life in the Early Years. New York, Cambridge University Press, 1996

Twemlow SW: The psychoanalytic foundations of a dialectical approach to the victim/victimizer relationship. J Am Acad Psychoanal 23:545–561, 1995a

Twemlow SW: Traumatic object relations configurations seen in victim/victimizer relationships. J Am Acad Psychoanal 23:563–580, 1995b

Twemlow SW: The roots of violence: converging psychoanalytic explanatory models for power struggles and violence in schools. Psychoanal Q 69:741–785, 2000

Twemlow SW: Modifying violent communities by enhancing altruism: a vision of possibilities. Journal of Applied Psychoanalytic Studies 3:431–462, 2001

Twemlow SW, Fonagy P, Sacco FC, et al: Premeditated mass shootings in schools: threat assessment. J Am Acad Child Adolesc Psychiatry 41:475–477, 2002

Twemlow SW, Bennett T: Psychic plasticity, resilience, and reactions to media violence: what is the right question? Am Behav Sci 51:1155–1183, 2008

Twemlow SW, Sacco F: Peacekeeping and peacemaking: the conceptual foundations of a plan to reduce violence and improve the quality of life in a midsized community in Jamaica. Psychiatry 59:156–174, 1996

Twemlow SW, Sacco F: A multilevel conceptual framework for understanding the violent community, in Collective Violence: Effective Strategies for Assessing and Intervening in Fatal Group and Institutional Aggression. Edited by Hall H, Whitaker L. New York, CRC Press, 1999, pp 575–599

Twemlow S, Fonagy P, Sacco F: Feeling safe in school. Smith Coll Stud Soc Work 72:303–326, 2002

Vaillancourt T, Brittain H, Bennett L, et al: Places to avoid: population-based study of student reports of unsafe and high bullying areas at school. Canadian Journal of School Psychology 25:40–54, 2010

Vernberg EM, Jacobs A, Twemlow S, et al: Developmental patterns in aggression, victimization and violence related cognitions. (submitted)

Wasley M, Gladden N, Holland S, et al: Small Schools, Great Strides: A Study of New Small Schools in Chicago. New York, Bank Street College of Education, 2000

7

Assessment of At-Risk Children

ASSESSING at-risk children is a central contribution of this chapter. This approach seeks to integrate various individual and social perspectives in order to create a multiple-impact strategy to prevent and intervene early in school violence and also to prevent teen suicides related to victimization of vulnerable youth in schools.

Risk Analysis, Suicide, and Bullying

Recent highly publicized suicides related to bullying illustrate the principle of the IN or OUT expression of aggression (see Figure 7–1 later in this chapter). We review the OUT direction in Chapter 10, "Risk and Threat Assessment of Violent Children." When aggression is turned OUT, this leads to school shootings. The IN direction is represented by suicide. The mechanics of prevention in both conditions involve identification of vulnerable or at-risk children and adolescents. Whether the direction is IN or OUT, there can be lethal consequences in either case. Recognizing and monitoring at-risk or vulnerable children is key to keeping our schools safe. This is the job of adults working with students and their families.

Patchin and Hinduja (2008) note that suicide is the third leading cause of death among youth ages 10–24 years. Younger people are more vulnerable than ever in modern society. The world of virtual reality is a percolator of shame that can inflame already vulnerable children to acts of self- or other destructiveness. Suicide is a desperate solution that is enacted whenever shame is allowed to brew within a vulnerable child in a social context that is not paying attention. Schools are the place where the shame is acted out, and the Internet creates the illusion of inescapability and ultimate exposure that can lead to the implosion of aggression associated with the humiliation, as the child immersed in texting, twittering, and instant messaging adopts the world of virtual reality as an illusory substitute for reality and its complexities. (We explore the addictive quality of this virtual reality in Chapter 10, "Risk and Threat Assessment of Violent Children.")

There is an eerie similarity between these facts and those that have been studied as causal factors in school shootings. In both suicide and homicide, there is clearly (with the aid of 20/20 hindsight) evidence of what the Federal Bureau of Investigation (FBI) refers to as "leakage," or warning signals sent by a youth prior to engaging in an act of violence at school. Similarly, in the suicides related to bullying, there is this same pattern of early-warning signals that were missed by the adults.

The recent suicides attributed to the impact of bullying have illustrated several elements critical to understanding the relationship between bullying and suicide. Two cases highly publicized in western Massachusetts have illustrated the need to understand the vulnerabilities of youth as revealed by their behaviors at school. In the first, Phoebe Prince of South Hadley, a 15-year-old Irish immigrant girl, committed suicide after being bullied at school and on the Internet (Oliver 2010). This case illustrated the power of bullying to propel self-destructive behavior, especially in vulnerable youth. News reports revealed that Phoebe's mother had met with the school and expressed her concern that Phoebe had been a victim of bullying in Ireland and was very socially awkward and easily targeted by a bully. The ongoing pressure stemmed from a romantic rivalry, allegedly with older students. The entire school body is reported to have been aware of Phoebe's relentless exposure to bullying at school and on the Internet.

The second case involved Carl Walker-Hoover, an 11-year-old African American boy who hanged himself in his aunt's closet after being bullied due to being seen as gay (BostonChannel 2010). Carl was picked on, and his mother also tried to engage the school in a solution prior to the suicide. Carl's mother appeared on the *Ellen* and *Oprah* television shows to discuss the bullying based on gender identity. Carl's mother is active in bully prevention in Springfield,

Massachusetts. Again, the role of shame (gender confusion in an African American child) and the school as abdicating bystanders can be seen in the evolution of this tragedy.

After such highly visible cases, the community often targets the youth(s) involved in the bullying. In South Hadley, nine students were charged criminally as juveniles and adults. Phoebe Prince's vulnerability has become a necessary way to defend against the criminal charges filed against the students. This will not result in any positive change in the factors that led to this tragedy. These cases reinforce the need for adults in a community to take charge of scanning the schools for early warning signs of students in trouble. The entire school in South Hadley knew of Prince being a sustained target; the adults knew she was vulnerable. Blaming the children misses the point. Involving adults and learning from other communities' mistakes builds community resilience and protective resources into the school.

Similar patterns can be found in a number of other recent cases reported in the news, in which families have spoken up about the impact of bullying on their child's suicide. In September 1998, Jared Benjamin High, a 13-year-old boy who was being bullied, committed suicide. His mother maintains a Web site (www.jaredstory.com) in his honor that acts as a clearinghouse for services and ideas about bullying and suicide.

"Sexting" involves the sending of explicit images using the Internet. Jessica Logan (Celizic 2009) and Hope Witsel (Inbar 2009) are examples of young people who hanged themselves after being humiliated by mass distribution of intimate visual images. The Internet was used to generate humiliation, triggering self-destructive ideas that become perceived as inescapable due to the power of the Web to connect youth 24 hours a day and 7 days a week.

The suicide of Tyler Clementi at Rutgers University illustrates that bullying does not stop at high school. In this case, the Internet was used to generate humiliation by streaming a gay sexual encounter. Identifying someone as gay is a very common way to bully and a notoriously sensitive issue for young people. The shame that resulted from this prank led Tyler Clementi (Lohr 2010) to jump off the George Washington Bridge. There is some indication that Tyler reached out through the Internet and reported his situation to a residential supervisor. The students involved in the Rutgers case were charged with invasion of privacy and possible hate crimes. The power of the Internet and the hyperconnectivity of the digital era have created a new landscape for proliferation of self-destructive ideas, plans, and actions that can lead to adolescent suicide.

This aggression is most prominently visible at school and through the eyes of the students. The analysis of risk factors ranges from individual personality dynamics and family dysfunction to larger issues of social contagion. No single approach is powerful enough to anticipate and prevent violence in every situation. The key element in creating the conditions necessary for a successful in-

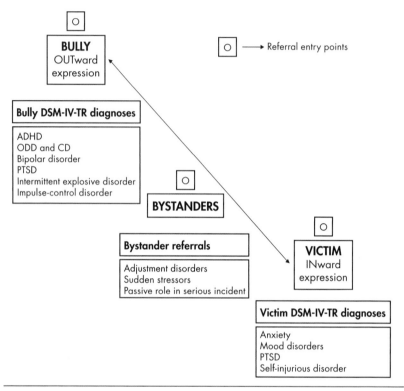

FIGURE 7–1.   Diagnosis of risk conditions leading to school violence: the referral landscape.

ADHD = attention-deficit/hyperactivity disorder; CD = conduct disorder; ODD = oppositional defiant disorder; PTSD = posttraumatic disorder. Diagnoses are based on DSM-IV-TR (American Psychiatric Association 2000).

tervention requires that the risk conditions be identified and protective factors be woven into the child's life starting at home, following him or her to school and into the community. The mental health professional (MHP) needs to develop a macro-understanding of the problem that also reflects a thorough understanding of the child's experience of the world (see Figure 7–1).

This perspective has two main endpoints in a continuum from victimizer or bully to victim or target. This can be seen as a range of expression for aggression from OUT (Bully) to IN (Victim), with the Bystanders distributed around the connecting line. High-risk children will be pulled to the endpoints of this continuum, and bystanders will become part of the surrounding population of children who lean either to one end or the other and who may be easily pulled in either direction, depending on the social context.

This referral landscape has a number of different portals, or referral entry points, that an MHP may encounter in a number of different capacities. Bullies are likely to be referred to an outside agency by a state agency or court and will frequently include children diagnosed with attention-deficit/hyperactivity disorder (ADHD), oppositional defiant disorder (ODD), conduct disorder (CD), childhood bipolar disorder, posttraumatic stress disorder (PTSD), intermittent explosive disorder, or an impulse-control disorder. These referrals are often made by members of the child welfare and juvenile justice system. Victims of bullies are typically referred by child protective agencies and child welfare services; parents may also make referrals to behavioral health clinics or private practitioners. Victims often include children diagnosed with anxiety or mood disorders or PTSD who are prone to acting out in self-defeating or self-injurious ways. Bystanders, like victims, may be referred by parents, school guidance counselors, or social workers. They may manifest signs of an adjustment disorder or behavior problems brought on by sudden stressors, or they may have been passive participants in a serious violent incident. Bystanders are often bored and impatient with an unsafe and violent school environment.

This landscape perspective is meant to offer MHPs a method to orient themselves to measuring risk in a way that allows for prediction and prevention of school violence and to give the at-risk child a happier home and school experience. School problems often manifest themselves in complaints and disciplinary actions. Teachers refer high-risk children for in-school support and may frequently refer such children for disciplinary action by the school administration. This offers a number of intervention and prevention opportunities. A high-risk child (e.g., bipolar) in a high-risk social context (e.g., unstable home) can enter school and be pulled quickly into the unhealthy social role of bully. The clinical challenge involves prediction of violence based on an analysis of individual and group risk conditions.

Case Example: Maria, an Aggressive Middle School Student

Maria was a 14-year-old Latina middle school student who entered an urban school late in the fall semester. Maria was living with her mother and three siblings. Her father was incarcerated for domestic violence, and Maria had moved from shelter to shelter until being placed in supportive housing with her family. On the very first day of school, Maria was suspended for fighting and was referred to the school social worker, who arranged for a meeting with Maria's mother. Maria reported that she had been very quickly targeted by a group of popular girls, who challenged her during lunch. Maria had no friends and was trying to fit in with other girls at lunch. Maria had been in psychotherapy since she was nine and had been prescribed a variety of medications, including stimulants and selective serotonin reuptake inhibitors. She had not been in treatment for the last year, due to multiple moves from various temporary protective housing services. The school social worker met with Maria's mother, who readily agreed to refer Maria for therapy. The therapist quickly referred Maria for a therapeutic mentor.

Maria became interested in martial arts and worked her way up the belt system without a single incident of violence. Maria's mother also reported that Maria had regularly suffered when adjusting to schools and was very easily provoked into fighting. In her life, Maria had witnessed a great deal of domestic violence and when she herself felt threatened, she quickly erupted into violence. The school social worker supervised a peer mediation program and began to involve some peers in helping Maria adjust to school after serving her 3-day suspension. The school social worker also referred Maria to a local clinical social worker, who visited the family's home and immediately connected to the school social worker. Maria was also referred to a psychiatrist and was eventually placed on a mood stabilizer and involved in an after-school dance program. Maria's mother joined the PTA and became active in supporting a program to promote safe dating and a positive school climate.

This case illustrates how a teenager with a high-risk personality, living under high social stress, entered a school without anyone considering how she would fit in and what could be done to make coming to school easier for her. Maria was, interestingly, part bully and part victim. She had attacked another girl based on feeling shamed at lunch. The school social worker was very alert and immediately recognized the risk factors and began to initiate an intervention that involved home, school, and community. The school already had been active in developing climate programs and had already established peer mediation and mentoring programs. This allowed for a comprehensive intervention that resulted in Maria being able to settle into the school and eventually feel safe and free to follow her passion, which turned out to be hip-hop dancing.

Table 7–1 illustrates the dimensions of how risk factors for aggression can become distributed or expressed. School violence can be viewed as behavior resulting from an interplay of personality characteristics and social context. DeRosier et al. (1994) studied African American children's (ages 7–9 years) playgroups and found "a dynamic relation between social context and the aggressive behavior of children" (p. 1078). This diagram is a landscape map to begin understanding the interaction between personality variables and social context.

Table 7–1 illustrates the interaction between the person and the social context revolving around a primary axis, involving the direction of the expression of violence: IN or OUT, victim or bully, murder or suicide. Other individual personality dimensions relate to the continuum of responses from submissive to aggressive. Also, there is an axis that involves a defensive style ranging from hypersensitive to numbed. Maria, for instance, was both aggressive and hypersensitive. Her response to entering a new school was reactive and unplanned, aggressive but not sadistic. She was quickly sucked into the bully role, due to an aversion to being masochistic; this

TABLE 7–1. Multidimensional risk assessment in school violence

Individual characteristics

DSM-IV-TR diagnosis: Axis I and Axis II
Social risk conditions: Axis IV (active pressure)
Personal strengths: Impulse control, social skills,
    educational accommodations, cognitive level

OJJDP pathways to serious and violent offending

Overt/aggressive	*Authority conflict (before age 12 years)*	*Covert/sneaky (before age 15 years)*
Bullying	Stubborn	Lying
Fighting	Disobedient	Property damage
Gang fighting	School avoidance	Fire setting
Rape	Truancy	Fraud
Murder	Running away	Theft
		Burglary

Social roles at school: Bully–Victim–Bystander

Protective factors

Involved adults
School and community programs
Peer acceptance and support
Antibullying programs
Social-emotional support
Wellness for teachers and students

Note. DSM-IV-TR=*Diagnostic and Statistical Manual of Mental Disorders,* 4th Edition, Text Revision (American Psychiatric Association 2000); OJJDP = Office of Juvenile Justice Delinquency Prevention.

is a common reaction for children who have witnessed domestic violence. The high-risk child is faced with a challenge from the moment he or she walks into a school. On her first day, Maria was catapulted into a social context that was not ready for her. Her sensitivities were not identified, and prevention was not possible. Early intervention, however, was successful, and future violence was avoided.

This multidimensional approach offers MHPs a number of ways to conceptualize the nature of a child's experience of going to school. Books (2007) highlighted a variety of issues in the care and treatment of homeless families. Yu et al. (2008) compared homeless and housed children and found that homeless children had more disruptive behavior disorders and lower cognitive functioning. Park et al. (2004) studied 8,251 homeless children in New York City and found that 18% of the children crossed over to the child welfare system after their first episode of homelessness. This study also demonstrated that the risks for behavioral problems were highest in homes with domestic violence and multiple shelter placements. In fact, the risks increased in relation to the ages of children the first time they were placed in shelters; the older the child happened to be, the greater the risk became for future aggressive behavior. We must also be mindful of the increasing number of children in a "post-welfare era" (Polakow 2003) that are homeless; schools and teachers are viewed as key supports for these children, who are experiencing "the social horror" of homelessness. Maria became homeless as a result of her mother's flight from domestic violence, rather than for purely economic reasons. Her style of coping was reactive, but her needs were clearly unmet, a circumstance that first manifested itself in the community in the form of school violence.

Table 7–1 also illustrates a conceptual framework to use in making risk assessments that use this multidimensional approach that integrates DSM-IV-TR (American Psychiatric Association 2000) diagnosis, active risk situations (often captured in the form of DSM-IV-TR Axis IV [Psychosocial and Environmental Problems] stressors), and individual personality strengths. Using the Office of Juvenile Justice Delinquency Prevention (OJJDP) model of three developmental pathways to serious and violent offending (Thornberry et al. 2004), the MHP can predict which pathway a child is at risk of following. These pathways represent the collective research on delinquency, showing how aggression and criminal behavior tend to unfold throughout a person's life cycle. These pathways are portals to the social roles that a child will be thrust into upon entering school. Such social roles are amplified by the impact of hyperconnectivity through the use of mobile devices, texting, networking, and the Internet.

Researchers have noted a strong connection between peer rejection and the appearance of violence (Kazdin 2003). The way a child is absorbed into the social fabric at school can become a matter of life and death. There are many examples of the relationship between bullying and suicide. Children at certain ages and with certain risk conditions have demonstrated that peer rejection and humiliation often fuel very extreme, out-of-character reactions. This is particularly true in suburban areas, where there is often a heightened awareness of social inclusion and exclusion.

This diagnostic picture would not be complete without representing the positive and protective influences that exist within the home, school, and community. The clinician needs to be aware of these protective factors, and if none exist, then recommendations need to be documented that such resources are needed to maintain normal social-emotional adjustment of children at school. Whether the approach used is based on family empowerment (as in wraparound services) or places the clinician at the helm of creating interventions, the basic formula remains the same. The values of striving for optimal balance in home, school, and family are the most crucial, followed by focusing on strengths and family involvement as shared values. It is also necessary to understand cultural diversity within the social context, as well as within the risk and protective factor profile.

Maria was Puerto Rican, and she had little social support because of moving so frequently from shelter to shelter. Traditionally, Puerto Rican families have strong extended kinships that offer backup support during high-stress periods. Maria, however, was quickly engaged by a Puerto Rican case manager, who became a therapeutic mentor and advocate that linked Maria to a high-interest activity.

Using our approach, Maria's case would be diagnosed as follows:

- *DSM-IV-TR diagnosis:* Axis I: ODD, PTSD
- *Social risk conditions:* homelessness, housing instability, witness to domestic violence
- *Personal strengths:* athletic, with a strong connection to her mother

Maria was not aggressive early in her life. She began showing aggression when her family began moving around to avoid domestic violence. She was more likely to be authority-avoidant but was easily pulled into a bullying role at school because her aggression was reactive. There was an active social work department and a peer mediation program, which allowed for quick response to the violent incident at school. There were no repeats of this incident at the school.

Maria became a functioning part of the school as a result of some quick action by an alert school social worker, who collaborated with a community clinician; both were backed up by a psychiatric medication program that supported Maria during critical times. Also, the community was involved in the intervention from a very early point. This problem was not an abstraction with a simplistic solution. Maria did not require any placement, despite an aggressive outburst that instantly reached the level of a juvenile justice problem. This action plan began because of an incident at school.

Risk Conditions

Assessment of risk conditions can be accomplished in a variety of ways, ranging from a DSM-IV-TR classification approach to one that stresses developmental pathways. These various methods are described to assist clinicians in the task of evaluating the social context of the child as part of creating a comprehensive treatment plan capable of responding to presenting problems in school violence.

Traditional Psychiatric Classification

There are a wide variety of traditional ways to categorize and conceptualize the risk conditions likely to impact on a child's behavior. The traditional psychiatric classification approach uses DSM-IV-TR to diagnose mental impairments, offering the clinician the tools to recognize how a mental impairment is likely to be manifested in a child's behavior.

Table 7–2 compares traditional psychiatric diagnosis (Simon and Tardiff 2008) with two other approaches—the OJJDP model (Thornberry et al. 2004) and Kazdin's (2003) framework—to illustrate points of similarity between the three models as the MHP grapples with different data and opinions when trying to assess and predict school behaviors.

In Maria's case, her PTSD and ODD had an OUT expression, so the MHP's intervention immediately staked out key action points involving the areas of home, school, and community. Maria's PTSD, combined with the high-risk stresses of homelessness and domestic violence, created a scenario of violence, erupting at school. In this case, the intervention was rapid and complex, offering services in multiple areas with a psychiatric and strengths-based approach (mentoring and martial arts) that stopped the reoccurrence of violence at school. Maria was not allowed to slip into a bully role to protect her social position within the school. The school social worker was able to use her position within the school to initiate an intervention that stopped the violence at school. She provided a balanced service plan that allowed for the family strengths of a strong mother–child bond to be blended with supportive school, home, and community supports. The program was eventually directed by the child's therapist and by a prescribing psychiatrist from a community mental health clinic.

This approach will also create opportunities for the clinician to interface with a school and to be of help in addressing climate issues that impact the child every school day. Cyberbullying, for instance, inflames what happens at school and makes the climate a causal aspect in the evolution of violence at school. A school climate is an aspect of modern children's social development, and we have witnessed a growing number of examples of how school culture and cyberbullying can have tragic results. The role of the Internet in a child's development is an increasingly important factor in how violence will be enacted in schools. The school will be the very first place that reflects the ugly realities of life within a community. If the community has given up on its schools, the children will feel it first. Racial tensions may increase, feuds may build up pressure, and the school may become the stage on which children act out their reactions to toxic psychological forces within the community.

Simon and Tardiff (2008) have outlined the DSM-IV-TR categories and how they may present as school violence problems. Mood disorders require immediate psychiatric evaluation. These problems can drive children to extremes in their school behavior. With elevated mood, there is an increased chance of the child having an irrational outburst or being hyperactive and disruptive. Depression, on the other hand, might create a victim mind-set, leading a child to become vulnerable as a target of bullying. This victim mind-set may be most useful in pre-

TABLE 7–2. Three approaches to assessment of risk conditions leading to school violence

Traditional psychiatric diagnosis (Simon and Tardiff 2008)	OJJDP developmental pathways (Thornberry et al. 2004)	Internalizing/ externalizing (Kazdin 2003)
Mood disorders	Early overt aggression	Externalizing disorders
PTSD	Authority conflict	Internalizing disorders
Substance abuse disorder	Covert activities	Substance-related disorders
Personality disorders Neurological disorders		Learning and mental disabilities
ADHD and disruptive behavior disorders (ODD, CD)		Severe and pervasive psychopathology

Note. ADHD=attention-deficit/hyperactivity disorder; CD=conduct disorder; OJJDP = Office of Juvenile Justice Delinquency Prevention; ODD=oppositional defiant disorder; PTSD=posttraumatic stress disorder.

dicting who will be at greatest risk from cyberbullying attacks. Children or teens with depressive or dysthymic conditions are more likely to turn to suicide to escape the ongoing shame and humiliation associated with this type of bullying. The home, school, and community boundaries blend into one inescapable reality for the child, who may become acutely depressed and act on these impulses by committing suicide.

There is little evidence to suggest that schizophrenia will be a major force as a risk condition in school violence. This may play a small role if there is an untreated, rare case of schizophrenia emerging in an early adolescent or late childhood. There are always risks associated with undiagnosed and severe mental disorders in children at school. Fortunately, the most severe conditions are usually diagnosed early and will have an early active treatment component involving a psychiatrist and a social worker. This may become an increasing problem as the student ages and enters a college or university.

Developmental Pathways to Conduct Disorder

Disruptive behavior disorders are characterized by high rates of noncompliant, hostile, and defiant behaviors, often including aggressiveness and hyperactivity.

DSM-IV-TR categorizes these behaviors under three broad headings: ADHD, ODD, and CD. Disturbances of conduct cover a wide range of behaviors manifesting somewhat differently at different ages in the same child across settings. A wide variety of treatment techniques have emerged in response to the diversity and prevalence of these problems.

Perhaps more than other problems of children and adolescents, disturbances of conduct are in the eye of the beholder. The acting-out behaviors of oppositional young people range from the irritating (yelling, whining, temper tantrums) to the frightening and terrorizing (physical destructiveness, interpersonal aggression, even murder). The literature on antisocial behavior is difficult to summarize due to conflicting definitions of the problem, often linked to the background of the scientists reporting the investigation. However, these heterogeneous behaviors appear to be elements of a complex syndrome. Accumulating epidemiological evidence suggests that a young child's annoying oppositional behaviors—for example, noncompliance and argumentativeness—are developmental precursors of more serious forms of antisocial behavior in adolescence. Although ODD and CD have been carefully defined in DSM-IV-TR, the treatment possibilities that have been researched have very rarely kept to these specific criteria, but instead focus more on children with the general characteristics already mentioned.

Empirical studies have shed light on the risk and protective factors for conduct disturbances in children (Kazdin 1995; Rutter et al. 1998). Risk factors include perinatal complications, poverty, large family size, overcrowding, poor housing, disadvantaged school settings, difficult temperament, parental history of criminal behavior or alcoholism, inadequate parenting (harsh, erratic, or inconsistent discipline), child maltreatment, insufficient restraint and supervision, unhappy marital relationship between parents (including domestic violence), dysfunctional family communication patterns with dominance of one family member, poor social skills, and poor school performance.

Risk prediction is a fraction, with "risk" factors being the numerator and "protective" factors being the denominator. Protective factors include high IQ; easy disposition; ability to get on well with parents, siblings, teachers, and peers; ability to do well in school; having friends; being competent in nonschool skill areas such as social problem-solving; and having a good relationship with at least one parent or other significant adult. Risk factors are cumulative (Rutter et al. 1981). Fergusson and Lynskey (1996) found that children with scores at the highest end of a 39-item social adversity index in middle childhood were 100 times more likely to experience multiple problems in adolescence.

Behavioral manifestations of conduct disturbance change over time and are powerfully influenced by a range of contextual factors, including characteristics of constitution, family, peer group, and even broader ecologies such as school and neighborhood. For example, parent–child relationships are inevitably distorted by early disturbances of conduct and in turn are aggravated by the parent's reaction (Coie and Dodge 1998; Hinshaw and Anderson 1996).

What other factors turn a child with CD into a violent delinquent or adult criminal? The link is well established (Frick and Jackson 1993), and studies suggest that something more than anomalous parenting may be involved. A number of other factors may play a part, including parental alcohol and substance misuse (Wills et al. 1994), maternal depression (Cummings and Davies 1994b), marital distress (Cummings and Davies 1994a), and parental antisocial behavior (Frick and Jackson 1993), as well as neighborhood risk (Attar et al. 1994). The critical proximal risk factor may be parental failure to monitor the child's activities. Aspects of the quality of parenting a child receives may mediate the effect of other risk factors. For example, marital distress may lead to conduct problems through frequent disagreement over child-rearing practices, absence of a parenting alliance, and interpersonal conflict in the presence of the child (Abidin and Brunner 1995; Jouriles et al. 1991).

The unfolding of childhood-onset disturbances of conduct is relatively well known. These problems manifest early, often in preschool, and continue throughout childhood and adolescence into adulthood (Hinshaw et al. 1993). The prognosis is more negative than in the case for a disturbance of conduct starting at a later stage of development (Loeber 1988; Speltz et al. 1999). The progression is from overt nondestructive problems to more destructive ones. Overt problems manifest earlier than do covert ones (such as lying and stealing), but new problems do not replace old ones; rather, they are added to the child's expanding repertoire of conduct disturbance (Frick and Jackson 1993; Lahey and Loeber 1994). ODD usually precedes CD by several years. Some ODD that leads to CD is associated with ADHD, but only children with more aggressive and delinquent behavior and family histories of CD are likely to progress from ODD to CD given an ADHD diagnosis (Biederman et al. 1996). Nevertheless, in long-term follow-up studies, hyperactive subjects were shown to have a fourfold elevation of juvenile arrest rates and a 20-fold elevation of adult arrest rates (Satterfield and Schell 1997). Among hyperactive children, the risk of becoming an adult offender is strongly associated with conduct problems in childhood and serious antisocial behavior in adolescence.

A good proportion of toddlers who go on to manifest conduct problems also show a disorganized attachment pattern in infancy (Lyons-Ruth 1996; Lyons-Ruth and Jacobovitz 1999). This attachment pattern is characterized by fear of the caregiver and a lack of coherent attachment strategy (Main and Solomon 1987), but the origin of this pattern is as yet poorly understood. While it is clear that children with conduct problems rarely, if ever, have secure attachment relationships with their primary caregivers, the precise nature of the association between attachment and disturbances of conduct is poorly understood. Thus, attachment difficulties may specifically create problems in affect regulation, mentalization, and social cognitive skills, which are known to be dysfunctional in groups with conduct problems.

A further key component of the etiology of disturbances of conduct is the deficit in social-cognitive skills that Ken Dodge and colleagues have repeatedly demonstrated in CD children (Coie and Dodge 1998; Crick and Dodge 1994; Mathys et al. 1999). Children with conduct problems have a variety of difficulties in processing social information: 1) encoding deficits (failing to pay attention to some social cues and being hypervigilant toward others), 2) attributional biases (frequently attributing hostile intentions where other children might not), 3) misinterpretation of social cues (in particular, misjudging affect in others), and 4) social problem–solving deficits (generating solutions for situations of conflict that are poor in quality and quantity). These children favor aggressive solutions to social problems (this may explain their frequent aggressive behavior) and do poorly at generating constructive solutions to conflicts. These disturbed patterns of social information processing are thought to be driven by knowledge structures, such as internal representations of social relationships and other schema representing social phenomena (Crick and Dodge 1994). Attitudes and beliefs that support coercion and overt aggression as acceptable, warranted, and effective forms of social behavior reflect a particularly pathognomonic knowledge structure found to characterize highly aggressive youth (Slaby and Guerra 1988; Vernberg et al. 1999).

Assessment of Risk Using Power Dynamics

Power dynamics, as previously mentioned (see Chapter 5, "Bullying Is a Process, Not a Person"), are unconscious group processes that become acted out in school through the social roles of bully, victim, and bystander (Twemlow et al. 1996) These roles exist as part of a school climate and are generally tied to a student. We have suggested (Twemlow and Sacco 2008) that these social roles apply to everybody and that they are fluid, meaning that everybody steps in and out of these roles. The problem, however, arises when someone, regardless of age and position, becomes locked into a role and blindly functions as a bully, victim, or bystander. Bullying has become, in many ways, a national obsession. States in the Unites States are rushing to pass laws to outlaw types of aggressive behavior, turning schools into courtrooms, with the principal forced into the role of judge in reported cases of bullying. Such laws have little hope of success.

There are two key strategies involved in the assessment of risk in school violence. The first is to work from the child outward to the school climate. A clinician may diagnose a client and document impulsivity. This child has to go to school and enter the social drama. The clinician can predict and plan supports for the child to enter one of the three roles in a power struggle (bully–victim–bystander). The impulsivity could be part of a bully dynamic, or it could be a reactive victim response based on a misread social cue. This is where collaboration between the outside clinician and the school becomes absolutely critical. The second approach works from the larger social context back to the child. Interventions that target prevention and peer social support can improve the entire school climate and can use natural leaders in the school to head off the negative power dynamics that can pull vulnerable children into unhealthy school behavior as either fixed bullies or fixed victims. School violence requires a bully and a victim, as well as a social context (bystanders) that allows, or even promotes, coercive behaviors by anyone in the school.

When the social roles of a power dynamic within a school become fixed, an individual is allowed to function as a bully or a victim without accountability, and the social climate becomes pathological. This bullying dynamic creates a group hunger for the display of violence through enactment of the bully–victim–bystander dynamic. Clinicians working outside of a school may not have the necessary information about this risk factor, so they need to take steps to connect to the child's school as part of the assessment and treatment planning process. Peers are the best source of early information about the formation of bullying and victimization patterns in a school. The community, in the end, is ultimately responsible for helping schools stay safe. When the community acts as a blaming bystander, a school is unsecured and may easily slip into a passive stance, tolerating increasing aggressive and violent behavior.

Table 7–3 outlines some of the characteristics of the social behavior in each of the roles of bully, victim, and bystander. There are clear patterns of social and physical behavior that can be seen played out with the school as the primary stage. A clinician can interview a child or caretaker to explore the client's view of the power structures at the school. This can be a very rich source of information. Some parents are acutely aware of the power dynamics and how they impact their child's social and emotional world. Understanding these power dynamics can create clear openings for services that can be used to prevent violence from erupting at school. We must remember that these power dynamics do not remain at school; they follow the child in virtual reality. The Internet is forcing the blended analysis of these power dynamics as they follow the child into his or own reality.

Bystanders run the risk of being pulled into bullying behaviors when the power dynamics in a school are not addressed. Being a bystander may feel safe for the youth and may bring a false sense of comfort to parents, but being a bystander can significantly increase the risk of children being pulled into bully or victim roles, especially when the bystander is also experiencing developmental changes, such as puberty.

TABLE 7–3.   Characteristic behavior patterns in social roles related to school violence

Bully	Pathological bystander	Victim
Impulsiveness	Either bully or victim (passive)	Submissiveness
Overt aggression	Situational problems	Anxiety
Early onset of trouble making	Developmental issues	Social withdrawal
Sadism	Substance abuse	Clinginess
Manipulation of weaker peers	"Groupthink"—passive involvement in trouble making	Hypersensitivity
		Sneakiness
		Social insecurity

Table 7–4 illustrates how bullying behavior might be expressed at various levels of development. In assessing a risk condition associated with a power role, it is critical to observe those behaviors that can fall into different categories of behaviors based on the child's developmental level. The clinician is challenged to assess these behaviors accurately. This is a critical link to prevention. Fighting is an easy behavior to respond to by law enforcement and school officials. It is a crime to assault someone, but much behavior called bullying is not that clear and falls between the category of a mental health problem and usual behavior.

Targeting Truancy and Other School Behavioral Problems

Truancy represents the gateway to disconnection from normal social peer interaction and the beginning of a pathway that can lead to substance abuse, delinquency, and teen pregnancy. Truancy prevention is an example of a larger-scale effort that by necessity involves parents, law enforcement officers, courts, and state agency case managers. Quick and creative responses to the earliest signs of truancy can have far-reaching benefit in preventing further delinquency. Again, these areas offer the clinician a chance to assess both the individual and his or her social context, including school, family, and community. One of the key symptoms of ODD is truancy, and it is frequently the first reason for a referral to a mental health clinician. Clinicians working in this area of mental health must be aware of the need to collaborate with home, school, and community in order to create the most effective interventions.

TABLE 7–4.　Developmental stages of bullying

Stage	How bullying can be expressed
Early childhood	Physical intimidation Verbal abuse Threats Stealing snacks or lunch Name calling
Middle school	Physical intimidation Beginning of inclusion/exclusion in social groups or cliques
High school	Social positioning Serious romance (often lovesickness) Self-destructiveness (eating disorders, self-cutting, substance abuse disorders)
College	"Failure to launch" (see Chapter 4, "Case Studies in School Violence") Identity diffusion (see Chapter 6, "Children Need to Feel Safe to Learn")

The clinician would be negligent to simply sit in his or her office and discuss any problem as an abstraction with the child and his or her family. While this isolated approach can be helpful in shifting family dynamics, stopping the truancy will be best accomplished by creating a tightly woven web of adult support and direction. The youth is signaling trouble by refusing to go to school. When that person is redirected back to school, there is an additional element of risk that exists for him or her to be victimized or join in the victimization of others. This point is where it becomes crucial for the clinician to function as part of a team who communicates and works together to respond to the situation. The clinician is charged with discovering the mechanics of the problem by exploring the roots of the imbalances within the home, school, and community.

Garbarino (1996) explained school violence as the result of a child being overwhelmed with stress; he likened this state to a bathtub filled to the brim and then overflowing at the slightest addition of water. This explanatory image of how children process stress and anxiety highlights the cumulative impact of stress in a system and the fact that children can only take so much before they begin to act out their frustration at school. The MHP needs to understand where the imbalances in the systems are and begin to collaborate in an effort to drain pressure, build supports, and monitor overall levels of stress. Table 7–5 is a summary of several quite different ways that school violence can start.

TABLE 7–5.   Common problems leading to a school violence referral

Predatory behavior in the home, school, or community

Learning disabilities, developmental delays, or pervasive developmental disorders

Autism spectrum disorders

"Problem of excellence" (see Chapter 1, "School Violence: Range and Complexity of the Problem")

Truancy

Parent-directed aggression

Teenage pregnancy

Gender and Risk

Assessing vulnerabilities in youth is a central part of preventing school violence. The outward expression of aggression is seen in males, with virtually all school shooters being male. Symbolic killers such as serial murderers are predominantly male. Conduct disturbances are strong factors in pushing boys away from direct self-harm and toward trouble. Klomek et al. (2009) studied the relationship between bullying and later suicidal behaviors in males and females. They found that females had a greater vulnerability to the impact of bullying than males when CD was controlled for; females tended to be at higher risk for suicide, while males tended to have this risk expressed as CD.

Kim et al. (2010) studied the differences in how boys and girls expressed overt aggression. Boys demonstrated higher levels of physical and verbal aggression than girls. McAndrews (2009), reviewing the literature on sex and cultural differences in physical aggression from an evolutionary imperative, found that males tended to be more aggressive.

Epstein and Spirito (2010) found that certain social factors wiped out gender differences in suicidality. Three factors were significant for both boys and girls: sex before age 13 years, injection drug use, and being forced to have sex. Smoking was associated with making suicidal plans in girls, and fighting was a risk factor for both girls and boys. Boys are aggressive earlier, but girls catch up with relational aggression and increased vulnerability to suicidal thinking and gesturing. De Boo (2010) described the important roles of temperament and problem-solving styles in determining the direction of aggression. Early vulnerability to mood disturbances in girls is also theorized as explaining why girls tend to have an inward direction of aggression rather than CD. Langhinrichsen-Rohling et al. (2009), in a comprehensive research review of suicide attempts, concluded that the traditional practice of using self-report of suicidal gestures might miss the male adolescent who makes fewer gestures but takes action more frequently than females. De Munck et al. (2009), in a study in Belgium, found that females clearly made more attempts at suicide. Males, as has been shown in other studies, have higher rates of self-injury from their suicidal behaviors. A link is clearly suggested between impulsivity and increased lethality for boys, while girls are likely to direct their aggression inward and display more behaviors and communication related to suicide.

As is the case in most predictions in violence, simply saying that girls are more at risk for suicide than boys and that boys will be aggressive outwardly is a dangerous oversimplification. Careful study of vulnerability requires assessing the social context and past history to determine risk variables in both boys and girls. Risk assessment is a highly individualized process with only broad consistency regarding gender.

Social Risk Conditions for Bullying at School

There are certain social risk conditions that need to be considered in conceptualizing a plan of intervention for school violence. These social conditions represent the typical qualities that attract bullies to victims, invite bullies to spread aggression and shame, and impact bystanders in ways that distract them from experiencing a safe and creative learning environment (see Table 7–6). These social conditions exist within every school at all levels from kindergarten to college. Students with certain psychological qualities or physical appearances will have an increased chance of being victimized within certain schools. Clinicians need to become aware of how these conditions might play out in the life of any one child at school.

Case Example: Leon, A Gay Boy Without School or Family Support

Leon was a 12-year-old African American male referred for psychological testing by his therapist, who was concerned that he was being bullied at school. The therapist was working with the family including the child and mother. Upon presentation, the child demonstrated strikingly effeminate behaviors, immediately preferring to brush a doll's hair in the interview room rather than playing with any of the more traditionally male toys. His mother was not open to discussing her son's gender presentation. There were also learning issues that were evaluated, and Leon was diagnosed with a nonverbal language disability.

In this case, Leon's gender presentation clashed with his family's strong religious affiliation. Furthermore, his school's student population was primarily

TABLE 7–6.　Social risk conditions for bullying at school

Victim

    Seen as gay

    New arrival

    Immigrant

    "Different" appearance

    Obese

    Shy

    Romantic rival of a popular girl or boy

    Physically disabled

Bully

    Tightly knit "popular" cliques

    Athletic acclaim

    Criminal involvement

    Early and persistent aggression

    Frequent change of schools and housing

Bystander

    Participation in cyberbullying

    Echoing the bully

    Mocking audience

    Participation in exclusion rituals online and at school

African American children who were particularly cruel in taunting Leon. The therapist was able to work with Leon's mother, helping her to see the potential risks to her son if she did not participate in a solution to the almost daily bullying Leon experienced. The mother took a first step by allowing Leon to sing in an all-female choir at the church. Eventually, the therapist worked with the school to have a touring play presented that stressed the value of tolerance and of individual differences. This was followed up by a program that produced posters supporting the message, encouraging students to become friends and not to use violence. Leon was referred for therapeutic mentoring that connected him to several area choirs, and he was able to enroll for voice lessons at the local community college. Some cultures are more tolerant of gay, lesbian, and transgender issues than others, but children will always find something to pick on, no matter who the target may be.

Protective Factors

It is the interplay of risk and protective factors that leads to violence in any setting. Besides individual protective factors, community protective factors can be found in all three key areas of a child's life: home, school, and community. The protection may be delivered through formal networks such as providers of behavioral health care, child welfare, or juvenile justice; through natural supports such as community activities, faith-based groups, and extended families; or through a blend of natural and formal networks.

The clinical challenge is to create as wide a perspective on a child's life as possible and develop interventions that pull from a diverse set of resources. School violence solutions are not simple, and there is a very powerful temptation to oversimplify the problem and the fix. This is particularly evident in bullying prevention, where simple solutions abound and programs promise solutions and offer quick answers to very complex problems. Collaboration and cooperation among the school, home, and community are essential.

We strongly advise clinicians to be aware of the variety and availability of resources in their communities and to make efforts to learn the eligibility requirements for them. (We elaborate on the role of the clinician in opening resource doors in Chapter 9, "Role of Medical Leadership in Unlocking Resources to Address School Violence.") Every school exists within the social context of a community. This community will offer a variety of different problems and resources to solve them. In the United States, individual states work with the federal government to support communities through a variety of programs. It is important to consider the eligibility requirements for these programs. For example, the special education laws offer children from 2½ to 22 years of age a wide spectrum of support services. States offer Women, Infants, and Children (WIC) nutrition program benefits and Head Start based on income, and day care vouchers can be accessed for families based on need. Clinicians need to have a general understanding of who qualifies for each program so that they can make effective recommendations and referrals.

Psychotherapy and substance abuse treatment services are also protective factors. They offer the child and family a relationship that can be used to solve problems that, if left unattended, can lead to aggression that will bleed into the school environment. Connecting a child in need to a regular behavioral health plan is often the role of protective service case managers who work with the state under court supervision. The delinquent and status offenses have for the most part been separated, with delinquency having its own state case managers who work with the criminal and not the family side of the juvenile court. These state case managers are always on the lookout for services that will help children control their aggression and be more successful at school. MHPs should be equally eager to connect with ongoing service streams for the referred child and family involved in a school violence problem. There is added benefit and economic efficiency in collaboration among professions in the battle against school violence.

KEY CLINICAL CONCEPTS

- At-risk children need to be monitored, because their life at school is a primary place where they will communicate their pain and trauma.

- Risk has two poles: bully, or outward expression of aggression, and victim, or inward expression of aggression.

- There are many portals of entry in the landscape of a school violence problem.

- Bullies often are diagnosed with CD, ODD, ADHD, or childhood bipolar disorder. Victims are more likely to be depressed, withdrawn, and anxious.

- School violence problems can be conceptualized from a number of perspectives, including the OJJDP pathways to delinquency (overt/aggressive, authority conflict, and covert/sneaky); DSM-IV-TR classifications; and social risk conditions such as homelessness, foster care placement, and domestic violence.

- School violence can be understood using traditional psychiatric diagnosis that will be common in many cases.

- School violence can occur at older grades, as Virginia Tech illustrates so painfully.

- The power dynamics of the bully–victim–bystander triangle need to be factored into any risk assessment. Fixed roles as a bully or victim can lead to an extreme buildup of pressure, with lethal consequences.

- Bystanders are at risk of being pulled into school violence problems.

- MHPs need to be active and unafraid of reaching into the community to intervene directly in school violence problems.

- Protective factors need to be calculated and taken into account in school violence interventions.

- MHPs need to collaborate with and be active members of teams developed to address school violence problems.

References

Abidin RR, Brunner JF: Development of a Parenting Alliance Inventory. J Clin Child Psychol 24:31–40, 1995

American Psychiatric Association: Diagnostic and Statistical Manual of Mental Disorders, 4th Edition, Text Revision. Washington, DC, American Psychiatric Association, 2000

Attar BK, Guerra NG, Tolan PH: Neighborhood disadvantage, stressful life events, and adjustment in urban elementary school children. J Clin Child Psychol 23:391–400, 1994

Biederman J, Faraone SV, Milberger S, et al: Is childhood oppositional defiant disorder a precursor to adolescent conduct disorder? Findings from a four-year follow-up study of children with ADHD. J Am Acad Child Adolesc Psychiatry 35:1193–1204, 1996

Books S (ed): Invisible Children in the Society and Its Schools, 3rd Edition. Hillsdale, NJ, Lawrence Erlbaum, 2007

BostonChannel: Mother says bullies drove her son to suicide. 2010. Available at: http://www.thebostonchannel.com/news/19141470/detail.html. Accessed December 6, 2010.

Celizic M: Her teen committed suicide over "sexting." Today Parenting, March 6, 2009. Available at: http://today.msnbc.msn.com/id/29546030. Accessed December 6, 2010.

Coie JD, Dodge KA: Aggression and antisocial behavior, in Social, Emotional, and Personality Development, Vol 3, Handbook of Child Psychology, 5th Edition. Edited by Damon W, Eisenberg N. New York, Wiley, 1998, pp 779–862

Crick NR, Dodge KA: A review and reformulation of social information-processing mechanisms in children's social adjustment. Psychol Bull 115:74–101, 1994

Cummings EM, Davies PT: Children and Marital Conflict: The Impact of Family Dispute and Resolution. New York, Guilford, 1994a

Cummings EM, Davies PT: Maternal depression and child development. J Child Psychol Psychiatry 35:73–112, 1994b

De Boo GM: Pre-adolescent gender differences in associations between temperament, coping, and mood. Clin Psychol Psychotherapy 17:313–320, 2010

De Munck S, Portzky G, Van Heeringen K: Epidemiological trends in attempted suicide in adolescents and young adults between 1996 and 2004. Crisis 30:115–119, 2009

DeRosier ME, Cillessen AH, Cole JD, et al: Group social context and children's aggressive behavior. Child Dev 65:1068–1079, 1994

Epstein J, Spirito A: Gender-specific risk factors for suicidality among high school students. Arch Suicide Res 14:193–205, 2010

Fergusson DM, Lynskey MT: Adolescent resiliency to family adversity. J Child Psychol Psychiatry 37:281–292, 1996

Frick PJ, Jackson YK: Family functioning and childhood antisocial behavior: yet another reinterpretation. J Clin Child Psychol 22:410–419, 1993

Garbarino J: Lost Boys: Why Our Sons Turn Violent and How We Can Save Them. New York, Free Press, 1996

Hinshaw SP, Anderson CA: Conduct and oppositional defiant disorders, in Child Psychopathology. Edited by Mash EJ, Barkley RA. New York, Guilford, 1996, pp 113–149

Hinshaw SP, Lahey BB, Hart EL: Issues of taxonomy and comorbidity in the development of conduct disorder. Dev Psychopathol 5:31–49, 1993

Inbar M: "Sexting" bullying cited in teen's suicide. Today Parenting, December 2, 2009. Available at: http://today.msnbc.msn.com/id/34236377. Accessed December 6, 2010.

Jouriles EN, Murphy CM, Farris AM, et al: Marital adjustment, parental disagreements about childrearing, and behavior problems in boys: increasing the specificity of the marital assessment. Child Dev 62:1424–1433, 1991

Kazdin AE: Conduct Disorder in Childhood and Adolescence, 2nd Edition. Thousand Oaks, CA, Sage, 1995

Kazdin AE: Psychotherapy for children and adolescents. Annu Rev Psychol 54:253–276, 2003

Kim S, Kamphaus RW, Orpinas P, et al: Changes in the manifestation of overt aggression during early adolescents: gender and ethnicity. Sch Psychol Int 319:95–111, 2010

Klomek AB, Sourander A, Niemela S, et al: Childhood bullying behavior as a risk for suicide attempts and completed suicides: a population-based birth cohort study. J Am Acad Child Psychiatry 48:254–261, 2009

Lahey BB, Loeber R: Framework for a developmental model of oppositional defiant disorder and conduct disorder, in Disruptive Behavior Disorders in Childhood. Edited by Routh DK. New York, Plenum, 1994, pp 139–180

Langhinrichsen-Rohling J, Friend J, Powell A: Adolescent suicide, gender, and culture: a rate and risk factor analysis. Aggress Violent Behav 14:402–414, 2009

Loeber R: Natural histories of conduct problems, delinquency, and associated substance use: evidence for developmental progressions, in Advances in Clinical Child Psychology, Vol 11. Edited by Lahey BB, Kazdin AE. New York, Plenum, 1988, pp 73–124

Lohr D: Did Tyler Clementi reach out for help before suicide? AolNews, September 30, 2010. Available at: http://www.aolnews.com/nation/article/did-tyler-clementi-reach-out-for-help-before-suicide/19655785. Accessed December 6, 2010.

Lyons-Ruth K: Attachment relationships among children with aggressive behavior problems: the role of disorganized early attachment patterns. J Consult Clin Psychol 64:64–73, 1996

Lyons-Ruth K, Jacobovitz D: Attachment disorganization: unresolved loss, relational violence and lapses in behavioral and attentional strategies, in Handbook of Attachment: Theory, Research, and Clinical Applications. Edited by Cassidy J, Shaver PR. New York, Guilford, 1999, pp 520–554

Main M, Solomon J: Discovery of an insecure disorganized/disoriented attachment pattern: procedures, findings, and implications for the classification of behavior, in Affective Development in Infancy. Edited by Yogman M, Brazelton TB. Norwood, NJ, Ablex, 1987, pp 95–124

Mathys W, Cuperus JM, Van Engeland H: Deficient social problem-solving in boys with ODD/CD with ADHD and both disorders. J Am Acad Child Adolesc Psychiatry 38:311–321, 1999

McAndrews FT: The interacting roles of testosterone and challenges to status in human male aggression. Aggress Violent Behav 14:330–335, 2009

Oliver K: Phoebe Prince "suicide by bullying": teen's death angers town asking why bullies roam the halls. CBS News, February 5, 2010. Available at: http://www.cbsnews.com/8301-504083_162-6173960-504083.html?tag=mncol;lst;10. Accessed December 5, 2010.

Park JM, Metraux S, Brodbar G, et al: Child welfare involvement among children in homeless families. Child Welfare 83:423–436, 2004

Patchin J, Hinduja S: Cyberbullycide: suicidal ideation and online aggression among adolescents. Paper presented at the annual meeting of the American Society of Criminology, St. Louis, MO, November 12, 2008

Polakow V: Homeless children and their families: the discards of the post-welfare era, in Invisible Children in the Society and Its Schools, 2nd Edition. Edited by Books S. Mahwah, NJ, Lawrence Erlbaum, 2003, pp 89–110

Rutter M, Tizard J, Whitmore K (eds): Education, Health and Behavior. New York, Krieger, 1981

Rutter M, Giller H, Hagell A: Antisocial Behaviour by Young People. Cambridge, UK, Cambridge University Press, 1998

Satterfield JH, Schell A: A prospective study of hyperactive boys with conduct problems and normal boys: adolescence and adult criminality. J Am Academy Child Adolesc Psychiatry 36:1726–1735, 1997

Simon R, Tardiff K (eds): Textbook of Violence Assessment and Management. Washington, DC, American Psychiatric Publishing, 2008

Slaby RG, Guerra NG: Cognitive mediators of aggression in adolescent offenders, I: assessment. Dev Psychol 24:580–588, 1988

Speltz ML, McClellan J, DeKlyen M, et al: Preschool boys with oppositional defiant disorder: clinical presentation and diagnostic change. J Am Acad Child Adolesc Psychiatry 38:838–845, 1999

Thornberry TP, Huizinga D, Loeber R: The causes and correlates studies: findings and policy implications. Juvenile Justice IX (1), September 2004. Available at: http://www.ncjrs.gov/html/ojjdp/203555/jj2.html. Accessed March 20, 2011.

Twemlow SW, Sacco F: Why School Antibullying Programs Don't Work. New York, Jason Aronson, 2008

Twemlow SW, Sacco F, Williams P: A clinical and interactionist perspective on the bully-victim-bystander relationship. Bull Menninger Clin 60:296–313, 1996

Vernberg EM, Jacobs AK, Hershberger SL: Peer victimization and attitudes about violence in early adolescence. J Clin Child Psychol 28:386–395, 1999

Wills TA, Schreibman D, Benson G, et al: Impact of parental substance use on adolescents: a test of mediational model. J Pediatr Psychol 19:537–555, 1994

Yu M, LaVesser PD, Osborne VA, et al: A comparison study of psychiatric and behavior disorders and cognitive ability among homeless and housed children. Community Ment Health J 44:1–10, 2008

8

Activating Community Resources Through Therapeutic Mentoring

WHEN using a multidimensional assessment and treatment planning approach to school violence, there must be a mechanism for reaching out into the community and activating resources that can be linked to youth who are in need. Simply stating that a young person would benefit from an after-school activity can easily become an empty element in a treatment plan recommendation. Many of the children who are disconnected from normal activities in the community will present increasing difficulties at school. The use of therapeutic mentoring and psychotherapy is an emerging new practice that recognizes the intimate and interconnected relationships between a child's home, school, and community. When a child's world is out of balance in any of these areas, then school is the likely stage for the enactment of the imbalance. The approach described in this chapter is based largely on our own extensive observations in a community mental health center in Massachusetts. The center is actually developing this program as part of a statewide remedy to a federal lawsuit, and it offers the opportunity to explore new approaches to solving school violence problems.

Mentoring—a broad term, to say the least—is one such new approach. Traditionally, this term refers to the use of an older, more experienced role model to engage a youth in a series of activities. The prototype of this would be the Big Brothers–Big Sisters program, in which young people who need a role model are assigned to an interested adult. Ideally, participants develop an unstructured long-term relationship that mimics that of a visiting older sibling or parent. Mentoring is also frequently used by schools and community programs, where it is referred to as "peer mentoring." Wyatt (2009), in a literature review, emphasized the role of peer mentoring in encouraging academic achievement in African American students. This approach applies the empowerment theory model to aggressive African American adolescents. Kamps et al. (1994) reported that mentoring was useful in improving academic skills; Thomson and Zand (2010) researched the quality of mentoring relationships, finding a strong relationship between positive mentoring experiences and most other relationship-based outcomes, such as friendships and relationship with adults. Rhodes et al. (2005), in a study of almost 1,000 children applying for a Big Brothers–Big Sisters mentoring relationship, reported that mentoring was a significant factor in reducing substance abuse, mainly when it included a long-term mentor commitment *and* parental involvement. Short-term bursts of mentoring without parental involvement had no impact on later substance abuse. In a study in Uganda and South Africa, several hundred children orphaned by AIDS were compared with a nonorphaned control group (Onuoha et al. 2009). Not surprisingly, the AIDS-orphaned children had much poorer mental health and more negative outcomes than the control group. There were, however, significantly improved outcomes in those children who had been mentored. In this extreme sample, the power of mentoring to help with unimaginable trauma is crucial.

Mentoring is also commonly used by adults in order to learn professional roles, especially in teaching. Riley (2009) reported on an Australian initiative that uses mentoring for all school leadership positions. Data from this report indicated that the health of both mentors and mentees improved. Schools often develop programs in their guidance departments that will involve peers, specifically in mediation. This adult-supervised use of students in mediation harnesses the power of peer influences in conflict resolution and can offer a very valuable protective resource for a vulnerable child at school. Adult mentors are often invited into schools to offer vulnerable or high-risk youth the opportunity to become involved with an adult role model during school activities. These adult mentors are often recruited to come into the school as a way to assist in helping students with reading and learning difficulties, social problems, or coaching of recreational sports activities.

Peer mentors are often selected by teachers or school administrators to become involved with younger students and to offer them assistance in education, recreation, and social skills modeling. Often, these peer mentors can be used as mediators with their own age groups, offering an alternative to violence for older students who become embroiled in ongoing conflicts within the school. These programs are based at the school and often are organized and supervised by school personnel, social work departments in schools, or guidance counselors who create positive ways for students to help each other at school. In this type of mentoring program, there must be a high level of screening on the part of the school to ensure that the mentors involved are not predators or unsuitable role models. Schools maintain the responsibility for ensuring that the adult mentors are involved in healthy and safe ways with the students. A number of adult mentors can be recruited using the Junior Achievement model of targeting retired businesspeople to work with students to teach them business skills. In Springfield, Massachusetts, Massachusetts Mutual life Insurance Company ran a program where executives would read to elementary school students and become learning and life mentors for the year. These programs have proved very effective when they are well-run and -supervised.

A large urban high school on the East Coast had a peer mediation and mentoring program that was run by the school counselor. Twelve students were selected and trained by the school counselor, who closely supervised and monitored all aspects of the program. Most of the conflicts mediated involved distortions of communication around what someone had said about someone else. Romantic feuds often turned into fights at school, and a pattern of bullying was present, also leading frequently to violence. These stemmed from ongoing targeting of certain physically and mentally disabled students. The peer mentoring program was born out of the ideas presented by the 12 original students. This program relied heavily on early detection of brewing conflicts. The school counselor received the first report of a problem. The student team would assemble and design an approach to get more information and would then try to set up face-to-face mediation of conflicts. As part of the program, a mentoring program was designed to pair up football players with disabled students who became the target of bullying. This program ran for 3 years and greatly reduced the eruptions of violence at the school.

Mental health professionals (MHPs) may become involved in assisting a school to develop such a program and may be helpful in offering training suggestions, supervision, screening, and peer mentor supports. This is a supportive role that could assist in a multidimensional treatment plan designed to assist a student who is alienated from his peer groups and frequently in conflict at school.

This program also illustrates implementation of a peer initiative that uses both mediation and a mentoring process. The power of these peer mentoring programs may lie in their capacity to mitigate the destructive impact of peer rejection, especially in high-risk African American students. Miller-Johnson et al. (1999) studied a dozen elementary schools, focusing on the long-term follow-up of over 300 children. What they discovered was a strong correlation between peer rejection and aggression and serious delinquency. The fuel for school aggression is shame; peer rejection can provide a dangerous source of unending shame at school and on the Internet.

There are many excellent program examples that illustrate the power and value of mentoring programs within schools that are well-designed and -supervised. If not properly supervised, school-based programs have a tendency to degenerate into distracting activities for oppositional students, who will create "conflicts" in order to avoid school participation. If the programs are not well-designed and -supervised, they can create as many problems for the school as they solve. Once again, the role of the MHP working within the school is essential in ensuring that this type of mentoring program is well run. MHPs who work within schools are advised to look for opportunities to develop programs that tap into this resource of peer-to-peer interaction. In researching bullying programs, we learned that by fourth or fifth grade, bullying prevention requires the involvement of peers organized into programs that can assist in reducing bullying by increasing tolerance and friendship within the school. We have no doubt that the power of peer influence is needed most in prevention and can also be used in each intervention of school violence within the school.

Therapeutic mentoring is a highly specialized service that can become part of a clinical treatment plan in certain types of models using Medicaid. The description of this service offers a glimpse into the future of working with Medicaid children. This description is meant to outline some possible systems of care or models for states to consider in funding Medicaid services for children. The approach outlined in this chapter is being piloted in Massachusetts and other states involved in federal lawsuits over Early Periodic Screening, Diagnosis, and Treatment (EPSDT) services to Medicaid-eligible children. In the case of *Rosie D. v. Romney* (2006), a group of families successfully challenged the Massachusetts state Medicaid program under the EPSDT standard. Perkins (2009) of the National Law Center has offered an overview of other federal EPSDT cases brought against state Medicaid programs for failing to provide the range of services that would allow children with emotional disturbances to remain at home and participate in community schools. Using therapeutic mentoring to provide Medicaid-funded community supports for people under the age of 21 is a powerful way to create a team around serious school and community violence problems. This model is likely to become available in the near future in many states.

This community-based wraparound model has increasingly been used in states that are reassessing how child welfare approaches children with serious emotional disturbances. Programs have included multitiered combinations of services such as in-home therapy, in-home behavior management for autism spectrum disorders, and therapeutic mentoring. High-risk children have the most difficulty in adjusting to community schools. When a family is struggling to manage a high-risk child in the community, the school is a critical element in maintaining stability in the community. If a child cannot function within special or regular educational settings, there is a reduced likelihood that he or she will be able to remain at home as opposed to being forced into residential placement.

Massachusetts is one of seven states that have challenged Medicaid to include services such as therapeutic mentoring within its reimbursement system. This is a new tool for MHPs to use in developing multidimensional treatment plans and a concrete way to activate community resources in the care of a high-risk child functioning in the community. Many states may not have this capacity, but there is a clear trend nationally for Medicaid to invest in services such as these to reduce higher costs that often result from a lack of support in the community, home, and school. Both the state and the families win. The use of a therapeutic mentor in this context is similar to a physician's use of a physical therapist. The medical practitioner will order the involvement of the physical therapist, will work closely with the therapist in establishing goals, and will then monitor and evaluate progress. A therapeutic mentor uses the same structure with a psychotherapist who is working as part of a larger care planning team.

The therapeutic mentor's job is to develop a relationship with the youth and assist in building the social skills that will support the child's ability to function properly in the community, especially at school. Sacco et al. (2007) have offered a cost-containment model of community-based psychotherapy in multiple-problem Medicaid families. When these services are not reimbursable through Medicaid, therapeutic mentoring returns to an isolated child welfare service. This application of therapeutic mentoring is useful but will not become as powerful a tool in the overall treatment planning if it is not closely supervised and directed by an MHP with a wider scope of involvement in the families coping with a high-risk child trying to function in a community school.

In the wraparound process, therapeutic mentoring can become a Medicaid-eligible service if it is structured as part of a care plan overseen and monitored by a senior MHP who directs the therapeutic mentoring activities in a way that targets specific symptoms identified as interfering with a child's school performance. This approach uses Medicaid funds and follows a strict model of medical necessity. Therapeutic mentoring is especially useful in treating problems with school violence, in which the therapeutic mentoring is used as a way of creating alternative activities and strategies designed to reduce aggression and promote more prosocial activities in peer groups and with authorities at school. Therapeutic mentoring may also take the form of a social service intervention funded through community monies, which does not require medical diagnosis and treatment planning but does involve many of the same components of social skills building.

Therapeutic Mentoring as an Adjunct to Therapy

Therapeutic mentoring refers to the coaching and concrete teaching of social skills that result in a child's participating in an activity within the community, school, after-school program, or any other suitable adult-supervised program. All therapeutic mentoring activities are time limited and subject to a managed care authorization process. The mentoring is designed to be a teaching tool that works in concert with therapy; it is not intended to be limited to the activity itself. The final step in the mentoring process is creating a sustainable connection between the youth and a community activity. In other words, therapeutic mentoring contact is designed to help create the skills necessary for the youth to participate in an activity within the community. All activities performed by a therapeutic mentor have as their goal both the teaching of a specific set of skills needed to join in community activities and the discovery of natural supports within the family and community for the child.

It is important to understand that therapeutic mentoring is a critical service delivered under the careful supervision of an MHP and requiring regular communication with the referring MHP. Therapeutic mentoring is part of a wraparound care process, or the community alternative to substitute milieu treatment facilities. The services typically evolve from what has become known as a clinical hub or a service delivery center, such as an outpatient clinic, an in-home therapy service, or an intensive care coordination team. These services are part of a larger treatment plan that is already attempting to target specific symptoms that impact the child's school performance socially and academically.

The heart and soul of the therapeutic mentoring intervention is regular contact between the treating MHP and the therapeutic mentor. The mentor's involvement might span 90–180 days, with weekly reports to the MHP. It is this close working relationship between the MHP and the therapeutic mentor that makes this approach such a powerful tool for activating community involvement in preventing and intervening in school violence problems. This intervention strategy moves community involvement from a sociological consideration to a specific therapeutic intervention that can be applied to school violence problems through a wraparound service delivery process that stresses outcomes. The primary outcome is a life-touching event, such as successful and peaceful days at school and increased achievement. Table 8–1 outlines the differences between a mentor and a therapist. Effective interventions require supervision that keeps these roles separate. The mentor is a social skills teacher; the therapist is actively engaging the child and family in therapy.

Therapeutic mentoring involves the use of several psychological processes that are critical in establishing stability in the community and reducing aggres-

TABLE 8–1.   Comparison of psychotherapist and therapeutic mentor roles

Psychotherapist	Therapeutic mentor
Develops therapy goal for mentor	Teaches client skills needed to reach therapy goal
Works directly with client, family, and school	Works with client in the home and community to practice skills
Uses therapeutic relationship to explore issues, memories, trauma, relationships	Uses mentoring relationship to model social skills in the community
Refers client for evaluations, medications, and other services	Provides regular feedback to psychotherapist on client's social skills development
Recommends programs and activities	Links client to activities in community

sion in the school environment. Fundamentally, mentoring creates a relationship that models secure attachment. When a child experiences difficulties at school, it is usually expressed through displays of aggression or school disruption. Mentoring redirects this misplaced energy by engaging the child in a relationship that creates a secure attachment, resulting in the child's learning skills that can increase mentalization. The mentor becomes a real attachment entity that can significantly contribute to containing aggression at home and school. When children have trusted guides through the many barriers to successful participation in community activities, they will be able to model themselves and practice the skills necessary to achieve more self-control and, ultimately, a balanced life. When a child's life is balanced, it is less likely that there will be eruptions of school violence.

Case Example: Louis, an Adopted Child Showing Aggression

Louis was a 4-year-old child who had recently been adopted by a young couple frustrated by years of trying to conceive a biological child. Louis was adopted when he was 3½ years old after living in a preadoptive home for 16 months. Louis's behavior at the preschool and at home began to show signs of early aggression. Louis was referred for psychotherapy and had received a child psychiatric evaluation. The treatment and evaluation indicated that Louis had attention-deficit/hyperactivity disorder (ADHD), and he was placed on Adderall XR. He was referred for weekly psychotherapy with a child therapist, who began to explore various trauma themes that had emerged over the course of the therapy. Louis frequently would engage in vigorous play that focused on feelings of separation, fear, and an aggressive response to any imagined threat.

This therapy continued for several months; however, Louis was unable to continue in early childhood education because the frequent calls (with complaints) from the teachers in the early childhood program had placed his mother at risk of losing her job. The removal of this option for Louis placed a strain on his adoptive parents.

Louis's therapist referred him for therapeutic mentoring with the specific goal of ending his aggressive behaviors both in school and at home. The therapeutic mentor began by developing a set of signals to help Louis stop an undesirable behavior on the spot. These social skills were tailored to his developmental age, and a program was instituted in which Louis began to learn how to make friends. The therapeutic mentor consulted weekly with the therapist to work on barriers Louis faced in accompanying the mentor into the community to begin practicing his skills. Eventually, Louis began to respond to the simple hand signals that the therapist taught his parents to use. A new family daycare provider was also included in the signal plan and was cooperative with both the mentor and the therapist in linking Louis's behavior at school with his rewards and behavior at home. Eventually, the mentor worked specifically with Louis on how to make friends, and consulted with the therapist on ways to encourage Louis to invite friends from his new school or family members to have playdates at home. Louis's aggression was clearly an indication of his anxiety; this was identified by the child psychiatrist, who then intervened to gradually taper and discontinue the stimulants and eventually all psychiatric medication.

This therapeutic mentoring intervention illustrates how a mentor focused specifically on teaching and modeling social skills practiced in the community as well as at school for a young child. The younger the child, the briefer and more effective the mentorship process needs to be. The therapist was regularly informed, and all MHPs were working toward decreasing the aggression Louis exhibited when he was at home and school. The therapeutic mentor remained focused on teaching concrete skills that were supported by the therapist, who worked with the family in school to develop ways to help Louis feel more secure and to fear separation less.

The second psychological process that is being used in the therapeutic mentoring intervention is the concrete application of the natural leader (see Chapter 5, "Bullying Is a Process, Not a Person"). Therapeutic mentors are not highly trained MHPs who take an abstract and clinical approach. The therapeutic mentor is more of a natural leader who is skilled at maneuvering around children: at school, in their homes, or in a community setting. These mentors are able to use natural leadership as a way to hook children into the healthy process of participating in high-interest activities and developing social skills by practicing them in real community settings. The MHP consults with the mentor and offers weekly dialogue to ensure that the mentor is creating the opportunities that the therapist identifies in a treatment objective as being in the child's best interest. The therapeutic mentor is typically supervised by another independent MHP responsible for the overall supervision of the mentoring activities, not for the overall therapy. The natural leader is not a global role that is fueled by a well-meaning individual from the community who randomly becomes involved with the youth and acts as a role model. The therapeutic mentor is part of a therapeutic team supervised independently and working collaboratively within a therapy treatment plan to reach certain goals.

Therapeutic Mentoring Activities

Therapeutic mentors provide training and education in positive alternative strategies or social skills needed to be able to cope with the stressors involved in participating in structured community activities, building peer relationships, and developing other skills needed to participate in community activities. Alternative strategies may involve approaches to control aggression and increase self-control. This involves practicing skills, such as waiting in line, playing as part of a team, developing tolerance for peer teasing, and coping with conflicts. These skills are strengthened during the therapeutic mentor's time with the child using real-life experiences that can be practiced in real time rather than in the abstract world of the structured therapeutic hour. The therapeutic mentor may have from 4 to 6 hours a week to assist in helping a child explore and practice new ways of being with peers and joining in on activities that previously have been impossible. Often children cannot participate in activities due to an eruption of symptoms such a temper tantrums, aggressive outbursts, withdrawal, or highly anxious and phobic behaviors.

Case Example: Tania, a Depressed and Socially Vulnerable Student

Tania was an 11-year-old African American girl living in a family with four brothers and two sisters. She was the second youngest in her family. There were three uninvolved fathers, two of whom were incarcerated and one who had no contact with the family. Tania's mother suffered from a number of medical conditions, including diabetes and high blood pressure. She was very religious and tried hard to provide for her children.

Tania's brothers were completely uninvolved with her daily life. Two of her brothers had already moved out and were not available to her, while her two other brothers had significant histories of delinquency and were frequently in and out of the home. Her sisters were jealous of the amount of time that Tania's mother spent with her. Tania frequently baby-sat for her younger sister and spent most of her time after school assisting at home with household duties.

Tania had become a victim of bullying at school. The kids at school would pick on her because of her unkempt appearance and her inability to keep up socially with them, especially in using the Internet or other mobile devices. After being taunted on a daily basis, she eventually responded by becoming depressed. The state protective services had intervened on a number of occasions throughout Tania's life, and she was eventually referred for supportive psychotherapy and appropriate medication. Her depression worsened, and she was falling behind academically to the point where a referral was made for special education. While Tania's mother was her legal guardian, this family was an open case with a child protective service agency.

Despite several years of psychotherapy, Tania became increasingly more depressed. At one point, she even failed to come home and was thought to have been kidnapped. She was found that evening by the police, wandering by herself in the park. This incident reignited the concern of the state agency, which again referred Tania for family psychotherapy. During the initial phases of treatment, the therapist referred Tania for therapeutic mentoring. The mentor began by meeting with Tania and her mother and arranging for a series of activities in the community to see if there was some way to increase Tania's exposure to other young people in a productive fashion.

The mentor arranged a series of exploratory activities with Tania, beginning at the local Boys and Girls Club. During this exploration, Tania displayed an unusual aptitude for shooting baskets. She was able to dribble and was quite good at free throws. The mentor was surprised and asked Tania where she had developed these skills. Tania reported that she had always loved basketball, and the main influences in her life were her older brothers, who spent a great deal of time on the playground playing basketball. When she was younger, Tania frequently would hang around them and take every opportunity to shoot baskets and play.

The mentor quickly seized on this and arranged for Tania to join the Boys and Girls Club. There was open gym session that began right after school and first involved her doing her homework and then being allowed to play basketball. A voucher was obtained with the assistance of the child welfare agency and Tania was enrolled in the Boys and Girls Club after-school program, which she attended 4 days a week. Eventually, Tania was introduced to a local Catholic Youth Organization basketball coach, who enrolled her in the fifth- and sixth-grade traveling team. Tania enjoyed immediate success and began to exhibit much more positive behaviors at school. The mentor also worked with her on developing assertiveness skills so that she could be less submissive at school. In addition, the mentor was helpful in assisting Tania in self-care and grooming. There was an immediate shift in her personal appearance and how she handled herself at school. As she became more successful at basketball, she also became less introverted and more focused on her schoolwork. She continued to be in therapy, did not require medication after her involvement in basketball began, and her grades improved dramatically.

The therapist consulted with the school and arranged for an opportunity to make a presentation to Tania's teachers. The role of bullying at the school was addressed by the therapist, who offered to consult specifically about Tania but also expressed her willingness to be involved in a committee that looked at vulnerable children and how they were being treated in the school. The principal was very responsive and worked with the school social worker and guidance counselor to develop a program that fostered friendship and essentially consisted of a type of peer mentoring.

A therapeutic mentor may engage in role-playing and behavioral rehearsal. These strategies can be tailored to the developmental age of the child and will evolve over time as the mentor and child practice these skills in the community. The most common types of social skills practiced are outlined later in this chapter (see Table 8–2 in the "Building Social Skills" section); the mentor will use both role-playing and behavioral rehearsal in teaching resilience and ways to overcome problems that the child may face when participating in a community activity.

The therapeutic mentor may also be involved in a more structured series of exercises designed to build social skills in the community. The mentor has the opportunity to practice these social skills by joining the child in community activities and using real-life problems and barriers as teaching experiences. In this way, the mentor creates a way to expose the child to social situations in which age-appropriate skills can be practiced. This process begins by exploring an interest the child has. The mentor then accompanies the youth to a series of after-school activities. Therapeutic mentors use a variety of tools designed to teach various-age children certain social skills. There are hundreds of different curricula available for specific ages and types of problems. The therapist identifies the social skill needed; the mentor identifies a teaching strategy and implements it weekly, with reports to the referring therapist and consultation with a supervising MHP.

The goal of the therapeutic mentor is to substitute high-interest activities supervised by adults in the community for passive and often self-defeating or self-destructive behaviors that are unsupervised at home or in the community. When a child enters adolescence, this need becomes extremely critical, since there are an increasing number of destructive peer activities that are easy to fall into during this specific time. The unsupervised adolescent with few social skills and no role models is an easy target for recruitment into peer groups that are engaging in drug use or other types of self-destructive behaviors. When an adolescent lacks social skills, the threat of becoming involved with destructive groups within the community, such as gangs, is greatly increased. Therapeutic mentoring is designed to build these skills early and offer them at any time during the child's development as an alternative to simply allowing the youth to live in the community without being able to join and participate in social-recreational activities.

Therapeutic mentoring also has a strong component of teaching youth how to resolve conflicts without the use of aggression. These skills can be easily transferable to school and may blend well with existing mentoring programs. Conflict resolution skills are a necessary component to having the ability to participate in a community activity. If a child or adolescent has difficulty managing conflict and fights every time there is a provocation, he or she will not be able to make use of the resources that exist within the community. Participating in normal community activities requires that the child or adolescent be able to respond to authority, manage conflict with peers, and play and participate prosocially in the activity offered. An example might be a youth who is terminated from a Boys and Girls Clubs after-school program because he is fighting. Community programs cannot tolerate this level of conflict. Being barred from participating in this type of community activity leaves no recreational options for the child except highly specialized activities supervised by clinically trained professionals. Unfortunately, such programs are expensive, not easily reached, and will contribute to the child's or adolescent's alienation from natural community supports, forcing him or her into programs outside of their community.

The therapeutic mentor creates a natural way to teach children and adolescents communication skills. When a mentor is participating with a youth in a community activity, he or she will observe many instances in which the child or adolescent displays a pattern of communication that makes it difficult for the child to be accepted or to join in a particular activity. Children may also be unable to ask for what they need, may complain about what they can't do, or may argue and resist supervisors who are attempting to maintain order. The mentor plays a key role in assisting children in developing the communication skills that can facilitate their ability to join in and maintain involvement in a social-recreational activity. The mentor is part of a care planning team, not just a random support that comes in and out of the youth's life. In weekly consultation sessions with the therapist, the mentor reports on progress and barriers to the acquisition of social skills.

There are weekly reporting requirements for therapeutic mentors to discuss their progress with the referring MHP. This weekly contact ensures that the mentor and the MHP are synchronized in their approach. There is also a requirement for the mentor to be supervised weekly by an agency MHP. This supervising MHP is responsible for all of the young people with whom the therapeutic mentor is involved within the course of any week. A therapeutic mentor may have up to 10 students who are part of his or her caseload, and this activity is supervised by an MHP who offers specific skills for the mentor concerning approaches to teaching conflict management, communication skills, and social skills.

Case Example: Stephen, an Aggressive Youth Living in an Online Virtual World

Stephen was a 14-year-old white male who exhibited aggressive behaviors at school on a weekly basis, including fighting, verbal aggression toward his peers, and failure to respond to adult direction. Stephen was suspended three times over the course of 6 weeks. A disciplinary hearing was scheduled to determine whether Stephen needed to be expelled for the protection of others at the school. Stephen had been in psychotherapy several times and had been discharged due to a failure to attend therapy sessions. Eventually, the school filed a Child in Need of Services (CHINS) petition, and the court became involved. As a condition of his probation, Stephen was referred for family therapy. Stephen lived with his mother, who was remarried, and there was a 6-year-old biological child from this new union. Stephen's biological father had been incarcerated for domestic violence and had moved away from the area after having been released from a county correctional facility.

The therapist soon discovered that Stephen spent virtually all of his time in online activities, namely role-playing games. He was not interested in athletics and refused to participate in any after-school programs. Although his mother had tried to engage him in a variety of activities, he displayed no interest in any of them.

The therapist made a referral to a therapeutic mentor, who began by meeting Stephen at his home and trying to understand ways to engage Stephen in helpful activities. Stephen refused to participate with the mentor, and several attempts were made to have the mentor meet Stephen at his home. The mentor became increasingly frustrated and communicated that to Stephen's mother rather than to the supervising MHP. The mentor began to feel ineffective in the situation. After several more weeks of unsuccessfully trying to motivate Stephen to accept mentoring, the mentor met with the therapist to discuss strategies. It was clear that the mentor had wandered into the role of therapist and had begun to engage the family in conversations about how to overcome Stephen's resistance. Therapeutic mentoring was discontinued, and the therapist assumed a more active role in working with Stephen and his mother.

Eventually, the therapist suggested that the entire family meet; a new time was arranged, and evening visits involving Stephen's stepfather and Stephen's younger sibling were scheduled. These sessions quickly revealed the points of conflict that existed in the family. Stephen felt excluded from the newly formed family and took every opportunity to fight for the opportunity to simply withdraw into his online virtual world. The family therapy proceeded for approximately 6 months and Stephen begrudgingly participated and eventually expressed an interest in building electronic devices. His withdrawal and aggression seemed to stem from a sense that he was not wanted, and he would provoke others rather than feel rejected.

The therapist suggested programs in the community that could match Stephen's interests. A different therapeutic mentor was engaged and eventually helped Stephen find a program in robotics offered by a local community college outreach program. Stephen developed a genuine interest in building robots, and eventually improved greatly in his work at school.

The therapeutic mentor is a critical part of the care planning team and must communicate and participate actively in any care planning event designed to maintain consistency in a multidimensional treatment plan. The therapeutic mentor is not isolated in the community but becomes part of the overall intervention team and is in a unique position to offer specific feedback about the strengths and weaknesses that the child or adolescent displays during the time spent in therapeutic mentoring in the community. Being an active part of the care planning team can amplify the power of what the mentor does and the development of strategies to keep the activities going for the child in the community.

The therapeutic mentor is also responsible for developing a repertoire of activities in the community that could be used as practice experiences to help a child or adolescent develop the skills he or she needs to engage in community programs. The mentor's responsibility is to expose the young person to a variety of after-school activities that could become a regular part of youth's schedule. Often, the mentor will have to explore a variety of activities in the community before finding an activity that matches the young person's abilities or interests. Therapeutic mentors have a role in motivating young people to participate in activities and also in openly supporting them in overcoming discouragement when they attempt to participate in an activity for which they do not currently possess the necessary skills to have fun and succeed.

Activities can be developed and children linked to them once the mentor understands what the child likes to do. There are a number of different activities that can engage children in a community. Some children are athletically inclined and can be motivated to participate in a wide variety of different sports and physical activities. Other children may benefit from programs such as Boys and Girls Clubs or other after-school programs that provide a wide range of activities such as swimming, playing pool, or other adult-supervised recreational pursuits.

Some children, of course, will have no interest in sports at all. They may be more involved with online activities and become addicted to virtual reality. Others are obsessed with music and spend all of their time collecting and arranging music and secretly want to become performers. These young people might be directed toward community programs designed to teach music or engage youth in performance activities such as plays or community theater. Many communities have performing arts groups that can be approached to arrange for young people to participate. Children's interests may vary from observing or supporting artistic productions to training for various types of performing or expressive arts. Many children are very artistic and quietly draw and develop beautiful expressive and creative artwork. These youth can be linked to museums or other programs in the community that sponsor artistic productions.

Therapeutic mentoring is an opportunity to reach out and help young people to explore their interests. It is extremely rewarding to discover strengths in a child that can be linked to a stabilizing force, offering a strong protective factor against the evolution of aggression and violence. School performance is connected to the overall balance a child has in his or her life. When a healthy community activity is pursued, less aggression will be carried into the school. Children will begin to develop more social skills as they participate more actively in the community. Their ability to tolerate peer pressure will increase; the therapeutic mentoring experience offers children the opportunity to learn important life skills, such as conflict management, mediation, making friends, and self-control skills.

The therapeutic mentor must reach into the child or adolescent's natural support system in the community or in the extended family. Many young people will stick with an activity when they are rewarded or feel reinforced by a valued member of their family or extended family or by community role models. For example, a mentor may enroll a student in a city basketball recreation program. The mentor will contact the coach and ask whether the student can participate; the child will try 10 or 12 games and at least as many practices. The mentor would then focus on gaining the interest of a parent, uncle, or other extended family member for assisting in transportation or watching from the stands. The therapeutic mentor becomes active not only in identifying the resource but also in fostering interest within the child's extended social network to sustain participation. The mentor can also work with the therapist to find this support while performing therapy.

The ultimate goal of the therapeutic mentor is the development of a true linkage that can be sustained by natural supports in the child's or adolescent's world. This recruitment of natural supports is a way to cement the linkages. The mentor helps build the skills in the child and adolescent but also works to create ongoing support for the youth's efforts to maintain participation in these activities.

After-School Programs

The therapeutic mentor should consider a variety of social activities that are available in the community and offer children and adolescents a way to productively spend their after-school and weekend time. These social activities may include church-sponsored dances, after-school social clubs, parent-supervised playgroups, or other social activities sponsored by either faith-based groups or community agencies. These social activities vary, based on the developmental stage of the child. For younger children, the therapeutic mentor seeks out social activities that may include supervised opportunities on a regular basis for children to play together under positive adult supervision. Often, this will require the activation of natural supports within the child's world and the development of a series of activities that could serve as after-school releases for the children. Parents might be approached by the mentor and assisted in developing a rotating schedule for after-school playgroups supervised by parents with similar interests in the neighborhood.

Recreational activities are the most common type of program available within most communities. These programs typically are offered by Boys and Girls Clubs, YMCAs or YWCAs, and other organizations such as the National Urban League or by churches. These recreational activities often are combined with homework help and offer adolescents the opportunity to socialize after they have done their homework. Frequently, they are structured activities that may range from shooting pool to playing games of flag football or soccer. These programs are also very inexpensive and may have federal subsidies that include transportation after school to the activity and then back home. After-school recreational programs may also involve a variety of supervised trips and activities. The YMCA may offer a supervised afternoon swim program in which children can learn how to swim and enjoy using the pool after school. These are not specific athletic team activities, but they are structured and organized recreational activities that offer children and adolescents the opportunity to play and have healthy fun.

Therapeutic mentors can be very effective in identifying children and adolescents with athletic interests and skills. Often, these youth are not able to participate in community athletic activities because of the difficulty in identifying an available resource, connecting the youth to the resource, funding the participation in the resource, and transporting the youth consistently to practices and games. Many young people participate in sports in an informal way and may spend considerable amounts of time hanging around a playground or park playing basketball, handball, stickball, or pickup games of softball or baseball. While these are good activities, they are not structured, adult-supervised, instruction-based activities. These informal playground activities are the precursors of a youth's participating in a high school athletic program, and developing these skills in the community will have a strong positive impact on the youth's ability to function during a normal school day at high school. Coaches of community teams often require that their athletes do well in school and develop the necessary self-control skills to be able to play as part of a team. When high-risk students can be engaged in a sporting activity in the community, this not only serves as a way to burn off excess energy, but it also promotes team participation and helps build self-control and social skills.

The therapeutic mentor plans athletic activities based on the age and level of skill of the youth interested in participating. Most cities and towns have recreational programs that sponsor seasonal activities, including basketball, baseball, and soccer. These activities will vary based on the community that the child lives in and are often the most economical, pragmatic way to foster a child's interest and participation in athletics. These activities often begin in third grade and are how children enter into the world of organized sports. These activities require that the mentor be knowledgeable of the sign-up times and any requirements that may be needed in order for the youth to participate. The town or city recreational programs tend to be less formal, involving young people from the same community engaging in competitive activities against each other. In this type of activity, the athlete does not have to be particularly well developed in order to participate. Mentors are frequently able to enroll their high-risk clients in this type of athletic activity, even if the young person does not have the developed skill to play the sport at a higher level. This is how athletic skills begin to show themselves, and the therapeutic mentor can launch a lifelong skill or hobby by connecting the youth to an athletic activity, beginning at the recreational level.

The third level of participation in athletics typically involves a higher level of skill. These activities are frequently referred to as "traveling teams." Skilled athletes try out for a place on the team that represents a city or town in competitions against other cities or towns. This level of activity generally begins between third and fifth grade and continues through high school athletics and eventually into college. If the youth has athletic interests or talent, the mentor can make a big impact through this approach.

Naturally, a mentor also must activate resources for children and adolescents who are not athletically inclined. Many young people are interested in expressive arts such as drawing, writing, painting, or computer graphics. Others may be interested in the performing arts, such as drama, music lessons, participation in a school or local band, and other creative activities. When a young person is not active in athletics and shows no interest in participating in sports, the mentor can begin to explore other alternatives. Young people with too much time on their hands after school will get lost in unstructured video game playing and Web surfing. We have seen more and more adolescents with developing Internet and video game addictions that occupy virtually all of their nonschool time. Eventually, this immersion in the all-consuming world of cyberrecreation begins to interfere with children's general equilibrium and ability to maximize their performance at school.

While video games and certain Internet activities may promote social functioning and develop visual-motor skills, the fact that they are time-consuming and not supervised by adults presents a special set of problems. Young people who get lost in virtual reality do not develop the social skills necessary to function in the real world. The therapeutic mentor may engage a young person in developing a social networking capacity. There are increasing numbers of programs that use the Internet to promote positive social interactions. These activities, however, comprise a small percentage of what is likely to occur when young people are left to their own devices online. The future is likely to present more opportunities for therapeutic mentors to engage an alienated young person in an Internet activity that will promote social cohesion, making friends, sharing life experiences, and building life and social skills.

A therapeutic mentor can also be helpful in exploring vocational and educational opportunities. As young people enter high school and begin to explore their futures, a therapeutic mentor might become involved with adolescents exploring alternatives to pure academic educational experiences. These may take the form of exploring vocational programs or involvement in after-school woodworking, landscaping, or pottery. The therapeutic mentors assist with the therapist in real-life vocational exploration by visiting and observing various types of occupational and vocational activities. Many older adolescents may be interested in military service also, and therapeutic mentors need to stay aware of the interests that emerge as part of this process.

Finally, the therapeutic mentor may become involved in helping a young person learn skills that can be described as activities of daily living, such as taking public transportation, applying for a job, or setting up a bank account. These are more case management–style approaches and are useful with adolescents who are trying to develop life skills despite the absence of natural supports to assist them in this process.

Phases of Therapeutic Mentoring

Once a therapeutic mentor receives a referral from a therapist working in a clinical hub with a specific therapeutic objective in mind, the first phase of a therapeutic mentoring intervention is engagement. The therapeutic mentor must immerse him- or herself in the child's or adolescent's home and school culture, family patterns, and community. While the therapeutic mentor's primary responsibilities lie outside of the school, the goal of the community intervention is to strengthen an at-risk child's overall social skills. Also, the child who has a balanced home, school, and community activity schedule is less likely to present problems at school.

Once the therapeutic mentor engages the child or adolescent on his or her own turf, the next phase of the intervention is an exploration of the individual's interests. In this phase, the mentor explores with the child or adolescent a variety of different types of activity options to identify high-interest areas or passions. Frequently, the child or adolescent has a high level of interest in some type of activity, yet may have low participation. In these instances, the mentor is guided by what the child expresses as an interest area and begins to build opportunities, identify skills, and locate the resources needed for the child's participation. This is not always as easy as it sounds; the mentor's challenge is to find a high-interest activity in which the youth will be able to participate. High-interest activities tend to be fun and offer the opportunity to build a strong and healthy mind and body.

Once an activity is identified, the mentor can look into the community to identify resources available to begin the exploration in the initial phases of introducing the child or adolescent to an activity. Once a resource is identified and matched with an interest, the mentor is faced with the challenge of ensuring that the child or adolescent has the skills necessary to participate in the social-recreational activity. This can be accomplished through activity trials in which the mentor accompanies the youth to a community program and assists in any transitions into the program, acting as a supervising support system. This support system may take the form of simply transporting and introducing the child to the activity director, or it may require that the mentor work with the child on ways to make friends, resist rude peers, learn to take turns, and other social skills. The end result of this phase of engagement is that the child is enrolled and engaged in the activity. Once this has happened, the mentor can then work to support continued participation.

The final phase of the linkage to a community resource often requires that the mentor invite and provide a way for natural supports to participate with the youth in the activity. This may take the form of ensuring that participation fees are paid, enlisting an extended family member in providing transportation or becoming a fan of an athletic activity, or teaching the youth living skills that could allow for independent access and ongoing participation in a healthy activity.

Building Social Skills

Therapeutic mentors, as we have mentioned, are charged with re-creating a socialization process that was interfered with by some series of events that may have occurred in the child's home, school, or community. The problem most frequently begins at home with a lack of involvement of predictable adults in a child's socialization experience. The child experiences a lack of secure attachment, which then leads to a deficiency in his or her ability to use self-reflection, contain aggression, and understand the social cues of others (Fonagy et al. 2002). A secure feeling of attachment is a must in order for a child to mentalize and contain aggression. These two skills are the critical foundation for the development of future social skills necessary to participate in both school and community activities. The teaching of these skills in a natural setting is a parental function. If the family is unable to provide these opportunities and no one else fills the role, then the child develops without the social skills necessary to participate in the range of activities necessary to prepare him or her to attend school and succeed academically and socially.

The normal developmental life cycle offers many opportunities for children to learn basic social skills. When these skills are not learned, there is an additive effect that often results in behavioral disturbances that most frequently become enacted at school. When a child or adolescent does not possess these skills, his or her behavior at school quickly reflects this unfortunate fact. School problems evolve and grow worse, since school is the key place in which social skills are practiced and reinforced. However, most schools are not equipped to teach children the fundamental building blocks they need to learn.

Social skills development also requires the active presence of positive role models to imitate. Social skills are learned when children witness adults behave in ways that illustrate the social skills necessary to accomplish life tasks. Many children and adolescents live in homes where role models are unavailable or dysfunctional (such as homes without biological fathers) and rely solely on a variety of role models that are not consistently positive, contributing to the development of symptomatic behavior rather than the development of social skills. The presence of positive role models is a necessary element in developing social skills. The clinical introduction of the therapeutic mentor is an attempt to reestablish some basic skills for a child whose behavior has been negatively impacted because of having either destructive or absent role models.

This situation is further complicated in the modern digital era, in which children and adolescents are exposed to a myriad of nonhuman images masquerading as role models. The clearest example of adolescents seeking attachment at all costs is their vulnerability to being recruited into criminal gangs or into drug dealing and use. The developing child or adolescent is exposed to models of gender interaction and adult living that involve self-destructive and coercive ways of behaving in social situations. Without positive role models, neither boys nor girls know how they are supposed to act in social settings. This will become a primary engine for the escalation of violence at school.

It is difficult for a child to develop social skills when he or she lives in a home that is not safe and is regularly exposed to overstimulation or toxic influences within the family or the community. Regardless of their social and economic level, children may live in families with absent parents, due to a number of factors, ranging from incarceration to overinvolvement in business or work. Regardless of why the adult is absent, the child experiences the same void, and thus does not develop the necessary fundamental social skills required to succeed at school. The child may also live in a home where parents are aggressive and frequently argue, creating an unsafe home environment. This also sets a tone that infiltrates the way the child understands and learns how to behave in social situations. When role models are aggressive with one another, it is quite natural for a child to reflect that behavior at school.

All social skills require that the child be able to respond to limits and boundaries. Playing on a team demands that a child be able to wait his or her turn, listen to the coach, or share the basketball and to respond to limits and boundaries. When limits and boundaries are not consistently built and reinforced at home, this creates an immediate clash at school. If the child lives in a home where limits are inconsistent and boundaries are fluid or nonexistent, he or she may have difficulty transitioning to a school where limits and boundaries are clearly defined and enforced by adult teachers. School conflict is a frequent behavioral eruption that results from providing mixed signals to children.

TABLE 8–2. Developmental social skill sets

Developmental stage	Social skill sets
Early childhood	Separating from parents Sharing Playing with others Making friends Accepting limits Self-organization Listening to others
Middle and junior high school	Fitting in with peer groups Reading social cues Managing conflicts Being sensitive to others Communicating well with peers Dealing with worries about popularity and personal appearance
High school and college	Avoiding self-destructive habits and activities Joining unsupervised after-school activities Demonstrating good work habits Managing time and money Driving safely Dating safely

Finally, children build social skills when they are rewarded for behaving in a way that reflects the acquisition of that skill. Children need to be validated and feel valuable when they participate gracefully in activities and demonstrate their social skills. A child needs to be praised and rewarded after using manners at home; this is a process that validates the child's use of that skill. Without this validation of social values, the child is not motivated to use these skills in other settings and is at increased risk of displaying a lack of these skills at school and in the community. Academic success is often rewarded by stickers and other tangible tokens of success. Social skills need to be included in this reward system.

There are a wide range of social skills needed for children and adolescents to be successful in a variety of settings, especially school. Table 8–2 illustrates some of the basic social skill sets that must be mastered at different developmental stages. Once the basic elements of social skills are developed, the door to building specific skills is opened in real time, reinforced by supervised practice in the community with the mentor. Specifically, children will begin to learn how to choose good friends, to behave appropriately, to accept being themselves and fitting in, to handle popularity, to deal with embarrassment, to cope with injustice, to display empathy, and to show respect. All social skills begin with the youth being able to exert self-control. The child or adolescent must be able to trust that adult role models will be reliable sources of guidance. This trust in adult mentors needs to be transferred to adults at school or in other community settings. Self-control helps young people to avoid conflicts with authority that can play out at school and spill over into the community—and often, regrettably, can result in removal of the child from his or her home, school, or community.

Conclusion

The use of a therapeutic mentor to activate community resources is a process that is likely to become an increasing part of interventions targeted to complicated problems such as violence; however, this approach is not yet available in all states. As the wraparound models have demonstrated in psychotherapy, the coordination of care is a critical element in addressing the complicated problem of violence. Therapeutic mentoring as described in this chapter is a Medicaid service that would apply primarily to children who live under the poverty level. These same skills are applicable in suburban homes, but these children are unlikely to be part of a Medicaid program. Suburban children who exhibit the need for this service will likely be referred to courts, which then may remove custody from the family and place it with the state agency. Frequently, this is done in order to have the young person receive Medicaid as a ward of the state and thus be able to access Medicaid services, such as therapeutic mentoring. In any event, therapeutic mentoring as a process is a treatment intervention that can be adapted to meet the needs of both urban and suburban problems, regardless of socioeconomic status.

Therapeutic mentoring can be an extremely valuable tool in coping with school violence. Interventions in school violence will require an increasing number of new and creative approaches to keep up with the evolving face of school violence. Therapeutic mentors exemplify a new practice pattern that may become a regular part of the MHP's strategies for intervening in complex school violence cases. This intervention strategy illustrates the interconnection of the home, school, and community. Strategies like this are what is needed to replace the walls of residential care. Only the most needy and out-of-control children and adolescents need residential care. All options in the community should be exhausted before uprooting children or adolescents and placing them in supervised community residential programs.

KEY CLINICAL CONCEPTS

- Therapeutic mentoring is a specialized program that offers a concrete way to reach into the community and teach social skills to youth exhibiting school violence problems.

- Therapeutic mentoring is a service offered as a statewide initiative in Massachusetts and exemplifies emerging new strategies for reducing school violence.

- Traditional mentoring is the use of an older companion who fills in for an adult role model. Therapeutic mentoring is a specialized application of a mentor and therapist who work to build social skills.

- Mentoring has been used in many contexts, including adult professional role models for teachers and doctors. Businesses also can provide adult mentors to schoolchildren for specific skill enhancements such as reading and math.

- Mentoring is especially important as an antidote to peer rejection, especially in African American youth.

- Wraparound systems of care offer the multitiered intervention structures needed to effectively intervene in school violence.

- In this model of therapeutic mentoring, the mentor works with a psychotherapist just as a physical therapist works with a physician, identifying strengths and weaknesses and teaching skills.

- The MHP is the coordinator of therapeutic mentoring interventions and is responsible for designing and supervising these interventions. These are medically necessary services reimbursed by Medicaid, not a general child welfare program.

- Therapeutic mentoring is not just playing sports or enjoying other activities; its goal is to teach the skills necessary to continue participating in healthy community alternatives to violence.

- Therapeutic mentoring requires weekly consultations between the treating therapist and the mentor. In addition, the mentor receives independent supervision from an MHP who oversees the planning of strategies to engage youth and teach social skills.

- Therapeutic mentors are natural leaders and teachers of skills, not highly trained MHPs—hence the need for close supervision by an experienced MHP.

- Therapeutic mentors use role-playing, structured activities matched to developmental level, exploration of interest, and resource research and development.

- Therapeutic mentors can work collaboratively with existing school mentoring or mediation programs.

- Mentors teach communication skills by modeling them in real-life community settings.

- Mentors are active participants in care planning meetings.

- Mentoring is a strengths-based exploration of a youth's interests.

- Mentors work with teens to help them develop ways to resist peer pressure to engage in self-destructive behaviors.

- Mentors work to involve extended family and other natural supports in the development of a community activity based on the child's identified interest.

- Therapeutic mentors are very actively engaged in athletic programs and try whenever an interest or skill exists to connect the youth to organized sports, beginning with YMCA and Boys and Girls Clubs.

- Mentors can be used to break Internet addiction, explore vocational possibilities, and teach life skills.

- The first step in mentoring is engagement; there must be a connection before any work can proceed on a mentoring goal.

- The second step in therapeutic mentoring is interest exploration — finding a high-interest activity. And finally, the mentor must locate community resources that will allow for real-life practice of social skills.

- School is where children will display their lack of social skills.

References

Fonagy P, Gyorgy G, Jurist EL, et al: Affect Regulation, Mentalization, and the Development of the Self. New York, Other Press, 2002

Kamps DM, Barbetta PM, Leonard BR, et al: Class wide peer tutoring: an integration strategy to improve the reading skills and promote peer interactions among students with autism and general education peers. J Appl Behav Anal 27:49–61, 1994

Miller-Johnson S, Coie JD, Maumary-Germaud A, et al: Relationship between childhood peer rejection and aggression and adolescent delinquency severity and type among African American youth. J Emot Behav Disord 7:137–146, 1999

Onuoha FN, Munakata T, Serumaga-Sake PA, et al: Negative mental health factors in children orphaned by AIDS: natural mentoring as a palliative care. AIDS Behav 13:980–988, 2009

Perkins J: Medicaid EPSDT litigation. National Health Law Program, October 2, 2009. Available at: http://www.healthlaw.org/images/stories/epsdt/1-EPSDT-Docket.pdf. Accessed December 7, 2010.

Rhodes JE, Reddy R, Grossman JB: The protective influence of mentoring on adolescent's substance use: direct and indirect pathways. Appl Dev Sci 9:31–47, 2005

Riley P: The development and testing of time-limited mentoring model for experienced school leaders. Mentoring and Tutoring: Partnerships in Learning 17:233–249, 2009

Rosie D. v Romney, 4101 F.Supp. 2D 18 (D. Mass. 2006)

Sacco F, Twemlow S, Fonagy P: Secure attachment to family and community: a college proposal for cost containment within higher user populations of multiple problem families. Smith Coll Stud Soc Work 77:31–51, 2007

Thomson NR, Zand DH: Mentees' perceptions of their interpersonal relationships: the role of the mentor-youth bond. Youth Soc 41:434–445, 2010

Wyatt S: The brotherhood: empowering adolescent African American males toward excellence. Professional School Counseling 12:463–470, 2009

9

Role of Medical Leadership in Unlocking Resources to Address School Violence

AS we have emphasized, school violence problems are not simple interventions. When aggression spills into the school and classrooms, the causes and solutions generally require a complex treatment strategy. The psychiatrist is often in the unique position of determining medical necessity or documenting eligibility for services or benefits. In this role, the medical professional is charged with opening the doors to resources that will fund the services needed to address the school violence problem. In this medical leadership role, the psychiatrist guides the plan even if the psychiatrist's direct care role is an otherwise relatively small part of the plan. Social workers in the school and community are likely to be the most hands-on parts of the plan; their job is made easier when the medical professional takes a leadership role in creating intervention designs and unlocking resources. This model stresses the value of the medical leadership in identifying the key dimensions needing services. By contrast, wraparound models take a different view of intervention leadership and place the "voice of the family" as the guiding element of the system of care. In fact, the wraparound process is fundamentally defined not as therapy, but rather as a coordinated care process.

The wraparound process is distinctly different from services such as therapy and medication management, which are defined by medical necessity. There is an emerging trend in states to include more community-based services under Medicaid services, as described in Chapter 8, "Activating Community Resources Through Therapeutic Mentoring." The wraparound system of care (Downes and Austin 2004; Oliver et al. 1998) is being used as a state template for remedies by Medicaid in court decisions.[1] The mental health professional (MHP) is well advised to understand the system of care that exists in the community and to adjust his or her perspective according to local guidelines.

The use of medically necessary interventions requires medical authorization by a practitioner and can be an excellent point from which to exercise medical leadership in designing a school violence intervention. When children experience emotional disturbances, their behavior will be seen at school. This behavior needs to be assessed and understood, with an analysis of the factors leading to the symptoms and diagnosis. Because the intervention is medical, medical leadership is the key to effective interventions targeting the complex underlying dynamics fueling school violence problems.

The approach outlined in this chapter places the responsibility for intervention leadership in the hands of the MHP and strongly encourages medical professionals to take more active leadership roles in school violence interventions. The focus is on helping the MHP understand how disability and entitlement benefits work in the United States, who is eligible, and what is needed to document eligibility and need. In addition, we have included an outline of the private and public options for health and disability insurance in the clinical formulation process. In many ways, these funding elements form the skeleton of a school violence intervention. The benefits will vary greatly in state programs that work with federal programs, but certain federal guidelines will be imposed on any state that receives federal reimbursement. MHPs must understand how these programs work in their own states. MHPs in other countries, even those who are natural helpers in remote rural areas, likewise need to learn how to ac-

---

[1]See *Rosie D. v Romney* (2006; www.Rosied.org), a Massachusetts federal case brought against the state's Medicaid program by parents of children in residential placement who believed that availability of in-home services could have prevented the need for the children's out-of-home placement. *Rosie D. v Romney* is one of a string of what are referred to as EPSDT (Early Periodic Screening, Diagnosis, and Treatment) cases. State Medicaid programs are being sued for failing to provide EPSDT services to Medicaid children younger than 21 years.

cess available benefits and services. Regardless of country, the MHP's role is to understand how to gather the resources necessary to assist a family in coping with child aggression that leaks into school.

The approach used in this book parallels the biopsychosocial approach of DSM-IV-TR (American Psychiatric Association 2000) in its recognition of the multiple layers of factors contributing to mental illness and, in this specific context, how a mental impairment may be interwoven into a complex problem acted out at school. These interacting levels of needs in a young person's life can be viewed as the main engine for the propulsion of school violence. This model expands the contributing factors described in DSM-IV-TR to include unconscious power dynamics, social roles at school, the interfacing of multiple systems, the role of special risk factors, and the value of family empowerment and building on strengths in the home, school, and community. The psychiatrist is challenged in this model to create a comprehensive intervention map. Medical leadership requires that the psychiatrist move beyond the simple prescription of medicine. School violence is a complex problem that likewise requires a multilayered solution.

School violence interventions need to begin with recognition of the destructive potential of interdisciplinary power struggles that ultimately do the child and family no good. Medical leadership cannot be authoritarian, as in a physician's written order to other members of a health care team. Medical leadership begins by identifying power struggles that exist or are likely to form as an intervention is planned, dissolving these power struggles, and functioning as a work group leader, regardless of one's role in the overall treatment team. Bion (1970) described the concept of "Negative K" (discussed further in Chapter 5, "Bullying Is a Process, Not a Person") as group conflict that is supported by ineffective leadership when there is no valued uniting group theme. We have seen this happen in interventions when social workers hate the physician or when teachers resist any help from the outside. Such conflicts can be seen as an impediment to designing and implementing an intervention. An effective leader is one who encourages clear boundaries, opens lines of communication, and is mindful of the shifting variables in treatment. This is a work group mentality in a multiple-dimension intervention.

Often, this intervention planning process is interrupted by a lack of resources to accomplish the support needed to solve a multifaceted problem. From a diagnostic point of view, the principle here is to "follow the money"—that is, find out how a family survives and what will be needed for services. This will create a need for the MHP to be aware of the avenues to open doors to recommended services. This understanding strikes at the heart of Maslow's hierarchy of needs (Maslow 1971), applying it to the ugly realities of modern social pressures. When a poor family struggles without normal social support, everybody knows what is needed, but sees no way to make it happen. This is where medical leadership can team up with other disciplines to search for resources. Medical professionals such as physicians, physician assistants, nurse practitioners, and licensed psychologists can provide medical documentation in disability cases. Often, for instance, medical signatures are needed to obtain or activate transportation or a referral for early childhood care. Documenting medical need is the key to supporting interventions in both the private and public sector. Medical necessity is the driving force behind behavioral health services funded by Medicaid or private insurance. Even in countries with socialized systems, the key component driving access to services is still medical necessity.

Understanding medical documentation of disability is of equal value for disadvantaged families and nondisadvantaged families with a disabled child. Both would require that the medical professional or licensed psychologist document medical evidence of the disability. For example, working parents of an autistic child who is having school problems will benefit from Supplemental Security Income (SSI), which will open the door to Medicaid for the disabled child. This step could greatly reduce the pressure on the family, highlighting resources that could be applied in the school and community. The types of community services funded by Medicaid typically are not covered in private insurance plans. Medical leaders need a working understanding of how services are funded in the area in which they work and for the population they serve.

Frequently, MHPs view forms for documenting medical need as an annoyance and a clerical unfunded mandate of providing treatment. It is easy to let these forms and applications pile up on a desk or in a mail slot, but dealing with this paperwork is a critical part of school violence interventions. Much of what results in school violence can be easily traced back to factors in the home and community. The treatment of violence requires the activating of resources as part of the coordinated treatment plan. Clinical recommendations for school violence need to have follow-through and will challenge the treatment team to produce the information needed to access the service. A thorough school violence evaluation needs to explore all avenues for accessing services. The MHP needs to know what is available for resources and then must ask what steps have been taken to access those services. It is of no value to make a diagnosis, identify the underlying need, and then just leave the task of finding and accessing services for someone else to handle. A medical leader will ensure that everything possible is being done to help the child and family; this is best done by example. When the medical leader is the first to complete a necessary form or perform an evaluation, then the team is energized by the medical presence. This style of medical leadership builds buy-in from all members of the treatment team as well as from the family of the high-risk or at-risk child.

The general types of resources we describe here will vary according to the practitioner's location; however, this outline will help create a template that can be used in a variety of situations. Whereas this chapter focuses on resources in the United States, the basic principles of funding services are the same anywhere, although the pathways to accessing them vary considerably. In the United States, many services are federally funded but are directed by "state plans," which are formal documents that define eligibility, service content, and methodology. Other services are strictly local, such as summer jobs, camps, recreation, sports, and outdoor activities.

The following case example illustrates how an entitlement benefit, early childhood services, disability, and special education can be used to help resolve a school violence problem. The medical professional initiates the process by addressing basic survival needs as part of solving a school violence problem, and then exerts pressure on the community to provide assistance. The MHP did not just prescribe and run; she stayed with the problem, made referrals, completed medical documentation, and offered medical input to two special needs programs as well as several early childhood intervention services.

Case Example: Zeke, a Boy From a Disturbed Family Helped by Coordinated Entitlements

Zeke was a 9-year-old white male attending a rural industrialized elementary school. Zeke was expelled for stabbing a teacher with a pencil and was referred to a psychiatric nurse practitioner in a group practice. Zeke's family had very recently been evicted from their home; they were living in a family shelter and were on a waiting list for permanent housing. Zeke was not covered by insurance, as his mother had just lost her job as a fast food worker. Zeke was the oldest of three children. His younger brother (4 years old) suffered from some type of global cognitive deficit, and his younger sister (2 years old) had a history of severe tantrums and had been asked to leave several family day care centers she had attended while their mother was working. Zeke presented as a bright, active, but easily frustrated child. His mother was exhausted from the multiple demands of caring for three difficult children while living in a temporary shelter, and she felt demoralized because she was unable to find employment. She was proud and did not want to take "welfare" and was attempting to survive on unemployment benefits. She had always worked and had never been unemployed for more than 3 months. Zeke's mother had been out of work for 18 months this time, however, and eventually admitted that she was drinking too much, staying in bed all day, and overwhelmed by her own feelings of failure. She reported that she had a history of mental health issues as an adolescent and was hoping that she could avoid treatment as an adult. She clearly was seriously depressed and unable to work, but too proud to admit it.

The nurse practitioner completed the evaluation and began Zeke on Adderall. The nurse practitioner recognized the complexity of the case and the need to stabilize basic resources as a necessary step in treating Zeke's aggressive outburst at school. Also, she understood the landscape and was influential in making the appropriate referrals and documenting the medical needs for a wide spectrum of services. Zeke's mother was eligible for Social Security Disability Insurance (SSDI) benefits because she had been working for most of her life. The nurse practitioner referred the family to the local community action agency, which helped Zeke's mother apply for SSDI and receive temporary Medicaid and short-term disability assistance with cash benefits and food stamps.

The community action agency also used Medicaid to refer the family for in-home support services as well as Women, Infants, and Children (WIC) nutrition program benefits, and a special education referral was made for Zeke's brother. An early intervention program with parent supports was obtained for the younger sister. Zeke's mother was free to fully cooperate with the school and the mental health clinic, which constructed a plan to increase support for Zeke at school, offer rewards, and present to him new and challenging courses in science. Zeke responded well to the stimulant trial. His mother received SSDI benefits and began retraining for a position in medical records management at a local community college. She eventually recovered from her depression with the help of a brief cognitive-behavioral group and medication. Zeke was accepted into a charter school that specialized in science and technology courses. Zeke's brother began attending an early childhood program, and his mother worked with the local autism support group. Zeke's youngest sister eventually responded to the parent and child groups; the mother learned new ways to control her daughter's temper outbursts. Zeke's mother eventually received Section 8 housing and found a four-bedroom apartment she could afford.

This case illustrates how to use entitlements that followed the family by virtue of income. There are also cases in which an odd health disparity exists, such as an upper-income family with private insurance that cannot access community services funded by Medicaid:

Case Example: Lauren, a High School Student From an Affluent Family Who Needs Medicaid Help

Lauren was a 15-year-old female in ninth grade from an upper-income, intact African American family. Her younger brother was very athletic and academically at the top of his class. Lauren, however, was failing despite displaying above-average potential, as evidenced by her junior high and elementary school achievement. When Lauren entered high school, she abruptly stopped achieving and started fighting at school, abusing prescription medication, and engaging in high-risk dating behavior. She ran away from home and was missing and unsupervised for 3 full days. After several failures in recovery homes and inpatient programs funded by private insurance, Lauren was out of school, prostituting, and engaging in petty larceny.

Lauren required detoxification, an integrated substance abuse program, and community-based services not available to her family. The MHP quickly understood the limitations of benefits and enlisted a clinic psychiatrist and psychologist in applying for disability, which would carry with it Medicaid. Without Medicaid, Lauren would not be eligible for many substance abuse services. The disability process was facilitated with a quick written and follow-up conversation with SSI reviewers. Eventually, Lauren was accepted into a Medicaid-funded methadone program with supportive intensive outpatient services that included educational tutoring. She stabilized on methadone, continued in substance abuse counseling, and returned to school. Lauren was able to complete high school and subsequently enrolled in a community college. She detoxified gradually from methadone after community college and began working as a substance abuse counselor.

In Lauren's case, the activation of Medicaid opened the door to long-term methadone maintenance treatment that included transportation to and from medical providers.

Entitlement or Benefit?

The first major distinction in assessing resources is to differentiate an entitlement from a benefit. A *benefit* is a private option that a parent will purchase or receive as part of employment benefits. Private health and disability plans are example of benefits. An *entitlement*, by contrast, is driven by income and assets. An entitlement is typically defined at a federal level and then applied in different ways from state to state. Entitlements create a certain group based on income or other group characteristics, such as Native Americans. A person is either entitled or not, based on hard characteristics and numbers. Once the person is eligible for the entitlement, then the state offers all those entitled the same benefits.

This distinction is not as simple as poor versus affluent. A child may be eligible for disability and receive SSI even if the parents do not qualify. School violence problems often require services best accessed through Medicaid; private insurance plans often do not offer families the services they need beyond medical care and some limited specialty behavioral health services.

Some states take alternative routes to qualify a child for specialized services as part of solving a school violence problem. Two examples of these alternative routes are 1) use of special education laws in public education (special education does not apply to private schools; see "Special Education" section later in this chapter) in public education, and 2) use of the juvenile court in status offenses. In both instances, children can qualify for services based on federal criteria. Any public school student, regardless of family income, is eligible for special education, which could offer school support services for academics as well as behavioral problems, such as school violence.

Child in Need of Services (CHINS) or Person in Need of Supervision (PINS) is a juvenile court procedure in which a court can intervene when a child commits a status offense such as running away, truancy, and oppositionalism.[2] All of these offenses are based on being a minor child who acts out beyond a parent's or caretaker's control. Many states have statutes to cover this type of problem, but others do not. If the MHP's state does have such a law, then this may be a resource to improve safety for an unruly adolescent, as well as to have the state provide Medicaid and partial guardianship. There is no income or asset requirements for CHINS or PINS; any parent or school in a state with this statute can make a referral to the juvenile court. If the judge finds the child in need of services, then the state can step in; usually this will include Medicaid and other state services connected to the child welfare system. Simply living in the state would entitle a family to access this resource.

There is a fair amount of diagnostic information involved in discovering the way benefits and entitlements can be used. Many people are too proud, or their doctors are too busy, to put all the pieces together to obtain a benefit or entitlement. Not all entitlements are welfare; some derive from geography. Citizens in certain areas are eligible for or entitled to certain benefits simply because of where they live. Education is a very good example. All citizens are entitled to a public education. All public school students are guaranteed, regardless of income, an accommodation plan to facilitate learning. Transportation is an entitlement for public education outside of certain distances set by the city or town. Certain recreational activities are open to all citizens at public facilities for little or no charge.

Resources can be grouped using Maslow's pyramid (Maslow 1943, 1971). The first two levels involve basic survival; this includes cash, food, and shelter. These resources are usually provided by a family who works and takes care of its basic needs. If a family is unemployed, disabled, or homeless, the children will have trouble adjusting to school. School adjustment problems cannot be effectively addressed if basic survival needs are not being met. It is here that intervention begins; the MHP needs to determine how the family survives economically, or "follow the money." When working in disadvantaged areas, this problem can halt an intervention in its tracks. The question is, what can be done to secure a life that guarantees basic survival needs? If the family is economically secure, then the question shifts to whether the parents are substituting money for time, affection, nurturance, and direction. This is a factor that the MHP needs to assess and include as either a strength or a weakness.

---

[2]For a perspective on CHINS, MHPs should check their local state provisions. A description of the CHINS process in Massachusetts is provided at www.clcm.org/chins.htm.

Disability

The medical professional is a necessary element in the documentation of disability for a mental impairment. This becomes an important ingredient when facing school violence problems. Medical leadership can step up using this approach and contribute directly to stabilizing the out-of-balance forces at home or in the community. Financial instability or occupational preoccupation of the parent or guardian can deprive a child of the necessary adult involvement to prevent aggression from leaking into the school.

In the United States, disability can be public or private, for the young or old, job connected or not, and physical, mental, or both. Many parents and youth may be eligible for disability benefits to address the complicated behavioral health problems that often underlie school violence. There is no distinction between physical and mental disabilities; both are powerful designations of disability protected under Section 504 of the 1973 Rehabilitation Act. The challenge in either case is to establish a person's eligibility and then to document the existence of a disability, which, again, is often the domain of a medical professional or a licensed psychologist.

The process of documenting a mental impairment has two parts: first, the MHP must establish the existence of the disabling condition (U.S. Social Security Administration 2008a, 2008b), and second, he or she must determine the individual's residual functional capacity (RFC; U.S. Social Security Administration 2008c). For establishing that a mental impairment exists, psychological testing is considered medical evidence, as are the reports sent to MHPs as a course of medical determination. There must also be evidence that the mental impairment is preventing the person from functioning in a work setting of any type. For children, the evidence needs to demonstrate that the child has been unable to function at school or in the community for at least 1 year because of a mental impairment. Tables 9–1 and 9–2 list the conditions that qualify as mental impairments for the purpose of determining disability in adults and children, respectively.

The two major divisions in disability are public and private. Most people pay into Social Security through payroll taxes. To qualify for Social Security Disability Insurance (SSDI) benefits, a person must have worked both long enough and recently enough (for a summary of eligibility requirements, see U.S. Social Security Administration 2011). If a person has not been working at that level, he or she is eligible for Supplemental Security Income (SSI), which is more connected to a federal and state match. The major differences in these two programs involve income and eligibility, as well as residency and asset ownership. SSDI is income-sensitive and not asset-sensitive. Also, with SSDI, a window is provided, allowing a person to be on disability and still work up to a certain level. The MHP should advise clients to obtain information relevant to their case from their local Social Security Administration office. Under SSDI, the dis-

TABLE 9–1. Disability evaluation under Social Security: adult mental disorders

Limitations on work that have lasted or are expected to last for a continuous period of at least 12 months

12.02	Organic mental disorders
12.03	Schizophrenic, paranoid and other psychotic disorders
12.04	Affective disorders
12.05	Mental retardation
12.06	Anxiety-related disorders
12.07	Somatoform disorders
12.08	Personality disorders
12.09	Substance addiction disorders
12.10	Autistic disorder and other pervasive developmental disorders

Source. U.S. Social Security Administration 2008a.

TABLE 9–2. Disability evaluation under Social Security: childhood mental disorders

Limitations that have lasted or are expected to last for a continuous period of at least 12 months

112.02	Organic mental disorders
112.03	Schizophrenic, delusional (paranoid), schizoaffective, and other psychotic disorders
112.04	Mood disorders
112.05	Mental retardation
112.06	Anxiety disorders
112.07	Somatoform, eating, and tic disorders
112.08	Personality disorders
112.09	Psychoactive substance dependence disorders
112.10	Autistic disorder and other pervasive developmental disorders
112.11	Attention-deficit/hyperactivity disorder
112.12	Developmental and emotional disorders of newborn and younger infants (birth to attainment of age 1)

Source. U.S. Social Security Administration 2008b.

abled person becomes eligible first for Medicare A and eventually for B and D. By contrast, SSI is an entitlement that is correlated to assets, income, and residency. SSI clients often become eligible for Medicaid. Once an asset surfaces, however, the entitlement stops. On SSDI, asset acquisition is allowed and does not mean the benefit has to stop. Also, SSDI clients can live anywhere; they are not bound to the state, as are individuals receiving SSI entitlements. SSDI clients may also receive dependents benefits. If a caregiver is disabled and on SSDI, his or her dependent children are entitled to a monthly cash benefit.

Some individuals may be covered by a private disability plan. This is common in municipalities and state governments. Private plans basically set their own protocols for determining eligibility and RFC, guided by state and federal rules. Veterans also are eligible for a variety of benefits based on status and service record. Combat veterans have access to disability that does not conflict with private insurance benefits but does affect entitlements.

When approaching a school violence case to screen for whether disability would be useful or appropriate, the medical leader should ask and find answers to the following four crucial questions:

1. Is there financial stress due to unemployment; has the caregiver been unable to work?
2. Is there a seriously disabled child who would independently qualify for SSI entitlement?
3. Is there a mental impairment interfering with a caregiver's ability to work?
4. Is there a source that will fund the services needed to prevent the child's aggression at school?

Often, the major reason to seek disability for a child is to obtain Medicaid. In addition, the problem of school violence is intensified by the financial stress experienced by caretakers. This situation is recognized in the Axis IV dimension (Psychosocial and Environmental Problems) of DSM-IV-TR. It is important to emphasize that the medical leader will typically *not* be the one helping the client fill out forms or accompanying the client to the Social Security or welfare office. Rather, it is the medical professional—who will be required to endorse the documentation of the mental impairment and the RFC. MHPs can obtain information and suggest that clients or case managers apply for disability online (at www.ssa.gov/disability).

RFC is a critical component of documenting a disability claim. MHPs are encouraged to follow available guidelines (U.S. Social Security Administration 2008c). The basic element of this analysis is establishing the ability to perform "substantial gainful activity" (SGA). This assessment documents the disability's impact on work-related abilities. Step 1 is establishing that there is a disabling condition; step 2 is to document its impact on SGA. The Social Security Administration standard for RFC is "consideration of the ability to understand, to carry out and re-member instructions and to respond appropriately to supervision, coworkers, and customary work pressures in a work setting." Mental impairments almost always interfere with a person's ability to function at work or (for children) at school.

Children are also eligible for disability through Social Security if they meet eligibility criteria regarding income and resources. Children of parents who re-ceive SSDI are also eligible for dependents cash assistance until the age of 18 years. If a child is disabled, he or she can apply separately from the parent for SSI, but the Social Security Administration will first need to determine whether the child is eligible under the formulas used to determine eligibility; the second component is the medical documentation, which is similar to an adult's process. Children of working families may qualify for the Children's Health Insurance Program (CHIP; see www.insurekidsnow.gov), which is designed for families who cannot afford commercial private health insurance.

There is also a type of disability related to a workplace accident that becomes compounded by depression. A common scenario in many families begins with the primary breadwinner becoming injured and disabled after years or decades of employment. Depression often sets in, but is not recognized as a factor in the dis-ability documentation. Parents may be struggling needlessly because their mental impairments have not been adequately diagnosed and documented. This can contribute to the breakdown of parental support, diluting the positive signals sent to the child from the home about behavior at school. Because of the many vari-ables, the MHP needs to understand the conditions that can be considered when applying for disability. This can build the treatment alliance as well as decrease the financial pressures on the family. Many parents can be helped to become stronger themselves in order to help contain their child's aggression or diminish their like-lihood of their child's becoming a victim at school.

Anybody who has been employed and pays Federal Insurance Contributions Act (FICA) tax will also have unemployment benefits and workers' compensa-tion insurance. In addition, many states offer short-term disability support. This is often used to assist substance abusers who have been released from treatment programs or detoxification centers. Each state offers different programs, and some may not offer this benefit at all, as the Social Security Administration has removed substance abuse from the list of impairments qualifying for a disability. States can use Medicaid to assist eligible individuals for short periods of time. Typically, however, this is a limited benefit and will be combined with cash sup-plements and/or food stamps.

Medicaid

A valuable and often underused tool in addressing school violence is Medicaid. There is a strange health care disparity in this area. Many private health plans have mandatory coverage for behavioral health but offer few to none of the specialized services available under Medicaid. If the family happens to be privileged, they can simply write a check, presuming that such services are available. Ironically, for the working class, especially for those of lower socioeconomic status (SES), there are fewer intervention options than if the family were homeless and on Medicaid. Many school violence problems stem from the disadvantaged populations covered by Medicaid. When school violence erupts in either a high- or lower-SES family, there are fewer options available through health insurance. If the school violence issues increase, insurance fades as a primary resource and either the child welfare or the juvenile justice system will move in to manage the child's or adolescent's out-of-control behavior erupting at school.

Medicaid varies greatly across the United States. Each state must create a state plan that defines the relationship between the state and federal Medicaid services managed through the Centers for Medicare and Medicaid Services (see www.cms.gov). There are two types of Medicaid plans: the clinic option and the rehabilitation option. The clinic option limits the state to nonresidential options for solving behavioral health. In other words, there is no payment for overnight stays under this state plan option. The rehabilitation option *does* pay for overnight stays and relies on the residential or milieu treatment options.

Most states in the United States have the clinic option. Under the clinic option, the state creates an entitled pool based on income; this formula is used to determine eligibility. This is purely about income, immigration status, and expenses. Once the state determines this population, then all are entitled equally to use certain benefits at a certain rate with certain providers. Waivers exist to allow states to have managed care of this public option, such as in the case of Value Options (see www.valueoptions.com), a managed care organization that specializes in managing Medicaid. Otherwise, the state has to play by the federal rules. The Medicaid provisions (Title XIX) of the Social Security Act (see www.ssa.gov/OP_Home/ssact/title19/1900.htm) govern the rules of how a state offers services and to whom. The state shares the expense of the Medicaid disbursement proportionately with the federal government. It is critical for MHPs to be familiar with how Medicaid operates in the areas in which they practice.

Medicaid's child health component, the Early Periodic Screening, Diagnosis, and Treatment (EPSDT) program, requires that children in Medicaid have regular well-child examinations and that Medicaid children age 21 years or younger be screened for health and mental health problems according to the standards established by the American Academy of Pediatrics. (The Robert Wood Johnson Foundation [Smith 2005] provides an excellent briefing on EPSDT.) This mandate is a very powerful tool in the hands of a medical leader. A child's physical and mental health needs must be documented and have medical backup to drive services; this is where medical leadership can lead to change in violent youth and their victims. It is rare that a student who is violent and is on Medicaid will not have some identifiable emotional disturbance. This is clearly a mandate of Medicaid law, yet there exists no such mandate for working-class or upper-income families. It is up to the parents and school to come up with solutions, since they cannot rely on private insurance. Therefore, these families will naturally rely more on services from public schools than on health insurance for specialized interventions. In extreme cases of school violence or truancy, the family may be forced to use the family court, probation, child welfare, or juvenile justice systems. Knowledge of how services are funded can equip the MHP with the perspective required to understand and respond to the needs of the case.

The experienced medical leader uses Medicaid to its fullest extent to address underlying causes of school violence. In order to apply Medicaid in situations of school violence, medical necessity needs to be established. The child's problem is translated from a socially deviant act at school into a medical condition such as oppositional defiant disorder (ODD), posttraumatic stress disorder (PTSD), or attention-deficit/hyperactivity disorder (ADHD). When root problems are addressed in this fashion, then Medicaid can be used (for poor children age 21 years and younger) under the protective umbrella of EPSDT to screen, prevent, and treat serious emotional disturbances. The MHP needs to be able to translate psychopathological problems such as behavior disturbances, truancy, and hyperactivity into medical symptoms of a diagnosable condition requiring medically supervised treatment. The medical leader can significantly improve the intervention with involvement at this basic-needs level. It is the senior medical professional's responsibility and duty to ensure that all bases are covered in responding to youth violence in a school context. Accessing Medicaid opens many doors, and the medical leader has the key. This is an excellent position from which to generate constructive action plans with multiple agencies and the child, family, and school.

Early Childhood Programs

Early childhood enrichment is a key ingredient for creating a successful student. (The National Education Association offers an excellent overview of the benefits of early enrichment in economic terms; see www.nea.org/home/18226.htm.) Early enrichment is the beginning of a prevention process that could reap rewards throughout the educational cycle. Early childhood programs are often the first place that a new parent interacts with the child's ecological system. Prior to this point, children may have been the sole focus of attention from their immediate family members, and now they have to transition to being one of many students in a larger system. They begin to build the social skills that will be needed to maintain self-control and self-discipline in later grades. This is the point where bullying prevention has the most value and can really contribute to good social skills around friendship. As an intervention point, early childhood programs offer an excellent opportunity to screen for problems such as impulsivity, aggression, or submissiveness very early in the developmental process. Early childhood programs can be an especially important component of interventions in families with children who have been diagnosed with neurodevelopmental disorders, autism, or intellectual disabilities. The special education laws apply to children ages 2½ through 22 years. Language and motor delays in children are common points of early entry into dedicated special education classrooms in American schools.

Head Start (see www.acf.hhs.gov/programs/ohs), a national early childhood program funded by the federal government, provides comprehensive education, health, nutrition, and parent involvement services to low-income children and their families. In addition, all poor children are eligible to receive WIC (see www.fns.usda.gov/wic/aboutwic), which pays for the survival supplies for U.S. children until the age of 5 years. Every country has some type of plan for ensuring that children's basic needs are met, thanks to the United Nations standards for the basic needs of children (United Nations General Assembly 1989). WIC is an income-driven federal grant program for which Congress authorizes a specific amount of funds each year. Table 9–3 is a quick-reference guide from the U.S. Department of Agriculture summarizing the WIC program.

Early childhood programs vary greatly, but they provide two major types of opportunities for the MHP. First, they offer an excellent screening and intervention point. Second, they offer some family support when an older sibling may be acting violently at school. The medical leader will scan the family and ensure that all their needs and risks are screened and that a plan is made to intervene. This is the level of intervention that is needed to respond to the core problems underlying school violence. It is well known that the early eruption of violence in school is a signal that a pathway is forming to crime, delinquency, and adult offending. The Office of Juvenile Justice Delinquency Prevention (OJJDP) offers publications that support this idea (see http://ojjdp.gov/publications/PubResults.asp?sei=31; also refer to Chapter 7, "Assessment of At-Risk Children").

The higher-SES version of early childhood enrichment is the overinvolved parent pushing and pressuring children to be "at the top." This can result in the children themselves becoming entitled and arrogant. When the parent dismisses signals from the school about the child's coercive behavior, the child becomes increasingly grandiose and may eventually become mean and violent at school. (This pattern is described in Chapter 10, "Risk and Threat Assessment of Violent Children.") Sometimes early enrichment can be overdone, and children are forced into crowded and pressurized after-school programs in academics, music, dance, and sport. The problem is not the lack of involvement of a caring parent, but the constant push to succeed, which leads to a "conditional love" formula. The child begins to believe that he or she has to succeed and excel in order to be loved. As the child develops at school, hostility against the school can build up

TABLE 9–3. Women, Infants, and Children (WIC) nutrition program

Population served

Target population is low-income and nutritionally at risk:

• Pregnant women (through pregnancy and up to 6 weeks after birth or after pregnancy ends)
• Breast-feeding women (up to infant's first birthday)
• Non-breast-feeding postpartum women (up to 6 months after the birth of an infant or after pregnancy ends)
• Infants (up to first birthday). WIC serves 45% of all infants born in the United States.
• Children up to their fifth birthday

Benefits

Supplemental nutritious foods

Nutrition education and counseling at WIC clinics

Screening and referrals to other health, welfare, and social services

Program delivery

WIC is not an entitlement program as Congress does not set aside funds to allow every eligible individual to participate in the program. WIC is a federal grant program for which Congress authorizes a specific amount of funds each year. WIC is

• Administered at the federal level by the Food and Nutrition Service.
• Administered at the state level by 90 WIC state agencies, through approximately 47,000 authorized retailers.

WIC operates through 1,900 local agencies in 10,000 clinic sites, in 50 state health departments, 34 Indian Tribal Organizations, the District of Columbia, and five territories (Northern Mariana Islands, American Samoa, Guam, Puerto Rico, and the Virgin Islands).

WIC services are provided in the following locations:

• County health departments
• Hospitals
• Mobile clinics (vans)
• Community centers
• Schools
• Public housing sites
• Migrant health centers and camps
• Indian Health Service facilities

Source. Adapted from U.S. Department of Agriculture, Food and Nutrition Service: WIC at a Glance. 2010. Available at: http://www.fns.usda.gov/wic/aboutwic/wicata-glance.htm. Accessed December 7, 2010.

and be supported by the parent. This will lead to signals that allow the child to disregard adults at school and use violence to reinforce his or her position.

Special Education

In the United States, one of the most powerful tools for managing school violence is special education. The Individuals with Disabilities Education Act (IDEA; see http://idea.ed.gov/) guarantees a free appropriate public education (FAPE) for all children with disabilities, and Children involved in school violence often have serious developmental or emotional disturbances that require substantial supports in order for the student to receive a FAPE. The special education laws provide for creation of a team that decides whether the student qualifies and makes a yearly plan to meet the student's special needs. Supports in this area are both academic and social-emotional. Once the team determines that the student has a special need, a plan with specific objectives is created to improve the student's chances of learning and succeeding at school (Boundy 2009). When the disability is social-emotional, there may be increased involvement of special needs students in violent scenarios in school as the bully, victim, or bystanders.

The special education process is, as one might imagine, complicated and very highly regulated. States are required to create a plan that meets the goals of the federal IDEA program. Section 504 of the Rehabilitation Act also allows a school to create a plan to respond to a medically documented disability. Schools typically deal with this when a student is physically handicapped and needs assistive equipment in order to access learning environments. When a 504 plan is applied to the social and emotional needs of students, a school can make adjustments that assist in reducing pressure by altering schedules, test taking, marking, dismissal times, and/or choice of teacher and providing special supports during the day. The medical leader is again at center stage in initiating the documentation to allow the 504 plan to be constructed at the school. When a medical professional documents the disability and recommends accommodations, the process can be informally done at schools. Accommodations for disability may be a quick and flexible option to use in combating school violence.

The medical leader may not be the most active participant in the special education process but has a powerful supportive role to play nonetheless. Educational professionals and school and community counselors and social workers are the frontline players at school. The medical professional's role is to support their efforts in documenting a need and creating a plan to meet that need. School violence does not just appear out of the blue at any age. There are always reasons for the violence, but the reasons vary. Diagnosis of the factors involved in school violence is like trying to hit a moving target. There is no one diagnosis or treatment. The intervention is a process. Special education and 504 interventions can be very powerful tools in reducing the incidence of disruption and violence at school.

Special education programs are for public schools only. Like Medicaid, special education is a partnership between state and federal initiatives. Special education requires that the school be financially responsible for services needed to provide a FAPE for all students with a disability. Parents are not financially responsible for services needed in special education, and children in private schools will not benefit from this federal program. The special education and 504 procedures are part of an educational approach known as No Child Left Behind, which is a program that targets disproportionately disadvantaged schools and provides for incentives and penalties based on their performance on state tests (see www2.ed.gov/policy/elsec/guid/states/index.html). The idea behind this approach is to provide schools with a way to measure their performance on state tests and to offer global academic assistance to underperforming schools. The special education laws (IDEA) and Section 504 of the Rehabilitation Act are action programs for specific intervention plans for individual students.

Special education can be the primary arena within which a school violence intervention is planned, implemented, and monitored. It may also be the primary source of support for working or higher-SES families with children in public schools. Private schools do not have the same service demands as do the public schools. Once a school receives money from the federal government, that school is obliged to observe the special education laws.

Juvenile Justice and Family Court

School violence cases often require that the MHP work with a family and the court through the juvenile justice system. This is true in many countries and in most U.S. states. When parents lose control of their children, they turn to the courts for help. In the United States, many states have adopted formal processes to deal with noncriminal but dangerous child and adolescent behavior known as *status offenses*. These are a matter for the court only by virtue of the age of the child and the seriousness of the offense. When a student crosses the line into criminal behavior, the juvenile court will intervene through another mechanism similar to adult court. The major difference between a status offense and a crime can be seen in the difference between bullying (which is dangerous but not illegal) and assault and battery (which is always criminal). From a DSM-IV-TR diagnostic perspective, this may translate to the difference between conduct disorder (tending toward more serious crime) and ODD (status offenses).

Zeke, from our earlier case study, was an example of a child with a conduct disorder. The teacher never filed charges and instead insisted that Zeke's family get help, instead of prosecuting the child for assault with a deadly weapon. Thus, children and adolescents can present with different levels of aggression and court involvement. The MHP needs to understand the exact nature of the child's or adolescent's relationship to the court; this involves discovering 1) whether a status offense or a criminal charge is involved, 2) whether the parent has retained custody of the child or custody has been placed by the court with the state, 3) what the terms of probation are, and 4) the specific status of the student at school.

In most cases, the juvenile will have a contract with the court through the probation department. This is where the MHP can exercise medical leadership in maintaining a focus on the underlying causes and medical basis for the eruption of violent, disruptive, or self-destructive behavior. This focus opens the door to medical and psychosocial interventions that use the community to support positive alternatives that build self-esteem and self-control rather than stress punishment and exclusion from the community.

Courts respect the power of the medical professional. The respect accorded to the medical field can be a source of envy and resentment for frontline workers in the fields of social work, psychology, and mental health counseling. School violence cases will often involve a high incidence of primitive behavior that forces helpers into conflicting roles through projective identification. This splitting "comes with the turf" in treating school violence. The medical leader needs to work on dissolving this useless power dynamic in the treatment team and role-model a shift in focus to the "best interests of the child" (Goldstein et al. 1996) and family. The medical leader also needs to back up his or her frontline troops and not just hide behind a prescribing function.

Probation agreements can be a very useful tool in bridging the gap between home and school, as well as in activating community involvement. The MHP can use these arrangements to structure treatment contracts and may even use the court as the "bad guy" looming in the background. This actually can be a very helpful dynamic so long as it is not overused. When a youth becomes experienced in delinquency and in navigating the juvenile justice or child welfare system, these "good cop, bad cop" approaches lose their therapeutic punch. Nevertheless, the involvement of the court can be a very powerful way to create a protective factor for the school as well as the child. When the community is violent, the juvenile justice system will be a larger part of the school violence problems referred to MHPs.

Using the court in cases with higher-SES families can be even more useful. Often, these cases involve two-parent families with an entitled adolescent who runs the family by threatening aggression. Parents try to take back control, but the teen is in charge. If this is not stopped at the status offense level, it has a good chance of resulting in delinquency. If the state has a status offense provision in family or juvenile court, MHPs are encouraged to support parents in retaking charge of their family and exerting control on their out-of-control adolescent who may be acting out at school and home. School violence often is the reason an adolescent is in the juvenile justice system. Truancy has a very high correlation with crime, drug abuse, and violence (Chou et al. 2006; Hallfors et al. 2006; Henry and Huizinga 2007). The goal of a community intervention in school violence is to create ways to prevent absenteeism and truancy, which are a known gateway to trouble and often begin with aggression at school.

The juvenile justice system will reflect the community's values. Some states punish more than they treat, while others treat more and punish much less. Regardless of the state, the MHP needs to understand how the juvenile justice system works.

Delinquency is a phenomenon of youth that is viewed in many different ways. Aichorn (1963) and Redl and Wineman (1951) offered psychodynamic models that see a youth's delinquent acts as symbolic of his or her internal and social conflicts. Theories on delinquency cover a wide spectrum, ranging from the internal and dynamic to the sociological and political. Regardless of which theory is accepted in a specific setting, medical leadership is key to blending community interventions involving delinquency and school violence.

Child Welfare

In the United States, mandatory reporting of child abuse has created the need to develop a system for intervening in and managing child abuse and neglect. States create policies that reflect federal guidelines and matching reimbursement. States also create laws governing how investigations are conducted, how interventions are made, and how interventions are created as part of child protection. The state may investigate a report, find no abuse or neglect, and close the case. The state may also immediately remove a child suspected of being in imminent danger. Then, usually within 72 hours, there is a hearing in juvenile or family court. If the state removes the child, it may place the child in either foster care or a program, or it may return the child, now under the state's custody, to the family or extended family. A service plan is developed, and decisions are made about the safety of a child in a particular home.

School violence often is acted out by children in the child welfare system. These are children who make the most obvious targets and will have the most pent-up aggression. The neglect at home may lead to an unkempt appearance and eventually to being targeted by peers. Alternatively, children who have become aggressive out of fear of an aggressive caretaker are likely to act out this aggression at school. This is most often seen in the younger grades, when children may have changing caretakers and may witness very intense aggression at home or in the community. Often, these vulnerable children are in the legal and physical custody of the state and live in foster care.

Sacco et al. (2007) described a style of intervention that stresses attachment to a clinic that offers long-term outpatient mental health services. This type of intervention uses Medicaid to intervene in child abuse and neglect families early in the cycle. Children who are in the child welfare system usually are high risk at school. They are easily lured to the extremes of peer culture as bullies or victims. If the child lives in foster care, then the contact person is a state agency case worker and the physical custodian is a foster parent. There is considerable variation in the level of involvement from the child welfare system. This is a factor the MHP needs to assess carefully and thoroughly. While the problems these children present at school are extreme, the level of supportive services may be expanded due to the state custody. Again, this is a variable resource, depending on the MHP's location.

Conclusion: 10 Intervention Truths

The community model featuring strong medical leadership described in this chapter can be applied in any setting. School violence intervention requires the backup of multiple agencies. While delivery systems differ from state to state, certain universal truths apply in activating community resources to respond to school violence:

1. The school needs a partner in control at home.
2. A family needs adults at school to be child-focused.
3. Bullying is psychological humiliation in all schools and at all ages.
4. An active child or adolescent is less at risk than an unsupervised or unattached child or adolescent.
5. Children need to have proper nutrition to learn at their best.
6. Children at risk of being violent at school have a natural support somewhere in the community.
7. Effective school violence interventions in older students need law enforcement help.
8. Truancy is often the gateway to crime.
9. Medical leadership can greatly enhance school violence interventions.
10. Adults need to control the climate at school.

In this chapter we have focused primarily on strategies for funding services or accessing resources. To make recommendations that are realistic and practical, the MHP needs to understand the available funding mechanisms and how to access them. When formal services are not available or are not funded for a particular child, the MHP needs to seek natural supports from the community and the school.

KEY CLINICAL CONCEPTS

- Medical leadership helps unlock doors and document medical necessity; this is a key supportive role for MHPs on the front line of service delivery.

- Many school violence problems stem from medical conditions that are treatable and preventable.

- The MHP is the central figure in this approach to violence prevention and intervention.

- MHPs need to learn what federal, state, and local resources exist. Every state is different, but the needs of the children and demands on the adults are the same.

- Interdisciplinary power struggles interfere with effective treatment of school violence problems.

- MHPs need to keep Maslow's hierarchy of needs in mind when analyzing a school violence problem. Safety is a primary need.

- Medical documentation of a parent's disability can be a critical step in securing basic subsistence requirements for a family. If there is this level of need, no intervention will work, and children's problems will surely spill into the school.

- Eligibility criteria and applications for disability and other programs are available online. MHPs can quickly refer to Web resources to move these processes along.

- Entitlements and benefits have different rules for eligibility, but both require documentation of disability. Medicaid is an entitlement; SSDI is a benefit.

- CHINS or PINS is a juvenile court process for status offenders commonly involved in school violence problems. Most states have these laws, although specifics vary from state to state.

- "Follow the money" refers to the strategy of learning how a family functions by tracing its income sources.

- SSDI is for adults and children. Physicians, nurse practitioners, and psychologists can offer "medical evidence," and the MHP can report as a treating clinician.

- Mental impairments have the same weight as physical impairments in disability law.

- Medicaid is a federal partnership with states to provide for the physical and mental health needs of eligible children age 21 years or younger.

- Early childhood programs offer a unique intervention point for school problems. Early detection is key to preventing violence.

- WIC is an early childhood nutritional and well-child care service available for all Medicaid-eligible children.

- Overenrichment in higher-SES communities can cause pressure and psychological damage to young children.

- Federal special education laws apply to public schools. There are many resources online that can quickly orient the MHP to these laws and how they can be used to solve school violence problems. "504 plans" refers to Section 504 of the Rehabilitation Act of 1973.

- The juvenile court system is a common player in school violence cases. MHPs are urged to collaborate with the probation and court systems in creating interventions for extreme school violence problems.

- School violence often involves children from the child welfare system who become ensnared as either victims or victimizers within unmanaged school climates.

References

Aichorn A: Wayward Youth. New York, Viking Press, 1963

American Psychiatric Association: Diagnostic and Statistical Manual of Mental Disorders, 4th Edition, Text Revision. Washington, DC, American Psychiatric Association, 2000

Bion W: Attention and Interpretation. London, Heinemann, 1970

Boundy KB: The Legal Framework for Meaningful Accountability. Washington, DC, Center for Law and Education, November 2009. Available at: http://www.cleweb.org/sites/default/files/IDA2009S11Boundy.pdf. Accessed March 20, 2011.

Chou L, Ho C, Chen C: Truancy and illicit drug use among adolescents surveyed via street outreach. Addict Behav 31:149–154, 2006

Downes D, Austin MJ: Wraparound services for homeless TANF families recovering from substance abuse, in Changing Welfare Services: Case Studies of Local Welfare Reform Programs. Edited by Austin MJ. Binghamton, NY, Haworth Press, 2004, pp 251–266

Goldstein J, Solnit AJ, Goldstein S, et al: The Best Interests of the Child: The Least Detrimental Alternative. New York, Free Press, 1996

Hallfors D, Cho H, Brodish PH: Identifying high school students "at risk" for substance use and other behavioral problems: implications for prevention. Subst Use Misuse 41:1–15, 2006

Henry KL, Huizinga DH: Truancy's effect on the onset of drug use among urban adolescents placed at risk. J Adolesc Health 40:9–17, 2007

Maslow AH: The Farther Reaches of Human Nature. New York, Viking Press, 1971

Oliver RD, Nims DR, Hughey AW, et al: Case management wraparound expenses: five-year study. Adm Policy Ment Health 25:477–491, 1998

Redl F, Wineman D: Children Who Hate. New York, Free Press, 1951

Rosie D. v Romney, 4101 F.Supp. 2D 18 (D. Mass. 2006)

Smith AD: Medicaid EPSDT and AOD Treatment Services: Policy Brief. Boston, MA, Resources for Recovery, February 2005. Available at: http://www.rwjf.org/files/publications/other/PolicyBriefFinal.pdf. Accessed April 1, 2011.

Sacco F, Twemlow S, Fonagy P: Secure attachment to family and community: a college proposal for cost containment within higher user populations of multiple problem families. Smith Coll Stud Soc Work 77:31–51, 2007

Section 504 of the 1973 Rehabilitation Act, Pub. L. No. 93-112, 87 Stat. 394 (Sept. 26, 1973), codified at 29 U.S.C. § 701 et seq.

United Nations General Assembly: Convention on the Rights of the Child, 20 November 1989. United Nations Treaty Series vol. 1577, p. 3. Available at: http://www.un-hcr.org/refworld/docid/3ae6b38f0.html. Accessed March 28, 2011.

U.S. Department of Education, Office for Civil Rights: Protecting Students With Disabilities: Frequently Asked Questions About Section 504 and the Education of Children With Disabilities. March 17, 2011. Available at: http://www2.ed.gov/about/offices/list/ocr/504faq.html. Accessed April 27, 2011.

U.S. Social Security Administration: Disability Evaluation Under Social Security (Blue Book—September 2008): 12.00 Mental Disorders—Adult. SSA Publ No 64-039; ICN 468600. September 2008a. Available at: http://www.ssa.gov/disability/professionals/bluebook/12.00-MentalDisorders-Adult.htm. Accessed December 7, 2010.

U.S. Social Security Administration: Disability Evaluation Under Social Security (Blue Book—September 2008): 112.00 Mental Disorders—Childhood. SSA Publ No 64-039; ICN 468600. September 2008b. Available at: http://www.ssa.gov/disability/professionals/bluebook/112.00-MentalDisorders-Childhood.htm. Accessed March 20, 2011.

U.S. Social Security Administration: Program Operations Manual System (POMS) Disability Insurance (DI) § 24510.006: Assessing Residual Functional Capacity (RFC) in Initial Claims (SSR 96-8p). May 16, 2008c. Available at: http://policy.ssa.gov/poms.nsf/lnx/0424510006. Accessed April 27, 2011.

U.S. Social Security Administration: Disability Planner: How Much Work Do You Need? March 29, 2011. Available at: http://www.ssa.gov/dibplan/dqualify2.htm. Accessed April 27, 2011.

10

Risk and Threat Assessment of Violent Children

EVALUATING threat or risk in a school is a common role for mental health professionals (MHPs). When someone in the school, a parent, or a law enforcement agency has concerns that someone might be planning an attack or presents an imminent risk of lethal activity, they typically turn to an MHP to evaluate that individual and the larger social context. This process will have tremendous variations for implementation in the school, depending on the country and the community within which the school exists. In the United States, students frequently present situations in which there is suspicion of threat or the risk of violence erupting. In many of the documented school shootings in the United States and Europe, the perpetrator attempted to communicate his intention well in advance of the attack. There are strong commonalities between a threat assessment for violence and a risk assessment for suicide. Since so many of the school shootings across the world end in suicide, it is not surprising that the dynamics of homicidal and suicidal behavior in schools are similar, suggesting that the clinically observable pattern of internalizing anger can lead to depression, followed by explosive rage.

This chapter will outline some threat assessment protocols that have been developed in the United States by the Federal Bureau of Investigation (FBI) (O'Toole 2000) as well as the U.S. Secret Service (Fein and Vossekuil 1997; Fein et al. 1995, 2002), using a case consultation model and, informally, our own consultations using a clinical profiling model (Twemlow et al. 2002a, 2002b). These agencies have studied the process of threat assessment intensively, working from different models of school violence, especially lethal outbursts with firearms.

In countries that are less formally developed than most Western nations in their school systems, the threats and risks may be considerably different. In countries with, for example, flaring ethnic conflicts, threat assessment from an individual within the school is actually quite uncommon. Instead, the threat and risk may be from warring ethnic groups or feuds that have evolved over long periods of time. In Kingston, Jamaica, a number of garrisons have had decades-long feuds that have resulted in Jamaica being in the top three countries in the world for per capita lethal violence (NationMaster 2010). The threat in a school in Jamaica comes from what is outside and reflects the community disorganization that has crippled Kingston.

Threat assessment is a notably broad term encompassing a wide spectrum of possible approaches, depending on the social context of the community where the school is. This chapter will outline an approach to assessing threats that relies on a single principle: a school needs to be protected by its community. This is not "simply" the job of the police force or the teachers. It takes an entire community to protect the school and to prevent children and teachers from becoming targets of random or planned lethal aggression.

Threat of lethal violence and risk of suicide share several commonalities. Both threat of homicides and risk of suicide involve the use of some type of note or communication about the motivation and symbolic meaning of the activity. There is a "leakage," or a pressure release in both suicide and school shootings in which the perpetrator communicates the intention to lash out for whatever reason. There is also a tendency for individuals who are either suicidal or homicidal to disconnect from their normal daily activities, including peer relationships. In both situations involving suicide and those involving school shooters, the student begins to act in radically different ways following certain triggers, usually involving shame and humiliation (real or perceived).

Both homicide and suicide are frequently responses to shame and to the perpetrator's perception of being humiliated. The psychological burden from this shame seems unlikely to end and feels intolerable. When a 16-year-old high school student breaks up with a boyfriend or is the target of sexting, she may think that her life is over and disconnect from her normal relationships. Tunnel vision then comes into play; the young adolescent loses hope, is unable to maintain a wider perspective, and may take her own life to end the shame and humiliation, a pattern typical of the "freeze, flight, fight, or fright" (Bracha 2004) fear-based stress reaction first described by Cannon (1915). This same pattern holds true in school shooters, who have repeatedly been profiled as students who feel persecuted and oppressed by others at the school and eventually shift from the victim role to the victimizer role, becoming their own versions of avenging angels (victims), often with fantasies of martyrdom.

A community must wrap itself around its schools and provide the expertise to evaluate and prevent violence, whether perpetrated symbolically against the school or internalized. As we have noted (see Chapter 5, "Bullying Is a Process, Not a Person"), Gilligan's (1996) concept of shame and its relationship to violence is a guiding principle for identifying trouble spots that may lead to eruptions of lethal violence. In Gilligan's view, preventing violence requires identifying shame and humiliation in its social context. This can be true on an individual basis or in small groups. Whenever an individual or a small group feels shamed, the probability for violence spikes. Even though the assessment of threat or risk is a highly psychological process, threat assessment cannot be accomplished simply by an MHP in his or her office. A thorough investigation of a bomb threat, for instance, will require the coordinated efforts of a team that should be in place prior to the appearance of that threat.

Schools need to prepare themselves by constructing a threat assessment team. The MHP has a key role in assisting law enforcement and school personnel in developing relevant information about the personality of the alleged perpetrator or understanding the family, community, and school dynamics that might be contributing to the difficulties that may motivate the eruption of lethal violence in the school setting. However, there can be many variations in the structure and process of a threat. Many of the elements discussed will be presented in a continuum in order to allow the MHP the opportunity to evaluate dimensions of threat within a variety of different cultural settings. Figure 10–1 outlines the factors that contribute to the social context of mounting threat and illustrates the dialectical connection among variables that could lead to lethal explosions of aggression at school.

Sources of Threat

Threats may occur from within the school or outside of the school. On June 11, 1964, in Cologne, Germany, at a Catholic high school, 11 people were killed and another 22 were injured by an attacker who identified with Adolph Hitler, felt cheated by the government, and had a history of schizophrenia (Wikipedia 2010). With a self-made lance and a flame thrower, he went on a rampage, ultimately committing suicide at the scene. In this case, we see that the source of

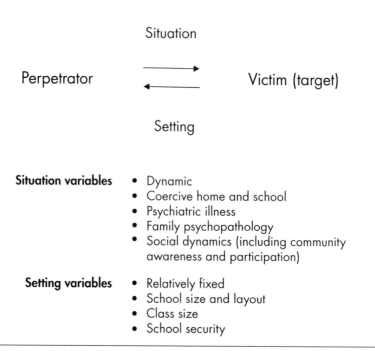

Situation

Perpetrator $\longrightarrow$ Victim (target)
                    $\longleftarrow$

Setting

Situation variables   • Dynamic
                          • Coercive home and school
                          • Psychiatric illness
                          • Family psychopathology
                          • Social dynamics (including community
                            awareness and participation)

Setting variables   • Relatively fixed
                          • School size and layout
                          • Class size
                          • School security

FIGURE 10–1.   The social system and threat.

Source.   Reprinted from Twemlow SW, Fonagy P, Sacco FC, et al: "Assessing Adolescents Who Threaten Homicide in Schools." *The American Journal of Psychoanalysis* 62:221, 2002. Used with permission.

threat for that school was external, with the school as a symbolic target, not the cause of the violence. On December 6, 1989, at the École Polytechnique in Montreal, Quebec, Canada (Listverse 2008), another shooter killed 14 females; his motivation was abstract, but he separated his victims by gender, primarily attacking women. His suicide note indicated that he blamed feminism for his misery.

In these cases and many more that have followed since, the school was a symbolic target for some unique psychological wound that caused deep shame and disruption in the life of an individual. This is a clear example of how the threat existed outside of the school and became acted out inside the school. Similar situations may be faced by schools in communities torn by ethnic violence or urban gang warfare. The threat may be presented by a rival ethnic group or gang. The school may be threatened by virtue of being primarily identified as committed to the education of the ethnic enemy. This type of symbolic targeting is, unfortunately, becoming more common and has spread to places of employment, churches, and school buses that carry children.

The alternative dimension in the social threat is an alienated student within the school who becomes disconnected and explodes into violence as a symbolic expression of his or her experience within the social structure of the school. Most modern school shootings, dating from the 1990s to the present, are examples of this type of process. The source is inside of the school—a student who disconnects from normal peer social interaction becomes alienated and feels terrorized by the social attacks of peers. In Erfurt, Germany, on April 26, 2002, 17 people were killed and 7 more were injured when a gunman dressed in a ninja-style outfit attacked a school from which he had been expelled (Listverse 2008). Again, the student's motivation could be seen as revenge for past injustices, a way to end his mounting misery, based on the perceived rejection and humiliation suffered while at the school. In this case, a legally owned gun was used and adults were targeted.

On April 20, 1999, Dylan Klebold and Eric Harris, students at Columbine High School in Colorado, erupted into violence fueled by feeling persecuted by the "white caps," or socially elite athletic students at the school. They went on a shooting rampage within the school, killing 12 students and 1 teacher and injuring 21 students before committing suicide (Wikipedia 2011a). On October 1, 1997, Luke Woodham, a 16-year-old from Pearl, Mississippi, killed two students and wounded seven others at his high school, as well as murdering his mother. His explanation was that he felt like an outcast. Woodham was "coached" by a group of alienated youth, the Kroth, who helped desensitize him to cruelty by guiding him to torture his dog to death. They were charged as accessories to murder (Wikipedia 2011b).

The Secret Service has developed a list of information to be collected as part of a threat assessment (Vossekuil et al. 2002; see Table 10–1).

On a less lethal scale, there are always outside threats from a school from enraged parents who feel that the school has done their child an injustice. Enraged parents are an omnipresent threat for all schools. Teachers may feel bullied and targeted by specific parents or groups because of their teaching styles or because of issues beyond their scope of knowledge in the child's home. In addition, attacks (mostly nonlethal) of teachers by students have become increasingly common.

A 15-year-old suburban boy was arrested by the police for attacking his mother. His father was abusive toward his mother, and the boy virtually had permission to physically lash out at his mother, modeling what he had seen between his parents. The boy was suspended from school after striking a teacher when she tapped him on the shoulder. He turned and struck her, almost as if he had forgotten he was not at home.

Students who transfer into schools and begin to act out on arrival offer another high-risk situation for teachers, who almost certainly will not be aware of the new student's previous history of gang membership or violent behavior, much less know about the student's difficult home circumstances. In other cases, teachers fail to recognize the stresses that students are under in their personal lives.

TABLE 10–1. Information needed to assess threats of targeted violence in schools

- The attacker's development of an idea to harm the target and progression from the original idea to the attack
- The attacker's selection of the target(s)
- The attacker's motive(s) for the incident
- Any communications made by the attacker about his or her ideas and intent, including any threats made to the target(s) or about the target(s)
- Evidence that the attacker planned the incident
- The attacker's mental health and substance abuse history, if any
- The attacker's life circumstances/situation at the time of the attack, including relationships with parents and other family members, performance in school, and treatment by fellow students

Source. Reprinted from Vossekuil B, Fein RA, Reddy M, et al: The Final Report and Findings of the Safe School Initiative: Implications for The Prevention of School Attacks in the United States. Washington, DC, U.S. Secret Service and U.S. Department of Education, May 2002. Available at: http://www.secretservice.gov/ntac/ssi_final_report.pdf. Accessed April 27, 2011. Public domain.

There are also threats present in every school from peer predators. Predator aggression may be sexual or nonsexual. Predators may be psychopathic children who seek out victims for their own personal enjoyment or who involve more submissive victims in criminal acts or self-destructive activities. Sexually reactive children are an example of how prior victims of sexual assault by adults can come to school and victimize others from inside of the school. This type of threat is difficult to assess; it frequently is well embedded into the social climate of the school.

> Patrick was a 13-year-old middle school student who was repeating the sixth grade because of truancy. He was placed in foster care because he failed to get up every day to go to school. While in foster care, he was molested by an older foster child repeatedly, under the threat of physical harm. When the foster parents discovered the boys "in the act," Patrick was placed in a diagnostic placement for 45 days and then returned home. When Patrick began the new school year, he began to force younger girls into unwanted sexual activity, threatening them with a variety of unpleasant consequences if they were to tell anyone. Eventually, a counselor learned of these acts from one of Patrick's victims, and Patrick was removed from the school, but not before he had molested seven girls in the sixth-grade class.

Young predators are often extremely likable and can easily evade the attention of an MHP seeking to assess the safety of a school climate. This is especially true in schools where the community has little choice in accepting students for public education. These students may be academically successful; however, their behavior presents an ongoing daily risk to the safety of other students and of teachers.

There may also be sadistic adults at the school who will create a threatening atmosphere through their interactions with the children. Such teacher-bullies are frequently embedded in a school and can build and fuel the engine of humiliation that impacts children (as discussed in greater detail in Chapter 5, "Bullying Is a Process, Not a Person"). They may target an individual student or may provoke either a parent or a student into an avenging act at the school. This threat is ever-present and, once again, is difficult to identify within a school.

Another form of predator is one who exists outside of a school. Schools are an open hunting ground for adult predators seeking symbolic targets for gratification of their perverse needs. Many of these compulsive and psychopathic predators see schools as a source of their victims. These outside predators may make their way into schools and may even be part of an assessment of threat. School administration needs to be able to screen personnel to ensure that such predators are not allowed access to the school. This is accomplished by extremely careful screening of volunteers, teachers, and administrative support and maintenance personnel.

Threats from the outside can also exist on the way to and from school. For example, in Jamaica, families are responsible for ensuring that their children have a way to get to school. The government plays no role in transportation; children are forced to find a way to get to school by linking up together and taking route taxis to and from school. This can be a terrifying experience if there are adults who prey on children or older children who are aggressive or behave sexually inappropriately toward children on their way to schools. Clearly, children who face such traumatic experiences while traveling to school will be in no state to behave calmly, much less study and learn, once they arrive. In more developed countries, children may also become targets for aggression or bullying on the way to school from other students or from members of the community. In the United States, a great deal of aggression occurs on school buses, which—by combining students of diverse ages from different neighborhoods—become a compression chamber for students to act out bullying behaviors such as inclusion and exclusion, teasing, taunting, and physical intimidation.

Individual Versus Group Threat

A school violence threat may be part of a pattern that involves an individual or a group. In both cases, the individual or group becomes disconnected from normal social structures and feels targeted and shamed. Isolation from normal social activities creates an environment within which the shame and humiliation can become compressed, evolving into a motivation that drives lethal behavior. The isolated victim may begin by discussing feelings of shame and the need for retribution with similarly humiliated peers. This may evolve into a group that becomes a defined and disconnected social entity, or it may begin that way until one individual remains fixated in this socially alienated space.

Threat can also be generated by a sadistic bully who is allowed to take control of the peer culture within any one school. One sadistic and psychopathic student can wreak havoc within a school if adults cannot contain his or her behavior. In such cases, the sadistic bully often works as part of a small and informal group of friends who play a bystander role in the evolution of the aggression or bullying within the school.

A school violence threat can stem from a predator living in a student's home who negatively influences the student's behavior to such a point that it bleeds over into school and the community. A student who is being aggressively or sexually abused at home over a long period of time can present a real source of threat within a school climate. The student may be so victimized that he or she will become the prime victim in the evolution of a violent act at school. The student may also react in the opposite fashion, becoming sadistic or aggressive and presenting a threat to other students. Predators at home or in the community represent a source of threat that needs to be assessed and monitored regularly.

Students may be pressured to join a group that exists inside or outside of the school. Groups organized around hate themes, such as skinheads or neo-Nazis, may have a strong influence on the behavior of a student at school or on his or her way to school. Urban gangs with drug distribution motives can often exert tremendous pressure on children entering middle school. Threatening recruitment practices are common in such gangs and need to be monitored by law enforcement personnel working closely with schools and MHPs.

Threat can also be generated by peer group gangs formed in a middle school in which recruiters act in small groups to involve students in their criminal activities. The aggressive peer group disconnects from the mainstream culture and uses the school as a place to distribute drugs, recruit new members, and assert dominance by using violence. Teachers are often limited in their ability to interact with students in such groups and may themselves become targets of aggression, property crimes, or other forms of intimidation. This is clearly a law enforcement issue and not one that is easily managed by schools alone. MHPs must understand this and not place themselves in a position of trying to take on the challenge of dealing with this type of criminal activity within the school.

The highest level of risk is presented by the "injustice collector" who feels superior to others around him and develops a sense of entitlement. The organized violent social group is a counterpart to this and may be either a peer group engaged in criminal activities or an alienated group of peers organized around perceived injustice or shame. In either event, the individual or the group becomes disconnected from normal adult containment and is allowed to escalate within the school setting, developing a threatening climate from which a violent act may be generated.

Bion (1959) emphasized that the group and its members are a single functioning unit that cannot genuinely be studied in isolation. From Bion's point of view, the group leader is endowed with the fantasies of the group's members. In a school characterized by pathological dependency, teachers and other staff may believe, for example, that the principal will take care of their needs and will mobilize police and school security to protect them, so there is little impetus for them to do anything within classrooms or within school organizations to ensure safety. Bullying creates a dangerous school environment, one in which a student who feels hurt and blamed can reactively attack as a form of self-defense or retaliation. Teachers can provide guidance in such situations that is often missing, especially in schools that overemphasize academic achievement or that underemphasize it and overemphasize maintaining safety.

Cyberbullying

In today's environment of seamless Internet connectivity, a single individual can impact an entire school culture through the use of cyberbullying. An individual can sit in his or her home and create a tremendous amount of shame in a school setting by attacking other students via the Internet. This can become a group function through the use of social networking and other ways in which inclusion and exclusion can be used by groups of students within the school setting to generate shame and humiliation, fueled by the relative anonymity of the Internet. The organized groups can become extremely destructive by using their online social networks as generators of shame and humiliation. These networks can share hurtful images, messages, and campaigns that are designed to assert their social superiority at the expense of weaker individuals (Kiriakidis and Kavoura 2010; Tokunaga 2010).

The Web offers a shield that can be used to generate hate and social aggression. This creates a blurring of the boundary between home and school. Bullying on the Internet and digital phones is inescapable; modern youth are haunted by the ever-present existence of virtual reality and texting. What happens at school follows the student home and is amplified across large groups of peers online. There are an increasing number of suicides resulting from the shame generated by sexting or the distribution of erotic digital images of romantic teen partners who break up and post private images for public view. The tragic case of Jessica Logan (Celizic 2009), who committed suicide after her ex-boyfriend posted explicit and intimate pictures taken during their romantic relationship, is an example. Threats can also be transmitted through vicious text messages that can cause extreme reactions in the intended victims, as occurred in the case of Phoebe Prince in South Hadley, Massachusetts, in 2010 (Kennedy 2010). Twemlow (2008) has pointed to the role of violent video games and Internet immersion in the Columbine school shootings:

> There has also been further research on Columbine, as the diaries of Klebold and Harris were recently made public. The research suggests that both were strongly influenced by first-person shooter video games, including "Doom" and "Quake." Some have pointed out that their interest approached the level of an addiction. Their parents restricted their computer use after a criminal trespass indictment, suggesting that this restriction may have precipitated the immediate attack on Columbine, by denying the "drug" and the sublimatory outlet it provided.
>   Immersion in the virtual world is immersion in the unreal world of melodrama. In this world, human relationships and problems are oversimplified. The user controls the input, with endless repeating reinforcing at the will of the user. Over time, the shooter's world is defined by virtual relationships, not real people. Pain and its consequences are tidied up.

There is little doubt that the Internet and cellular phones have created new ways to compress and distribute shame and humiliation. Students obtain phones and Web access from a very early age, for many beginning in elementary school. This virtual world is peer-run and insulated from adult supervision. Many parents try to monitor their children's Internet use, but most simply cannot keep up with their children's activities in a plethora of virtual social worlds.

Impulsive Versus Planned Activity

Aggressive behavior within schools can be seen as reflecting a continuum. At one end is an impulsive eruption of violence, often the result of a feud concerning romance, criminal turf, or perceived verbal shaming. Impulsive actions can also involve vandalism or delinquent acts perpetrated in the school or around the school. For example, fire setting is an impulsive act that may be part of the larger delinquent behavior of a small group. The more impulsive types of violence are more often seen in urban public schools, where there are higher rates of poverty, crime, and serious addiction and more dangerous neighborhoods.

The other end of the continuum is represented by a planned and targeted lethal act by an individual or group seeking vengeance for a perceived humiliation or a series of shaming events associated with or generated from the school. This pattern of violence, which is deliberate rather than impulsive, is exemplified in the large-scale school shootings that are mainly a suburban school phenomenon. The repeated devaluation of a single peer group is often the origin of these high-profile cases. These groups are targeted by the larger school community,

TABLE 10–2. Characteristic patterns of violence in lower- versus higher-SES schools

Urban (lower-SES) schools
Shame-based impulsive reactions to perceived public humiliation
Crimes of passion
Romantic feuds
Clashes between cultures and/or races
Presence of organized street gangs

Suburban (higher-SES) schools
Planned revenge/retaliation after long-term exposure to shame
Targeted/planned acts
Indiscriminate targets
Prolonged social aggression

Both lower- and higher-SES schools
School toleration of social aggression and bullying
Intense social pressure to fit in and be seen as powerful
Increased availability of/access to firearms, aggressive Internet/other media, drugs

Note. SES = socioeconomic status.

and the humiliation is compressed through the dismissiveness of the adults within the school setting. The net result is a pressure cooker that allows the formation of groups that pull away from normal social containment and evolve into potentially lethal home-grown terrorist groups attacking the school.

Table 10–2 offers a rough overview of general tendencies in the expression of violence at school. These are not rigid categories, but rather are overlapping trends that are characteristic of different types of schools.

Forming a Threat Assessment Team

Clearly, threat needs to be assessed from a multidimensional perspective. We strongly advise MHPs not to attempt this task on their own (Twemlow et al. 2002a, 2002b). The development of a threat assessment team is a necessary prerequisite to adequate assessment of a school threat. It should be readily apparent to the MHP that multidimensional threat assessment is a task beyond the scope of a single person's capacities and vision.

The FBI and the Secret Service agree that a multidisciplinary team is required for threat assessment. For example, when an investigation of a home computer is needed during a threat assessment, law enforcement is usually at the forefront of this part of the assessment and needs to work closely with a team member from within the school, as well as an MHP (Twemlow et al. 2002a, 2002b), in order to obtain a wider view of the nature of the threat. Thus, the threat assessment team should have representatives from at least three areas: education, mental health, and law enforcement.

There are a number of formal and informal approaches to filling these three functional positions in creating a team. In regard to the educational component, all schools have a principal or vice principal who is responsible for the overall well-being of the school. This educator is the leader of the group that is threatened. There may be informal structures within the community that may need to fulfill this function for the school. The school could be a rural village school that may need the elders of the community to play the roles of the protectors of the school. Teachers are valuable resources in this area and often have the frontline awareness of what is happening day to day in the school. This perspective needs to be thoroughly represented in any attempt to assess threat within the school.

For the mental health component, an MHP from outside the school is a valuable asset to any threat assessment team. School counselors inside the school can team up with an outside expert to provide a thorough assessment of personality, family, and community dynamics. It is this outside MHP who plays a valuable role in assessing the variables that may be embedded within the school.

The third component in a threat assessment team is law enforcement. It is critical to be able to investigate elements of a threat that go beyond the realm of an MHP or educator. For example, many indicators of threat can be found by reviewing a student's home computer, investigating the criminal activities of a student in the school, or assessing lethal potential from organized groups outside the school. If the threat is seen as involving an organized criminal gang within the school, or if the signals of threat take the form of increasing vandalism, small fires, graffiti, and other "quality of life" crimes, investigation is the job of law enforcement; their participation in analyzing threats is essential to gathering the scope of information needed to make an accurate threat assessment. Conversely, if the threat comes from an alienated group of students who feel they are being left out of the mainstream of the school, assessment of the individual personalities and social dynamics by an MHP working with an educator may be the best initial approach. Moreover, in some situations, calling in the police too early can be unnecessarily alarming to parents and the community, as well as potentially damaging to the child involved, as the following example illustrates.

> We encountered a fourth-grade boy who was reported to the principal of a public charter school by an enraged parent who had received a macabre poem promising death and other violent actions against that parent's daughter. The poem contained lines such as "Because of love, you will die and I won't cry." It also made reference to stalking: "I watch you; you can't escape my love." The school reported the incident to the police, who visited the boy's home but found no evidence of stalking or weapons collection. The student did not have access to a

computer at home. The mother of the threatener asked for a psychological evaluation after her son was suspended for 3 days. The psychologist interviewed the student and his family. The poem had been a peer prank that was not meant to target that specific girl. The boy was socially inept and a follower. He had participated in the writing of the poem titled "Love and Death" on the school bus, and he clearly identified himself as the author. The evaluation pointed to the student being a victim of group pressure to participate in a joke that went bad; he was sufficiently victimized to take a risk to get attention. The family was referred for counseling, and no criminal charges were made. The student, once intermittently explosive, is now in the sixth grade and shows no signs of violence.

Conducting a Threat Assessment

Two distinct models of threat assessment have emerged from the work done by the FBI and the Secret Service. These models differ in their orientation to important variables to assess in the evolution of a threat.

The FBI model (O'Toole 2000) stresses personality variables and takes a so-called profiling approach that identifies a type of person that past experience has found to be at risk of erupting into lethal violence. Profiling of school shooters was accomplished through detailed interviews of school shooters who survived the attacks, as well as long-term interviews and conferences that brought together schools that had experienced shootings with FBI profilers and international experts. By contrast, the Secret Service model (Fein et al. 2002) takes a more action-focused approach, beginning with the threat and evaluating what concrete actions have been taken to plan the threat, acquire materials, or recruit accomplices. One way to summarize these differences in approach is to say that the Secret Service focuses on WHAT action has been taken, whereas the FBI focuses on WHO is taking it; however, there is much overlap in the two approaches.

Threat assessment typically begins when there is some sign that an individual or group has expressed an intention to strike out and hurt someone else, or another group of individuals. In the United States, this phenomenon is quite complex and can range in intensity from an elementary school student who makes a list of children to kill to a community college student who constructs an elaborate plot to blow up his school and attack his or her teachers. In other countries (especially when there is a more agricultural community and less formal educational structures), violence may be more likely to stem from generational feuds or personal vendettas that can brew for months or years before being acted out at the school. This type of threat is frequently related to long-standing grudges and clashes in communities that are struggling for basic survival, as we saw in Jamaica (Twemlow and Sacco 1994). In some countries, there are extensive protocols and highly complex legal processes that create civil opportunities to hold schools accountable for keeping children safe. In other countries, threats to survival stem from either ethnic tension or grudges.

Regardless of the context, there is a need for the MHP to assume the role of conducting an investigation into whether there is a threat. Threats of self-harm need to be taken seriously every time. Such threats may not all be part of a person's plan to hurt themselves; however, they all represent an extreme form of thinking that has a high probability of presenting a risk or threat to an individual or group.

Approaching the question of whether a threat exists has some universal principles that can be customized to virtually all schools or communities. The first step in assessing any level of threat involves contacting the child's custodian—that is, the parents or primary caretakers. This custodian assessment is either performed by an MHP working within the school or subcontracted out to a community MHP. The custodian assessment may also begin by making arrangements for someone in the school administration to contact the parents or caretakers to inform them that the child has become involved in a situation that presents a potential threat to his or her safety. Often this initial contact with the parent can offer many rich clues into the social context and whether the individual making the threat is in a fertile environment to present a real threat of direct action at school.

It is at this point that a threat assessment team can be most efficient. The team may be quite informal, or it can become highly structured and develop specific protocols that will outline steps that all agree will be essential for a quick, fair, and sensible response to various levels of threat coming from within the school or in the community.

Assessment of a potential threat requires the coordinated efforts of three disciplines: law enforcement, education, and mental health. Investigating a person's home usually falls within the realm of law enforcement and involves the seeking of court permission to enter and seize items that might be relevant to the investigation. It may also involve enthusiastic collaboration by a worried parent or caretaker. Similarly, law enforcement is usually the first responder when a specific threat is made concerning the use of an explosive in a school. Law enforcement's investigation of a home setting is a specialty that is outlined in two documents developed by the FBI (O'Toole 2000) and the Secret Service (Fein et al. 2002). Detailed outlines of how to approach the home setting and how to search for evidence of preparation for an attack are available to assist law enforcement (O'Toole 2000) and to protect the rights of both the individual and the larger community.

The search begins with assessment of Internet-connected devices and provides an opportunity to trace whether someone is engaged in actively researching weapons or methods for committing large-scale violence. This search clearly is not the job of an MHP, but rather is in the realm of law enforcement. This stresses the point of the need to develop collaborative strategies between disciplines in responding to violence. There cannot be turf-related battles when it

TABLE 10–3. Levels of threat

Level I (low)	Indirect and vague
	Details inconsistent and implausible
Level II (medium)	Direct and specific
	Details plausible
	General indications of place and time
	No definite indications of preparation
	May say, "I am serious"
Level III (high)	Direct and specific
	Details plausible and possible
	Steps have been taken to prepare
	Has means, method, and motive

Source. Reprinted from Twemlow SW, Fonagy P, Sacco FC, et al: "Assessing Adolescents Who Threaten Homicide in Schools." *The American Journal of Psychoanalysis* 62:223, 2002. Used with permission.

comes to sharing of information and the development of theories relating to threat assessment.

The next step involves gathering as wide a spectrum of evidence as possible to determine the context and the nature of the threat. In addition, as much data as possible need to be gathered concerning the person making the threat and the potential victims. A safety plan is essential to ensure that all precautions are taken to act as if there is a threat until an extensive investigation can be conducted. There are clearly different levels of risk that are identified and can be used in this initial phase of assessment. These levels will be clear to the MHP responsible for assessing suicidal risk. The type of thinking involved in making a threat is eerily similar to that of someone who is suicidal. In fact, in school shootings in the United States and around the world, the most likely outcome for the person making a threat is a suicide or attempted suicide. The "avenging angel" either destroys himself or places himself in a position where law enforcement is forced to use lethal force to protect the hostages. In any event, the net result is that the behavior is predictable and can be evaluated.

The levels of threat presented in both the FBI (O'Toole 2000) and Secret Service (Fein et al. 2002) guidelines are very similar to the way a clinician evaluates suicide potential: does the student have means, method, and motive? Ratings of threat involve a three-level scale, with Level I being mildest and Level III being the most specific or severe (see Table 10–3).

A Level I threat is a general expression of a wish to destroy or hurt an individual or group. This level of threat is often found in younger children and may be an expression of growing frustration due to a number of factors, such as learning disabilities, social disadvantage, or child abuse. A Level I threat can be easily identified because it is only verbal and does not show behaviors consistent with the threat. Think of the typical angry outburst from someone who is chronically unhappy with the way he or she is treated at school. There may also be lists from children wishing that they could destroy a certain group of peers whom they see as socially humiliating. This is happening at increasingly earlier ages because of acceleration of children's consciousness due to the Internet and other connectivity devices.

A Level II threat is more serious and involves the expression of a more highly specific and targeted threat. This might be the naming of an individual with mention of a specific weapon to be used and may also involve a person taking action in the form of research, recruitment, or targeting of a victim. This is a more specific and plausible expression of an intent to do harm to someone else. At this level of risk, there clearly is a law enforcement component and there needs to be some type of intervention that protects any known victims or separates the individual making the threat into a therapeutic context for the reestablishment of control.

A Level III threat is a critical level of evaluation. At this level, there is a clear, distinct, plausible activity expressed by a person toward the targeting of a victim or group of victims. At Level III, the person has demonstrated the ability to access the materials to construct a lethal device, has conducted specific research for carrying out a plan for a lethal attack, has developed strategies for targeting victims, and has sent messages created before or after completion of the act. At this level, it is clear that the individual or the group is organized around the idea of disconnecting from normal social values and attacking the symbolic target. This is a very credible and serious level and definitely needs to involve and include law enforcement. This is an extremely high level of risk and is statistically quite uncommon. Nevertheless, closer studies of school shootings around the world clearly suggest that this level is reachable for many young people. As fewer resources become available to identify and prevent the conditions that lead to social humiliation and alienation, these threats become real. There is an eerie pattern as to how school shootings have unfolded around the world; many of them revolve around symbolic dates (e.g., Columbine, which was planned to commemorate the birthdate of Adolph Hitler).

In 2001, a California community college student was discovered in the final stages of planning an attack on his school. He was caught when an alert photo development clerk noticed that he had taken pictures of himself and all the materials he had collected for the attack. He had researched the materials and their acquisition on the Internet; he had amassed detailed maps of the school, had selected specific targets, had written a postattack essay, and had made an audiotape explaining his actions. This was all accomplished in his family's home without anyone noticing and with no other "leaks" or indirect communications. There was little need to further analyze this case to establish the threat. The police responded to the photo clerk and, upon investigating the young man's home, found clear evidence of his plan.

Keeping in mind the cautions we have already clearly identified, although the analyst may feel most comfortable assessing the inner world of the child making a threat, his or her role as a member of an interdisciplinary team requires a mutual sharing of responsibilities with team members taking (and even emphasizing) other approaches.

The creation of a safety plan is a set of steps that is taken after information is gathered and initial assessments are made. In Level I threats, schools can use a variety of approaches that involve community MHPs and become part of a strategy that is taken over by the parents. If the parents are cooperative in a Level I threat, it is then possible to create a therapeutic response to the expression of frustration and aggression contained in the threat. This may involve weekly individual or family psychotherapy, psychiatric consultations, brief inpatient or residential state programs, or a combination of these community and mental health interventions.

Case Example: Henry, the Bully-Victim; Is He a Killer?

Henry was a 15-year-old boy referred to me at the insistence of the principal of a parochial school he attended, although his parents thought the referral unnecessary. Beginning about a year before, Henry had decided, as he said, to get people's attention even if he could not be popular (his mother said that Henry's friends "put up with him"). He decided to get attention in other ways. He had noted the publicity surrounding the Columbine tragedy and was openly jealous of the attention focused on this carefully engineered slaughter. Henry liked playing video games, particularly violent ones, and he specified the video game "Doom," which he called "a splatter game." He also liked listening to hard-core rap music. These interests were the antithesis of what his parents desired for him. In May of the year of referral, he had downloaded some printed material from a Web site on how to make pipe bombs and developed a hit list of individuals who had bullied him—including some drawings indicating how he would shoot them. His family physician had put him on Zoloft (sertraline), but there was not much change in his behavior, and he was in danger of being expelled from school (after having been suspended for a total of 13 school days in the previous year).

Although Henry described himself as endlessly bullied and picked on, the pattern that he demonstrated in his relations with peers was what we would describe as bully-victim; that is, like a provocative victim, he would often act passively, provoking others into responding to him in a bullying way, and then he would bully back.

His parents were both religiously and politically conservative; his mother was working as a librarian, and his father was a car salesman who was on the road a great deal of the time. His father also presented an openly aggressive manner, with keen interest in the brutal aspects of ice hockey, and was the proud owner of an extensive collection of guns and knives. As an only child, many of the family's wishes and expectation were invested in Henry. Discussions with teachers indicated that, as one teacher said, "when the predator is looking for prey, Henry is it." He was described as an open target, as if he were inviting abuse. The bullying included sexual taunting and taunting for being held back at kindergarten (at the request of his parents, who at the time did not think their son was emotionally mature enough to progress with his peers). Henry had been on Ritalin (methylphenidate) for many years for attention-deficit/hyperactivity disorder (ADHD) and had been a high-performing student, although at the time of referral he was doing poorly at school.

When I met with Henry, he spoke mostly about how unpopular he was, how he did not have girlfriends, and that he envied people who were athletic and handsome, even though he himself was not an unattractive-looking boy; he was somewhat gangly and rather clumsy for his age, but had nice features. As he began to trust me, he spoke more of his worries, the major one being that his father constantly put him down and called him stupid, as if he could not learn. I had an opportunity to observe his father in action; Henry's mother, although quite aggressive in her own right, adopted a very passive stance with her husband and would often burst into tears, especially when he was sarcastic with Henry. When Henry bullied back, he picked mainly on girls, since he was stronger than they were, and of course this did not increase his popularity among other girls, boys, or schoolteachers.

The parochial school he attended had a serious problem with coercive power dynamics; that is, there were many power struggles at the school that were denied by the staff, with a rather naively positive attitude taken in spite of some quite serious fights at the school. References to faith in God and religion were often used to avoid dealing with the fundamental power struggles.

In the middle of this morass of negativity and cynicism, this depressed young man would brighten visibly when he spoke of how good a salesman he was; he had sold a great deal of cookies and candles to raise money for the Boy Scouts and had received a prestigious award. An insurance agent friend of his father had said, "He speaks like a lamb and sells like a lion." The attempt to identify with his father's strength as a salesman was very clear, but when Henry would speak about this in family sessions, his father would sarcastically downgrade his actions, almost as if he were envious of them.

Henry felt that the diagnosis of ADHD had always made him different. He hated going to the nurse to get his Ritalin, since he was often called "crazy" by his peers. Yet, in class, he often acted like a clown, making noises to draw attention to himself. He would rather have the teacher report him and suspend him than receive no attention at all. In spite of his "I don't care" attitude toward his schoolwork, I learned over the period of assessment that he often obsessed for many hours over homework and then, of course, was sleep-deprived. At night, he tried to drown out troubling homicidal thoughts by playing his boom box loudly, and then he would nod off in the classroom the next day.

On one occasion, he attracted the attention of a Drug Abuse Resistance Education (D.A.R.E.) police officer. When asked what he liked to do in his spare time, Henry said that he liked to play violent video games to take his anger out in them. The officer reported him, and again he felt misunderstood because he thought that he had been taught it was good to get his anger out. His mother conveyed quite clearly that she was frantic that her efforts had produced a "monster," and Henry conveyed this to the officer, whispering to me, in his presence,

"How did we produce a child as sick as this?" As the contemptuous abuse at home and the peer bullying and stigmatization by teachers and administration and resource officers at school mounted, Henry became increasingly sadistic, destroying property and overtly bullying children who were limited intellectually or had physical deformities. He openly expressed satisfaction when he could dominate and hurt them, thus appearing even less likable and more sadistic.

Psychoanalytic evaluation revealed a boy with many as-if personality traits. The intensity of Henry's rage at his father's bullying and his mother's passivity resulted in a pathological identification with a perversely exaggerated twin identity, which both expressed his rage by embarrassing his father and adopted his father's phallic destructive interests. His personality lacked depth and conviction, except in the long nights of cyberfantasy, rap music, and trying to do his homework. As Kernberg (1984) emphasized, Henry's defective sense of self was clearly protected by a pathological paranoid grandiosity enacted at night in the privacy of his room, while during the day he retreated to an as-if passive victimization. Meissner (1988) called this the victim-introject.

Henry responded quite well to psychoanalytic expressive-supportive psychotherapy and aggressive physical outlets (martial arts) that were used with him in a therapeutic way. He was transferred to a public school setting where he felt less oppression from organized religion and from the more-affluent children. He did quite well in this setting; his self-esteem improved, and his need to receive copycat recognitions, both by adults and peers, decreased. As he became less and less needy for attention, he became more attractive to girls and was able to have normal dating relationships. The initial transference to me was quite stereotyped; he clearly did not expect help from anybody, as if he had virtually given up on adults or any source of help (as had the school shooters). His one outstanding skill was selling; it was an attempt to mimic in a normal twinning way, and to achieve some support for his growth and development from his father.

Family therapy was very helpful in teaching Henry's father to avoid contempt and bullying and to encourage his parenting skills. Henry acted out, in the transference, his well-known pattern of having to please the male, and he became fairly open about his expectations that women were worthless, passive, and weak. His oedipal defeat, actualized in the home setting, was able to be more normally traversed when he began to be able to see defects in his father and take them less personally, as the negative oedipal fixation was resolved. As he became less murderously angry, he also lost interest in karate, but thanked me for making the referral, which he felt had helped him. His interest in violent video games gradually changed, and he seemed to reenter a normal adolescent identity search. His parents, however, did not do well as he improved, and they ended up in a cold and hostile relationship, although the holding of the therapeutic relationship helped Henry traverse the marital distress without boundary diffusion and immersion in their psychopathology. I continued seeing him until he finished high school; after that, as expected, he left his distressed home at the earliest opportunity.

There may also be a school component in the response to a Level I threat; it may involve some type of disciplinary activity or some inclusion in supportive or creative peer socialization approaches. There are a host of possible ways in which a youth with this level of confusion who makes a threat can be reworked back into the community. (For an example, see Sacco and Larsen 2003.) In Henry's case, the threat assessment was awkwardly applied, while psychotherapy was expertly used and resulted in the student's reentering the school and completing a community college education.

Responding to Level II threats is more complex and will require the involvement of probation or some other type of law enforcement activity. In a Level II threat, there is clear intention to do harm. These threatening activities can be seen as either delinquent or criminal acts or an indication of a mental health or substance abuse issue. Simply referring a Level II threat to a community resource (such as therapy) and quickly returning the student to school may fail in protecting the school from possible eruptions of aggression from that individual making a Level II threat.

There are a number of approaches in the juvenile justice system geared toward communicating that certain behavior has crossed the line and could result in serious imprisonment. This is an approach that is best combined with a rehabilitative strategy that includes educational enrichment, mentoring (see Chapters 7, "Assessment of At-Risk Children," and 8, "Activating Community Resources Through Therapeutic Mentoring"), and after-school activities. These approaches are powerful and can involve the family. If the family is incapable of supporting this type of intervention, then state intervention may be required to ensure that all adults take the evaluated Level II threatening behavior seriously and not place the larger community at risk.

In a Level III threat, a real dilemma exists and has become a crisis. At this level, a person is probably within 72 hours of committing a lethal act. Evidence is collected that supports a criminal charge; the response to this may be primarily through the correctional system. There are a variety of alternative methods of responding to this type of threat, however. It is essential to remember that the most effective response is not assessment, but rather a prevention approach that encourages peers to report to adults when threatening behavior is expressed in the school. If an overly punitive zero-tolerance approach is taken, peers are less likely to be open about communications that might be early indicators of an impending threat to a school within the community. Responses to Level III threats need to have as their primary focus the protection of the school and of the larger community; however, an effort should be made to create the most humane response to the individual making the threat. Intervention at this point could allow the individual to remain in society without forced incarceration for long periods of time.

Clinical Profiling

The classic FBI approach to threat assessment (O'Toole 2000), which uses demographic and psychological profiles of violent perpetrators in similar cases, is one that is quite familiar and has many parallels in the field of mental health. DSM-IV-TR (American Psychiatric Association 2000) is a type of clinical profiling approach in which groups of characteristics are defined to form a diagnostic syndrome. They clearly do not define an individual, but they do cluster symptoms in such a way as to allow for a descriptive formulation of problems. The FBI gathered its information by interviewing school administrators and counselors from schools where shootings had occurred. A personality type did emerge from this profiling experience that can be a useful guideline in the hands of clinical MHPs.

The Secret Service approach (Fein and Vossekuil 1997; Fein et al. 1995, 2002) holds that no one individual personality type is more likely to commit a threatening act. While that may be true, and there are certainly many instances where false-positives may occur, a skilled MHP can help to understand the general type of person most likely to engage in such acts.

The individual who commits a school shooting can often be described as a grandiose "injustice collector." This type of individual feels superior to others around him and frequently makes complaints. This is in contrast to the more oppositional and defiant student, who will make trouble rather than constantly feel aggrieved by a sense of being misunderstood and mistreated. The pattern of feeling cheated and humiliated will be present in many types of threat assessment areas. Government agencies and religious groups frequently are attacked, and school shootings are occurring in older grades and post–high school (college) settings. There is a common element in many of these shootings that is rooted in this personality style of an irritated and grandiose individual who believes that the world has wronged him or her. This type of person can leave school and become involved in workplace violence or other random attacks on symbolic targets.

When this type of individual is forced to participate in a social system that is dismissive and allows humiliation, we have the beginnings of a dangerous social context for the incubation of violence. When a person is sensitive to injustices and feels easily bruised by shame and humiliation, a dangerous cycle begins. The ongoing shaming will fuel fantasies that become extremely violent. The victim feels persecuted, unheard, and isolated and subsequently disconnects from normal peer and authority social structures and escapes into a violent fantasy world. The essence of this world is retribution and the creation of an identity of an avenging victim. The Internet is an ideal environment in which to incubate this type of disconnected individual.

When people "escape" into virtual reality, they encounter many opportunities to gain information that can be used to fuel their violent fantasies and eventually to create the means and opportunity for the creation of plans, and any genetic or environmental predisposition to mental health problems becomes similarly aggravated. Attachment trauma can be easily reactivated. The fact that many school shootings result in suicide at the scene may indicate that the mechanisms of isolation and detachment from normal sources of social support are quite similar. There are other eerie similarities between suicide and the evolution of a school shooter. In both cases, the individual who has withdrawn into disconnected and isolating violent fantasies often sends out signals, usually to friends. These signals will increase in frequency as the individual moves closer to implementing a plan of lethal activity (O'Toole 2000). Again, this potentially deadly aggression can be targeted against the individual him- or herself, in the case of suicide, or against a symbolic target—the school—in the case of the shame-based humiliation personality.

An analysis of the home lives of many of the school shooters (O'Toole 2000; Twemlow 2008) revealed that their parents can often be characterized as dismissive. There was a pattern in the families of the school shooters where the shooter was viewed within his family as the "king of the roost." Families were thought to be fearful of the individual making the threats, who frequently was quite aggressive at home and felt tortured and tormented. Many parents were also distracted by their own problems or the strains of work. These families were also likely to have registered firearms, and the school shooters frequently used them in their rampages. Parents would frequently try to indulge their misbehaving child, creating a dismissive family environment where the individual could continue to isolate himself in his violent fantasy at home, assisted by unmonitored Internet access.

Families were frequently seen as being protective of the individual making the threat (O'Toole 2000; Twemlow 2008). The dismissive parents would frequently point fingers at the school, blindly protecting their child in any school dispute. The family rarely was active in the school (in the form of participation in parent groups) and thus was "dismissing" the value of school activities and unconsciously siding with the child. Families of school shooters were also likely to allow the youth far too much freedom at home. The school shooters were given privacy beyond what was reasonable and frequently would become aggressive if their right to be secretive was challenged by the parents, as illustrated in the case of a child in a two-parent home who was involved in a nonlethal school shooting. The child had literally created a tunnel of sheets so that the father would not see the sadomasochistic pornography, neo-Nazi propaganda, and transcript of the 15-year parole hearing of Charles Manson on the walls of the bedroom. The father meekly lived under the same roof as his child, yet never saw nor questioned the cover-up of these obvious clues of trouble in his own house (O'Toole 2000; Twemlow 2008).

Clinician Safety: Assessment of Personal Risk

The unexpected death on September 3, 2006, of Dr. Wayne Fenton, a division director at the National Institute of Mental Health (NIMH) and a prominent schizophrenia expert, illustrates the tragic irony of risk assessment, especially among experts. Dr. Fenton was seeing a patient with paranoid schizophrenia during the weekend at the special request of the patient's father. The renowned psychiatrist was mercilessly beaten to death in his own office. This case has raised many important questions about how MHPs should deal with high-risk consultations in the confines of their offices, often away from any easily available help.

With school-age children, awareness of personal risk may come up in the form of assessing an adult-sized adolescent who has been sexually mature for many years and is quite aware of his or her rights and the vulnerabilities of the MHP. Many experienced therapists are unaware that this type of attack can occur even with a patient the therapist has known for several years. The other problem is the question of our collecting reliable and valid evidence for serious attacks on clinicians. According to the Department of Justice (Friedman 2006), mental health workers have an annual rate of nonfatal job-related violent assaults of 68.2 per thousand, compared with a general rate for physicians of 16.2 per thousand. There is conflicting evidence regarding the prevalence of violence in mentally ill people. Strict mental illness, as such, contributes very little to violence in the population overall. Estimates of 3%–5% or lower have been made (Friedman 2006). Furthermore, it is important to note that substance abuse disorders account for the majority of violence in mentally ill populations.

Psychotic thinking that influences behavior, a history of violence, and significant concurrent substance abuse are psychiatric conditions with the highest risk of violence. A prevalence study of older adolescents also suggested that the presence of Cluster A and B personality disorder traits, together with paranoid, passive-aggressive, or narcissistic personality traits, had the highest association with violent behaviors (Johnson et al. 2000).

To enable a clinician to conduct a useful interview under potentially dangerous conditions, four main elements are needed (Twemlow 2001). The first element, *self-awareness,* especially awareness of early signs of fear and of transference and countertransference, works together with skill in establishing a therapeutic alliance and adopting a stance that conveys empathic attunement to the sources of the patient's anxiety. Safety checklists do not replace this important step.

The second element is *clinical knowledge of the psychiatric diagnosis and prior assessments,* such as psychological tests that have been made. These offer the clinician an opportunity to identify risky behavior or tendencies. The third element is *clinician self-care,* including attention to the client's personal, physical, and emotional needs, along with self-defense and de-escalation talk-down skills that MHPs should include as part of their own self-care inventory. Finally, *provision of a safe environment,* particularly an office environment with attention to obvious issues like seeing such patients during office hours with help and protection, and, if necessary, an arrangement of office furniture that ensures easy escape and the avoidance of objects or articles of clothing that can be potentially provocative or hazardous. The MHP needs to pay special attention if he or she is practicing in a setting with a violent young adolescent, who often will act before thinking, let alone speaking.

Certain automatic prejudices may sometimes influence the MHP in making these assessments. For example, the idea that violence is much more prevalent in men than in women, although true in prison populations, where the majority of inmates are male, is certainly untrue in hospital populations, where hospital incidents of violent behavior are shared equally between genders (Platts and May 1998). Awareness of the language and colloquialisms of the patient is critical. In certain cultures, it may be important to have an evaluator who is of a similar culture or who understands the cultural role of the family and the importance of cultural myths and language. For example, an African immigrant psychiatrist mistakenly decided to use Haldol (haloperidol) for a patient because the patient had said he wanted to "get this monkey off his back," referring to his wife, whom he was in the process of divorcing. If a child is violent, it will be very difficult to read individual nonverbal cues. By nature, violent individuals are suspicious of conveying anything to you, seeing this as a potential loss of control.

Although there is some evidence that command hallucinations are not an accurate indicator of violent behavior (Hellerstein et al. 1987), these symptoms are still considered an important part of an assessment of immediate violence risk. It is important to be nonconfrontational and very open in what one does, including avoiding note-taking altogether or else taking notes that the patient can see. The Hare Psychopathy Checklist (Hare 2003), which places strong emphasis on violence history, has outperformed sheer violence history as a predictor (Gray et al. 2003). What can be said about psychological scales? Their results should not be ignored, but of course there are no 100% reliable predictors of violence; therefore, such scales should be used as confirmation only. The value of scales depends on the therapist's knowledge of the populations surveyed, how the scale is standardized, the sample size, and whether the patient is on the extremity of a scale score, just to name a few of the many possible variables. Commonly used instruments include the Violence Risk Appraisal Guide (Quinsey et al. 2006) and the Historical/Clinical/Risk Management–20 (HCR-20) violence risk assessment scheme (Webster et al. 1995, 2009; updates also available at http://kdouglas.wordpress.com/hcr-20).

False-positives are very common; unfortunately, so are false-negatives. If in doubt, when the MHP is attempting to establish the risk for impulsive violence in a patient, he or she should not hesitate to use a trusted and experienced colleague as a consultant. Figure 10–2 is a decision tree that illustrates one way of assessing an individual patient who is being seen in an MHP's office as part of a threat assessment initiated by school referral.

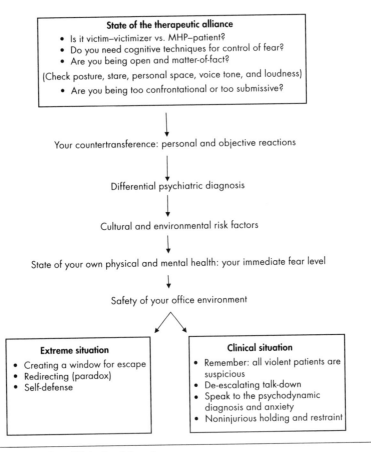

FIGURE 10–2.   **Risk decision tree.**

Conclusion: Climate Change in the School Social Context

We attended the Leesburg Conference,[1] which offered the opportunity for personnel from 18 schools that had experienced shootings to meet with experts and FBI profilers for a week to reflect on what may have been happening in the

---

[1]The Leesburg Conference, held in 1999 and sponsored by the Critical Incident Response Team of the FBI's Behavioral Sciences Unit, involved 18 schools that had experienced school shootings, experts on various forms of violence, school personnel, attorneys, police, and FBI profilers. The conference findings were reported in previously cited FBI references (O'Toole 2000).

schools and the shooters' worlds. The majority of the conference's participants agreed that most suburban schools contain a student who would fall within the category identified as being at high risk for this behavior by this group of schools that had experienced shootings. There was vigorous debate about the role of athletics in the evolution of the school environment that created the elite social group of athletes viewed as the enemy by the Columbine shooters.

There were also many contradictory communications about the roles of athletics and the "in-crowd" phenomenon as they related to any specific shooting. In some instances, privileged athletes did play a role in fostering a coercive environment. It was not a consistent pattern across all of the school shootings, since other intensely competitive activities like forensics and debate can create similar reactions over focus, yet there seemed to be a more common element. The concept of a dismissive school environment was hypothesized to explain how schools could be distracted by everyday demands of being academically strong and athletically well developed. Communities expected their schools to be places that children could attend and excel at athletics, forensics, debate, or other activities.

Schools can analyze their own climates and begin the process of making them more peaceful. We believe that every school has a climate that is unique to itself; thus, each school's social system, even within the same district, is unique. This requires that the adults create simple, sustained programs geared toward identifying coercive patterns of behavior, bullying, repeated victimization, and availability of positive outlets. This participation and awareness that young people form groups that can be destructive are necessary components of a successful program. Our recent research in Jamaica proved that content is less important than process in developing violence prevention programs (Twemlow et al., in press). Adults at all levels of a community need to become actively involved in strengthening their schools' climates, offering a positive, safe, and creative place for the community's children to be educated.

KEY CLINICAL CONCEPTS

- Threats to schools can originate from inside the school or from the outside. The school may also be a symbolic target.

- Threat of lethal violence and risk of suicide share several commonalities. Both homicide and suicide may be responses to shame and to the perpetrator's perception of being humiliated.

- A school violence threat may involve either an individual or a group. In both cases, shame and resentment from feelings of being ostracized can become compressed, evolving into a motivation that drives lethal behavior.

- Cyberbullying (including texting, sexting, and sharing of photo-graphic images) represents a new and extremely destructive form of social aggression.

- Aggression at school can be impulsive and reactive or planned and predatory.

- Affluent and lower-SES schools differ in how threat is expressed. In lower-SES schools, the threat is often in the context of criminal adult gang activity. In higher-SES schools, threat often takes the form of social aggression involving exclusion and humiliation.

- Threat assessment teams should include at least one educator, one law enforcement official, and one MHP from inside or outside the school.

- The FBI and the Secret Service have developed detailed ap-proaches to threat assessment of school violence.

- A three-level system is used in threat assessment to rate risk:

  — Level I: mild — improbable

  — Level II: moderate — probable but not likely

  — Level III: serious with specific target, means, and motive

- There is a strong similarity between threat assessment of school shootings and that of suicide. In addition, many school shootings result in the suicide of the shooter at the school.

- The classic profile of a school shooter is a grandiose "injustice collector" who feels persecuted and eventually shifts from the vic-tim role to the victimizer role of "avenging angel."

- In assessing a student who has made a threat, the following factors are important: 1) previous warning communications, 2) ambiguous messages, 3) availability of guns, 4) victimization by social groups or individuals, 5) concern expressed by adults or peers, 6) mimicry of media figures, 7) changes in emotions and interests, and 8) fam-ilies low in emotional closeness and knowledge of the adolescent's life.

- Clinicians need to be alert to personal safety risks. When conduct-ing a threat assessment under potentially dangerous conditions, four main elements are needed: 1) self-awareness, especially awareness of early signs of fear and of transference and counter-transference; 2) clinical knowledge of the psychiatric diagnosis and any prior assessments; 3) clinician self-care, including attention to the client's personal, physical, and emotional needs, along with self-defense and de-escalation talk-down skills; and 4) provision of a safe environment.

References

American Psychiatric Association: Diagnostic and Statistical Manual of Mental Disorders, 4th Edition, Text Revision. Washington, DC, American Psychiatric Association, 2000

Bion W: Experiences in Groups. Basic Books, New York, 1959

Bracha HS: Freeze, flight, fight, fright, faint: adaptationist perspectives on the acute stress response spectrum. CNS Spectr 9:679–685, 2004

Cannon WB: Bodily Changes in Pain, Hunger, Fear and Rage: An Account of Recent Research Into the Function of Emotional Excitement. New York, D. Appleton & Co., 1915 (see http://www.archive.org/details/cu31924022542470)

Celizic M: Her teen committed suicide over "sexting." Today Parenting, March 6, 2009. Available at: http://today.msnbc.msn.com/id/29546030. Accessed December 6, 2010.

Fein RA, Vossekuil B: Protective Intelligence and Threat Assessment Investigations: A Guide for State and Local Law Enforcement Officials (NIJ/OJP/DOJ Publ No 170612). Washington, DC, U.S. Department of Justice, 1997

Fein RA, Vossekuil B, Holden BA: Threat Assessment: An Approach to Prevent Targeted Violence. Research in Action (NIJ/OJP/DOJ Publ No 155000). Washington, DC, U.S. Department of Justice, 1995

Fein RA, Vossekuil B, Pollack WS, et al: Threat Assessment in Schools: A Guide to Managing Threatening Situations and Creating Safe School Climates. U.S. Department of Education, Office of Elementary and Secondary Education, Safe and Drug-Free Schools Program and U.S. Secret Service, National Threat Assessment Center, 2002. Available at: http://www.secretservice.gov/ntac/ssi_guide.pdf. Accessed December 7, 2010.

Friedman R: Violence and mental illness: how strong is the link? N Engl J Med 355:2064–2066, 2006

Gilligan J: Violence: Reflections on a National Epidemic. New York, Vintage Books, 1996

Gray NS, Hill C, McGleish A, et al: Prediction of violence and self-harm in mentally disordered offenders: a prospective study of the efficacy of HCR-20, PCL-R, and psychiatric symptomatology. J Consult Clin Psychol 71:443–451, 2003

Hare R: Psychopathy Checklist–Revised, Second Edition. Toronto, ON, Canada, Multi-Health System, 2003

Hellerstein D, Frosch W, Koenigsberg H: The clinical significance of command hallucinations. Am J Psychiatry 144:219–221, 1987

Johnson J, Cohen P, Smailes E, et al: Adolescent personality disorders associated with violence and criminal behavior during adolescence and early adulthood. Am J Psychiatry 157:1406–1412, 2000

Kennedy H: Phoebe Prince, South Hadley High School's "new girl," driven to suicide by teenage cyber bullies. New York Daily News, March 29, 2010. Available at: http://www.nydailynews.com/news/national/2010/03/29/2010-03-29_phoebe_prince_south_hadley_high_schools_new_girl_driven_to_suicide_by_teenage_cy.html. Accessed December 8, 2010.

Kernberg O: Severe Personality Disorders: Psychotherapeutic Strategies. New Haven, CT, Yale University Press, 1984

Kiriakidis SP, Kavoura A: Cyberbullying: a review of the literature on harassment through the Internet and other electronic means. Fam Community Health 32:82–93, 2010

Listverse: Top 10 worst school massacres. January 1, 2008. Available at: http://listverse.com/2008/01/01/top-10-worst-school-massacres/. Accessed December 7, 2010.

Meissner WW: Treatment of Patients in the Borderline Spectrum. Northvale, NJ, Jason Aronson, 1988

NationMaster: Murders (per capita) (most recent) by country. 2010. Available at: http://www.nationmaster.com/graph/cri_mur_percap-crime-murders-per-capita. Accessed December 7, 2010.

O'Toole ME: The school shooter: a threat assessment perspective. Federal Bureau of Investigation, National Center for the Analysis of Violent Crime, 2000. Available at: http://www.fbi.gov/stats-services/publications/school-shooter. Accessed December 7, 2010.

Platts WE, May JR: Defending against violence in hospitals. J Healthc Prot Manage 14:1–7, 1998

Quinsey V, Harris GT, Rice M, et al: Violent Offenders: An Appraising and Managing Risk, 2nd Edition. Washington, DC, American Psychological Association, 2006

Sacco FC, Larsen R: Threat assessment in schools: a critique of an ongoing intervention. Journal of Applied Psychoanalytic Studies 5:171–188, 2003

Tokunaga RS: Following you home from school: a critical review and synthesis of research on cyber-bullying victimization. Comp Hum Behav 26:277–288, 2010

Twemlow SW: Interviewing violent patients. Bull Menninger Clin 65:503–521, 2001

Twemlow SW: Assessing adolescents who threaten homicide in schools: a recent update. Clinical Social Work Journal 36:127–129, 2008

Twemlow SW, Sacco F: Psychodynamic approach to reduction of violence in Montego Bay. Psychiatric Times, Vol 9, No 2, 1994, p 36

Twemlow SW, Sacco F: Peacekeeping and peacemaking: the conceptual foundations of a plan to reduce violence and improve the quality of life in a midsized community in Jamaica. Psychiatry 59:156–174, 1996

Twemlow SW, Fonagy P, Sacco FC: Assessing adolescents who threaten homicide in schools. Am J Psychoanal 62:213–235, 2002a

Twemlow SW, Fonagy P, Sacco FC, et al: Premeditated mass shootings in schools: threat assessment. J Am Acad Child Adolesc Psychiatry 41:475–477, 2002b

Twemlow SW, Fonagy P, Sacco FC, et al: Reducing violence and prejudice in a Jamaican all-age school using attachment and mentalization approaches. Psychoanal Psychol (in press)

Vossekuil B, Fein RA, Reddy M, et al: The Final Report and Findings of the Safe School Initiative: Implications for The Prevention of School Attacks in the United States. Washington, DC, U.S. Secret Service and U.S. Department of Education, May 2002. Available at: http://www.secretservice.gov/ntac/ssi_final_report.pdf. Accessed April 27, 2011.

Webster CD, Eaves D, Douglas KS, et al: The HCR-20 Scheme: The Assessment of Dangerousness and Risk. Burnaby, BC, Canada, Mental Health, Law, and Policy Institute, and Forensic Psychiatric Services Commission of British Columbia, 1995

Webster C, Bloom H, Augemiri A: Violence risk assessment in everyday psychiatric practice: twelve principles help guide clinicians. Psychiatric Times 26(12):1–4, 2009

Wikipedia: Cologne school massacre. November 2010. Available at: http://en.wikipedia. org/wiki/Cologne_school_massacre. Accessed December 7, 2010.

Wikipedia: Columbine High School massacre. May 2011a. Available at: http://en.wiki- pedia.org/wiki/Columbine_High_School_massacre. Accessed May 4, 2011.

Wikipedia: Pearl High School shooting. April 2011b. Available at: http://en.wikipedia. org/wiki/Pearl_High_School_shooting. Accessed May 4, 2011.

11

Effortless Wellness and Other Afterthoughts

WHO would not want to be well? It seems a self-evident truth, one endorsed by all medical organizations, and most recently by health insurance companies, who even pay for it. The World Health Organization (1948) considers health to be more than the absence of disease, but rather a state of optimal well-being. So instead of merely curing illness, we now may achieve wellness, which (according to the American Holistic Health Association [2003]) requires "balancing the various aspects of the whole person"—physical, emotional, mental, and spiritual.

The American Holistic Health Association (2003) offers a Wellness Quiz consisting of the following questions: "Do you wake up with enthusiasm for the day ahead?" "Do you have the high energy you need to do what you want?" "Do you laugh easily and often, especially at yourself?" "Do you confidently find solutions for the challenges in your life?" "Do you feel valued and appreciated?" "Do you appreciate others and let them know it?" "Do you have a circle of warm, caring friends?" "Do the choices you make every day get you what you want?" The quiz ends with the statement, "If you answered 'no' to any of these questions, congratulations! You have identified areas in your life that you may want to change." A similar organization, the American Holistic Medical Association (www.holisticmedicine.org), has a medical focus combined with the integration of health-promoting strategies from other cultures, such as acupuncture, but has more recently also embraced wellness concepts.

Violence is obviously very far from wellness and will not be cured by exercise, diet, or feeling better about oneself. What, then, establishes wellness? The answer depends on complex personal and situational factors that are different for everyone. Typical of our individualistic American society, setting and achieving individual goals is deeply ingrained in how we think. The problem is that all too often we are not thinking in terms of collaboration and being a piece of the puzzle that is an open social system. People must accept that they must adjust in concert with all the other individuals in their worlds as each social system changes. If we don't feel interdependent and connected passionately to the community, we have very little likelihood of achieving optimal well-being individually—or even a much lesser state, the absence of violence in our school system.

> A young man came to my office a few years ago with a clear clinical history of dysthymia. He had been referred to a managed care agency provider, who gave him a written list of things to do and think about that would "cure" his depression, including daily exercise, positive affirmations, reframing his negative thoughts, getting a hobby, and so on. When he had returned a month later feeling no better, the therapist simply told him, "Okay, but this is still all you need. When you are ready to follow the written treatment plan, your symptoms will clear up!"

With his detective-like mind in the early days of his writings, Freud was perplexed by patients who would not change themselves, in spite of a detailed explanation of the reasons for their mental illness and its obvious negative impact on their lives. He became impatient, dogmatic, and at times angry about it all, and yet it remained a mystery to him. He discovered that the answer to the problem is captured in a phrase he coined, "unconscious resistance." Human beings consciously resist change for many different conscious reasons, but the hidden, unconscious reasons are the core problem; change threatens their transferences by arousing deep and primitive fears. It is said that Freud discovered this while standing in for a mentor of his who had become too attached to his patient, the later-famous "Anna O." While his chief, Breuer, was taking a second honeymoon (impelled by his wife's jealousy about Anna O. and the time her husband had spent with her), Freud, the student, discovered that Anna O. had fallen in love with Breuer, which she demonstrated by responding to Breuer's care (hypnosis) with miraculous results, provided that he hypnotized her every day. She even had a pseudocyesis when Breuer was away! Freud called this *transference*; the transference is of earlier or current feelings or ideas about relationships (in Anna O.'s case, earlier sexual love for her father) to those who are current reminders (triggers) of those other relationships (in this case, Freud's chief, the well-known and brilliant neurologist Josef Breuer).

The technique of looking carefully at the unconscious of our patients remains an essential part of psychiatric care to this day. Karl Menninger, arguably the founder of American psychiatry, wrote a book called *Man Against Himself* (Menninger 1938). His view of the unconscious was that the battle between unconscious self-destructiveness and human survival was an urgent one, demanding that we all be aware of the unconscious choices we make between survival and death. Modern medicine is now giving us many useful tools to manage change, and has produced a concept of wellness that could be achievable if combinations of conscious "cognitive-behavioral therapy," and unconscious "psychoanalytic therapy" treatments were used in harmony with other extraordinary developments in the genetic understanding of individualized appropriate drug selection, neuroplasticity, brain dynamics, and neuroscience. We may be moving rapidly to truly individualized treatment in a psychopreventive biosocial fashion, but this is still prevention after the proverbial chicken has flown the coop.

One expectation of optimally healthy individuals is that wellness would be *effortless.* They would simply integrate healthy actions and thoughts into their day-to-day activities, go to the gym, and behave constructively without a second thought. To do well, one must wake up to the extraordinary preciousness of being well in oneself. Many individuals have been inspired to wellness by a serious illness and or a near-brush with death (Kelly et al. 2007; Twemlow et al. 1982). A close call can awaken us to the urgency and immediacy of the value of life itself. Sometimes this experience is felt to be religious in the literal or sacred sense. More humorously, a great samurai once said that one should live each day as if a fire is raging in one's hair! It is what one might call waking up, coming out of the trance of life, or coming face to face with the light of pure reality. Not all of us (especially children) have had this "opportunity," nor would we actually want to have a near-death experience.

How, then, can we provide an environment in which we can learn to be well effortlessly and painlessly? As with everything else, it begins in the cradle. Children learn a lot through imitation. They imitate parents and parent surrogates in great detail, not just in broad brushstrokes. They automatically imitate modes of eating and talking, like and dislikes in food, accents and mannerisms, ways of managing conflict and trauma, and values, and they do it mainly unconsciously. Sometimes it's a trivial matter; for example, one day I noticed that one of my daughters was eating in a European way, although she had never been outside America. She was imitating her father. But think of a child who has been brought up to think that physical violence is a way of solving problems through imitation of his father's physical approach to his mother and his policy of beating up those who disagree with him. That child then goes to school and beats up other students, and ends up in serious trouble.

What Is Psychological Wellness?

In general, the literature on wellness deals variably with the topic, often focusing on things one does for oneself to remain well: having healthy attitudes, eating organic foods, getting aerobic exercise, avoiding addictive substances and habits—the list is literally endless. While all of these things are part of wellness, a resistant individual in Freud's sense will have great trouble doing any of them and may prefer instead to be a couch potato just because it's easy and it feels safe and familiar. The pleasure principle underlies the human behavior that moves us in that direction: we want to indulge our impulses and we want to do that whenever we want without regard for the welfare of others. The reality principle, where we have to recognize the reality that other people exist, is not easy for us to adopt and accept.

We know that the infant from birth is amazingly open to learning; besides acquiring language, infants are immensely influenced by parents' modeling, especially during the first 5 years of a child's life. Values learned in childhood may become habits of thought that persist throughout life. If one assumes that values such as physical wellness, eating healthily, exercising, and avoiding addictions will be resisted by long-standing irrational habits of thought, then modeling healthy behavior by parents is essential. But the parents themselves may not be sufficiently inspired by the idea of wellness, and they, too, may have a wide variety of ways to rationalize the meaning of life so that there isn't any real point to being well—for example, people will never change, it will be too costly, why try—and so the problem becomes a vicious cycle, continually renewing itself. There are two flaws in these rationalizations, however.

The first flawed assumption is that a change in a macrosystem, such as the population of a large school district or a city, requires *all* individuals within that system to change. However, behavioral studies indicate that this is simply not true. What we *don't* know for certain is what percentage of a population needs to change in order for that change to be reflected in the population as a whole in some significant way.

Research done with transcendental meditation (Brown and Edelson 1990) derives a concept from physics, suggesting that if 1% of a chemical solution changes, there will be visible macromolecular changes in that solution. This idea was applied to a variety of small towns where at least 1% of individuals meditated. The reports, composed during a phase of great public interest in transcendental meditation (between about 1970 and 1980), strongly suggested that such cities became much less violent and that overall crime rates declined. Although the validity of this literature has been sharply questioned (Carroll 2010), whatever the actual percentage of a macrosystem may be that needs to change is not going to be anywhere near 50%. So why not begin wherever we are, and see where we can go with wellness? We referred earlier (in Chapter 5,

"Bullying Is a Process, Not a Person") to an experience we had in Jamaica, where a "Tuck your shirt in!" chant was set to reggae music and quickly became very popular in the school. It had a remarkable effect on children's levels of tidiness and reduced violence in the school; kids were too busy being tidy to fight! Current literature suggests a number of innovative ways to create a craze. In *Switch: How to Change Things When Change Is Hard*, by Chip and Dan Heath (2010), a slightly modified table of contents gives us a series of clues: Direct the Rider, Find the Bright Spot, Script Critical Moves, Create a Destination, Motivate the Elephant, Find the Passion, Shrink the Change, and Shape the Path: Tweak, Rally the Herd, Build Habits, and Follow Through.

The second flawed assumption by those who prematurely give up on pursuing a heathy lifestyle is that wellness cannot be made palatable to children. Most gyms, for example, ban children under the age of 12 because of the potential risk of harm from improperly using the exercise machines. How about a child-friendly gymnasium? How about integrating schooling with home care? For example, offer schooling for children from the age of 2 years and onward. This would provide an alternative to child care and would enable children to learn languages quickly, as their brains are ready for language early. Such a measure would also allow socialization into effortless wellness thinking to happen. Of course, this also implies massive change in the training of teachers in social and emotional development, as well as intellectual education. Yet we have seen far too many situations in which a school will choose to build an athletic stadium rather than provide essentials for learning, like air conditioning in classrooms.

Could there be another missing piece in this jigsaw puzzle? In our opinion, success in achieving wellness goals has a great deal to do with how a nation's leadership selects priorities for the population. For example, Norway has been more successful than any other country in reducing bullying in schools, with the credit for that success largely due to a research psychologist, Dan Olweus (1993). His research is widely known and extremely well done. In fact, it prompted a Norwegian government manifesto (Zero Bullying) to be instituted in September 2002. Follow-up studies (Roland et al. 2010) showed lasting changes in Norwegian schools after the manifesto, opening up a sensible theory: if a government can be persuaded to list a series of basic psychologically healthy attitudes as primary policy priorities, such as managing bullying in the home, the school, and the workplace, a U.S. manifesto could follow suit, placing the focus where real and long-lasting good can be done in a proactive (rather than reactive) way.

A nonexhaustive list of matters that would ensure the wellness of children and for which immense amounts of data exist include the following:

1. *Be a "good enough" role model for your children.* Nobody's perfect, but children can respond to trauma without lasting damage if supported by their parents, especially when children are young (Vaillant 1977/1995). Many be-

lieve that coping with trauma and conflict is part of growing up. (An excellent book for parents by Steven Marans [2005] spells this out in user-friendly language.) Evolution and the way the human mind works has prepared children perfectly to learn from adults; what we have to do is model emotional health for our children, including how one develops a sense of oneself, what some would call an identity. Being comfortable within yourself, knowing who you are, even if you can't specify it in detail. These factors do not require an encyclopedic study, nor do they require medical visits. They do require family discussion and the sort of things that families discuss, such as setting priorities for what children consider important as they grow up. It is crucial to note that children well into young adulthood are highly impressionable, without much discrimination. Then, in adolescence, the parent is like a totem; children develop an identity by challenging the totem. Yet we still have to find coherent ways of establishing a wellness theme to take advantage of this impressionability of children. We pay far less attention to children's learning and wellness than we do to the cure of physical illness in older adults.

2. *Watch what your children watch in the media.* Don't just monitor how much sex and violence they may be exposed to, but pay special attention to reality television and to the range of commercials focused on children as young as 18 months. When children have questions about the validity of what they are looking at or how representative it is of human behavior, be prepared to discuss it.

3. *Watch for and take care of any subtle variations in your children's intellectual skills; don't deny them.* Take care of problems as early as possible, because the discovery of mild learning disabilities, dyslexia, social skills deficits that exist in the autism spectrum disorders, and mild impairments in visual and auditory learning can vastly affect the self-esteem of highly intelligent and competitive young people, who end up trying to hide the defects (often quite successfully) with issues like drug dependence presenting as a primary problem. Having intellectual deficits can be more socially disadvantageous (in terms of associated stigma) than having a bona fide psychiatric illness.

4. *Discuss the human mind and its various stages with your children.* What are dreams, and why is the night so often scary when you are little? How does a security blanket and imaginary playmate help young children feel safe? What are the stages of life? What is an adolescent and why are children's moods so variable during adolescence? What is a young adult and why do they constantly change what they believe in or what they want to do? What are the priorities and responsibilities for a fully grown adult? What is a midlife crisis, and why is it a crisis? What happens when you get older? These are all moments in the normal life cycle, explained and described in a classic and beautifully written passage in Erik Erikson's *Childhood and Society* (Erikson 1963).

5. *Care for the environment (what today is called "living green").* The countryside is a great deal more than what Edward O. Wilson in 1984 cynically called "the space between cities to a city dweller." The ecosystem imprints itself on the human mind, either by its presence, for those brought up in a rural environment, or by its absence, for those brought up in a large city. Nature should be a part of every child's life—not just taking care of it, but understanding *why* one takes care of it. Many believe that the ecosystem is a critical part of normal ego development and that awareness and love of nature creates a respectful mind-set that includes safe feelings and care about what goes into one's body.

6. *Encourage your children to think things through.* Thinking about thinking (mentalizing) and solving problems has been related to helping people maintain their intellectual integrity throughout maturity and old age. It is very important that all children, as part of growing up, learn to think through problems, learn to live with problems for which solutions are not known, and learn to collaborate with others in creating solutions where possible. Christopher Lasch, in *The Culture of Narcissism: American Life in an Age of Diminishing Expectations* (Lasch 1978), took us to task for being too self-absorbed. Thinking through involves recognizing and valuing interdependence, not independence.

7. *Do good for others.* We have touched on the idea of being altruistic from time to time in this book. As one Zen master said to a student who asked how he could help himself, "Help others." We found this to be an extremely useful attitude to take in managing school violence and in motivating the helpful bystander into altruistic actions. Philosophers have long debated whether or not altruism is an absolute quality or egoistic. We can accept the fact that there is an egoistic quality to altruism, so that practically speaking, being altruistic doesn't mean being a saint. Altruistic companies (like Hallmark Cards), strongly suggest that helping others and being good to employees can be financially profitable, as well as improve the quality of life for many. There are psychotic forms of altruism where the grandiosity in the individual is clear, and there are religiously fanatical do-gooders who are really trying to get you to do good in order to help them complete part of their religious obsession. We are not speaking about doing good in any of these ways, but merely realizing that when you do good for others, you do good for yourself; if everybody helps everybody, then the job gets done. Evolutionary psychology suggests that altruism in the form of attendance to one's own relatives ("kin altruism") or reciprocal altruism where you do good for others with goals similar to yours (to help them succeed or to help you succeed) is essential to human survival. Existing data strongly suggest that altruism is worth encouraging in your children, not in a fanatical or religious way, but merely as a part of what we have called "effortless wellness."

8. *Use leisure time for leisure.* Maybe this sounds simple, but in our hard-working society, having fun without regard for concrete work benefit is extremely difficult. European cultures see work as work and leisure as why you work and what you dress up for and enjoy. A colleague of mine lecturing in Norway felt a little overdressed in his suit and tie when his introducer was in shorts and unshaven, as were most of the professional audience. Determined to be culturally appropriate, he later dressed down for the evening banquet without tie and wearing slacks and a sports jacket. He walked into a room in which his hosts were all in formal wear and tuxedos! Workaholism is killing us as a nation and immensely injuring our families. Do your children have to be shut out of your professional life and cared for by an expensive nanny? No. Take your children with you where and when possible. Mine did ward rounds, assisted me in surgery, and visited hospitalized patients on their own. They were part of the practice.

This list can go on and on. Please add to it. Is the new generation any different? There seems to be general agreement that this is the case, but perhaps not necessarily—just indulged, lazy, and overly self-focused?

The Rise of the Millennial Generation

A CBS News story broadcast in May 2008, titled "The 'Millennials' Are Coming" (Safer 2008), observed:

> There are about 80 million of them, born between 1980 and 1995, and they're rapidly taking over from the baby boomers who are now pushing 60. They were raised by doting parents who told them they are special, played in little leagues with no winners or losers, or all winners. They are laden with trophies just for participating and they think your business-as-usual ethic is for the birds. And if you persist in the belief you can take your job and shove it.

What data exist to support this view? A research study conducted by MonsterTRAK (now MonsterCollege) and the Michigan State University Collegiate Employment Research Institute (Chao and Gardener 2008) followed 10,000 young adults between the ages of 18 and 30 years; 700 managers who employ young adults were also surveyed. Questionnaires were used to compare these young adults' attitudes toward work and managers' views of these young adults, particularly how they perceive them at work and what they are doing to attract and retain them.

In a much less dramatic way than the CBS story, the findings suggest support for the story; young adults are less interested in money and much more interested in good health benefits, job security, and their chances for advancement and promotion. Managers are more pessimistic than young adults are of themselves, and they perceive them to be less focused on work as a central life interest, compared with their own ratings of themselves. In other words, young adults did not indicate that work was a central life interest for them. Managers generally perceive today's young adults as believing themselves superior to others and yet not having clear goals for themselves. Sixty-four percent of managers felt that retaining young adults has become more difficult in recent years, and managers have often hired consultants to learn to manage this particular group of millennials, using organizational feedback about performance or awards for performance in the form of praise, bonuses, and mentoring relationships with senior organizational members. Young medical school graduates, for instance, realize that medicine provides "only" a good middle-class income, but they are okay with that, as long as the medical practice provides interesting patients, and the workday ends at 5 o'clock!

Clearly, for many millennials, their other life activities are as important to them as their work. What relevance does this have to stopping school violence? We think it offers a very hopeful angle. The millennials are clearly not participating in the compulsive work ethic that places the United States among the hardest working in the world, after South Korea and Japan. Perhaps the millennials will be more in control of themselves, especially more able to draw the limit at compulsive working. Imagine a young person in a high school who focuses his or her attention on personal health and happiness through exercise, yoga, or meditation, rather than a group of children utterly overwhelmed by the horrors of survival itself, with few psychological coping skills. We feel that schools can assist in improving the quality of children's lives, including their personality, outlooks, and beliefs, by setting up wellness centers, for instance. From this study of the millennials, it appears that many young people are quite ready for such wellness centers and may be even enthusiastic about them.

Overcoming Resistance to Change: Toward Successful Implementation of School Antiviolence Programs

As Vernberg and Gamm (2003) wrote in their articulate summary paper, most scientists who have worked in school systems to implement social interventions agree that it is very difficult to enact any social change without a culture that accepts that change. If *culture* is defined as traditional ideas and values that are learned, shared, and transmitted from one generation to the next, such ideas and values represent ways groups of people have learned to respond to life's problems (Sue and Sue 1999). Vernberg and Gamm (2003) suggested that there are beliefs in U.S. society that encourage aggressive behavior, thus creating barriers to effective violence prevention. Olweus (1993) proposed that bully–victim interventions rest on the fundamental belief that children have the right to be spared oppression and repeated intentional humiliation at school and at home. The problem is that even though almost everyone would agree with that statement, public policies and actions and privately held beliefs are likely to contain many contradictions of it. Many institutionalized forms of violence are used in the service of social control, including blacklisting, interrogation, torture, and corporal punishment (which is still legal in schools in 20 U.S. states [Kennedy 2010]).

Children develop through observational learning. If they have observed their parents using intimidation, ridicule, or aggressive behavior, they will tend to imitate this behavior. Inconsistent discipline is common in the family backgrounds of children who are aggressive toward their peers (Hodges and Perry 1996). According to teachers' reports, some parents admit to teaching their children to fight those who wrong them and are insulted when such lessons are questioned (Futrell 1996). Racism, homophobia, and other forms of prejudice can be inadvertently encouraged by legislative action. In 2001, a conservative Christian group in Washington State successfully stalled state legislation that would require schools to write policies against bullying and train employees and volunteers to stop harassment. The coalition argued that the proposed legislation would prevent students from exercising their constitutional right to condemn homosexuality and thus should be blocked (Bickler et al. 2001).

Simplistic interpretations of social Darwinism argue against protecting individuals with less-desirable qualities such as physical weakness, learning problems, or unattractiveness. Those who perform poorly in sports, business, education, and other highly competitive areas tend to be treated as outcasts, deserving pity but not protection. A significant number of individuals believe that teasing and bullying problems at school perform a useful function in mentally "toughening up" children and that such problems are simply a phase that children need to go through in order to be able to survive in a competitive world. A survey by Everett and Price (1995) found that the two main reasons adolescents reported carrying weapons to school were 1) to impress or gain acceptance from friends and 2) to feel important. Aggressive young people often hold the belief that victims have done something to cause their own troubles. By the time victims are thoroughly beaten down, they actually tend to believe that themselves (Kennedy 2010) and feel they deserve the punishment they get (Vernberg et al. 1999). These pathological beliefs are deeply ingrained in sick and violent societies and schools.

Wellness Centers in Schools

A number of larger high schools and wealthier schools do have mental health services for children available within the school. Sometimes crisis-related services are available, as in the New Trier school system in Chicago, Illinois. In that large high school, containing about 4,000 students on two campuses, 10 social workers are maintained full-time to provide crisis intervention. Dealing with illness and promoting wellness is, as we have shown, a complicated issue. Our view of wellness centers is that much more is needed than merely placing people in groups to promote healthy ideas. Such centers should also be available to help at-risk children manage some of their psychiatric problems, seamlessly molding them into effortlessly well citizens. Nancy Guerra's (2003) work is developmentally based; wellness suggestions are linked to developmental strategies, which we support as a critical focus for wellness centers, together with matching individual needs to the services. The various yardsticks Guerra uses to indicate healthy development (as opposed to compromised development in violent at-risk youth) are similar to ours. These capacities, while basic to all human relationships, develop at different rates from birth through adulthood, manifesting themselves in different ways at different points in development.

We would also add to this list classroom and school norms, which we feel are developed from children's interactions and interpersonal behavior. For example, bullying, community and gang violence, and the carrying of weapons are closely linked to the developmental strategies children practice to maintain an image of strength in their peer group and establish where they are and want to be in the dominance hierarchy—that is, the authority they have in their peer group. These risk factors (in addition to impulse control, empathy, and the development of positive peer relationships) can be modified by school-based programming. The DART (Linking Development and Risk Together) approach Guerra developed suggests a guide but not a method for service delivery with the goal of promoting a culture of wellness. The theory behind this, and it is an easily supported one, suggests that health and wellness become part of the regular dialogue between students, teachers, and parents. Wellness then becomes as important in many respects as intellectual skills, in turn fostering conflict-free learning and mastery (see Table 11–1).

Such centers could be shared by smaller schools or provided in the larger schools with 24-hour wellness hotlines and an interactive Web site, both of which could be set up at minimal cost. The activities of a center's staff need to be clearly defined, so that each staffperson can become a mentor, tutor, or counselor/surrogate parent to a child. The wellness center would be responsible for general health promotions at the schools, including management of the health education curriculum, which is now an established part of school curricula in

TABLE 11–1. Wellness initiatives at school

1. Involve all ages.
2. Promote positive attitudes, compassion, and tolerance.
3. Offer an alternative to unhealthy peer groups.
4. Strive to promote a positive school climate.
5. Offer a safe way for students to communicate a peer's psychological distress or threat to harm him- or herself or someone else.
6. Reward peer and adult activity that promotes wellness and reduces stress or coercion.
7. Encourage athletes and coaches to foster collaboration and winning peacefully, focusing subtly on helping socially awkward children.

many states. The center would also arrange and sponsor after-school activities and other programs that require cooperation from other community agencies, such as police athletic leagues. The wellness centers can further act as a more comprehensive health assessment center, working in conjunction with school nurses. Research has shown that school health nurses are a rich source of information about at-risk children (Vernberg et al. 2011).

The concept of effortless wellness—while on the surface a paradox—implies that a program of healthy behaviors can become as painless as any automatic practiced imitation behavior, such as brushing one's teeth or washing one's face. This requires help and modeling by parents and very early childhood practices that are influenced by preschool and early school and kindergarten interventions. The role of inspirational leadership—especially that of natural leaders—in processes like instilling good, healthy habits is also part of the equation and must be supported. Natural leaders (as defined in Chapter 5, "Bullying Is a Process, Not a Person") who can reach out to others and who feel that the outcome of the work they do is for the good of the community as a whole rather than for their own self-aggrandizement are vital parts of such wellness centers.

The unusual capacities of such natural leaders (whether children or adults) implies that they are *resilient* or hardy. Resiliency is an area of research that is growing in complexity and range. In those identified as possessing this trait, resilience can be seen as a form of invulnerability, in that despite having had difficult childhoods, these individuals go on to do well in their adult lives. Hauser et al. (2006) conducted long-term follow-up studies of resilient children, most of whom originated from very disturbed homes, and found that many were self-reflective and self-motivating, with persistent ambition, yet they tended to have fluctuating levels of self-esteem. The ideal type of resilient young adult—what Hauser and colleagues call a "consistent conformist"—is somebody who conforms to peer standards; everybody wants such a person on their team, because they simply click well with others. Such individuals have the highest resiliency and the lowest degree of hostility. They have few psychiatric symptoms, low rates of substance abuse and criminality, and high ego development, with many close friends and relationships and secure attachments, although their self-esteem is unstable. The research of Hauser et al. (2006) has shown that consistent conformist, high-resilience children are above the 50th percentile in positive development (good team player, hardworking) and below the 50th percentile in negative development (lazy, erratic, moody).

It would seem from these definitions that natural leaders fit this profile, and thus, while not necessarily needing a wellness center for their own development, could become excellent leaders in such centers if recruited and could work closely with any programs on the school campus. Such recruitment would give natural leaders a way of integrating the work they do with important group work that maintains a nonviolent school climate. The work of Maddi et al. (2002) on hardiness highlights a similar concept. *Hardiness* is defined as commitment, control, and challenge that facilitates the management of stress by turning stressful circumstances into growth-inducing opportunities rather than debilitating experiences. In the research of Maddi and colleagues, hardiness was correlated with vigorous mental health.

"Effortless" wellness centers have a number of very powerful advantages over traditional mental health clinics in schools. There is a natural prejudice against seeking help for psychological distress. Many children deeply resent the stigma of the "short bus" that is often used to transport special education students, since it marks them as different from the kids who ride the big bus. Inner-city students will shy away from anything that creates the possibility of being perceived as weak. Wellness programs can have a "hook," such as self-defense or forensics and debate, which can attract the students necessary to promote social wellness at school. Wellness programs in higher–socioeconomic status (SES) schools need to stress ways of helping others, such as teaming up with disadvantaged schools. These activities need to be made interesting and fun and then applied within the school itself. Such a focus on altruistic activities and making a positive contribution separate these centers from those that concentrate solely on "at risk" indicators.

In the Jamaica project we referenced earlier (see Chapter 5, "Bullying Is a Process, Not a Person"), the self-sustaining component included creation of a business to distribute the students' artwork online. The project is now ongoing and benefits the schools, taps into higher-SES students' sense of altruism, and is an online social forum that can be used in building school pride and spirit rather than predatory bullying. This is an example of wellness in action. Participation in this type of project could positively target the climate of the school, offering alternatives to simply preaching against and punishing the evils of bullying.

Offering teachers a chance to rest and relax in a wellness setting could energize them and reduce stress for everyone. Program activities could expand be-

TABLE 11–2. Characteristics of a peaceful school

1. Everyone feels safe.
2. Children cooperate.
3. Adults model positive behaviors/attitudes and school spirit.
4. Adults work together for children's benefit—parents and teachers, community and school.
5. Helpfulness, cooperation, and altruism are encouraged and rewarded
6. Competition is not exaggerated.

yond the school day (a program well suited for inclusion in grants), including offering a wide range of extracurricular activities during after-school hours.

Wellness centers are a way schools can show students and teachers that their health and well-being are valued. These oases from stress do not have to be heavily funded, but can be developed using existing time and resources. This creates a concrete way for the community to reach into schools with mentors, time, and money. Shared wellness with the community and schools enhances the quality of life for every citizen. Schools are often used in community activities such as voting, swimming, and open gym time for adults. Wellness would be, in a sense, the reverse process; a community enhances a school by reaching in and promoting wellness. The ideal goal for all of this work is summarized in Table 11–2. This is neither an enforced social conformism nor a pacifist's paradise, but rather a group of individuals with a high quality of life, able to compete without cutting each others' throats or ending up addicted to substances and drowning in work.

Conclusion

Time and time again, community and school buy-in is inspired by those with leadership and comprehensive, passionate common sense. An example would be the vitality project in Albert Lea, a small town in Minnesota (Buettner 2010). The project was successful because several thousand residents participated and improved their overall health and life expectancies significantly by working with each other on well-designed, enjoyable exercise routines that were the focus of friendly competition. The mental health professional can have a similar leadership role in wellness centers in schools. People generally see mental health professionals as concerned primarily with mental illness. This new role will change that. A new challenge for the mental health professional, while not mandatory, in the school setting would be a vital activity such a professional needs in order to play an important role in stopping school violence.

William Menninger, co-founder of the Menninger Foundation, has summarized the "symptoms" of emotional wellness; these are listed in Table 11–3.

TABLE 11–3. William Menninger's criteria for emotional maturity

1. The ability to deal constructively with reality
2. The capacity to adjust to change
3. A relative freedom from symptoms produced by tensions and anxieties
4. The capacity to find more satisfaction in giving than receiving
5. The capacity to relate to other people in a consistent manner with mutual satisfaction and helpfulness
6. The capacity to sublimate, to direct one's instinctive hostile energy into creative and constructive outlets
7. The capacity to love

Source. Menninger WC: Criteria of Emotional Maturity. Copyright 1966, The Menninger Clinic.

KEY CLINICAL CONCEPTS

- Wellness is the state of optimal well-being balancing all aspects of the whole person.

- Violence is the opposite of wellness.

- The unconscious plays a major role in wellness.

- Wellness should be natural and effortless, not a rigid regimen.

- Wellness needs to be modeled by adults and offer open spaces to exercise and balance stress.

- Wellness involves healthy mental attitudes as well as physical health and fitness.

- Wellness involves habits learned during childhood when imitating parents.

- Communities need to overcome resistance to change and barriers to creating peaceful schools and promoting wellness.

- Wellness centers at school offer a positive alternative to the disease model with a clinic focus.

- Natural leaders promote wellness.

- Mental health professionals can assist schools from the outside in creating wellness.

References

American Holistic Health Association: Wellness from within: the first step. 2003. Available at: http://ahha.org/ahhastep.htm. Accessed December 8, 2010.

Bickler R, Jenkins S, Lea B: Editorial—Anti-bullying bill is aimed at saving young lives, not promoting homosexuality. Yakima Herald-Republic, May 7, 2001. Available at: http://www.highbeam.com/doc/1P2-18441733.html. Accessed June 20, 2011.

Brown R, Edelson D: The Maharishi Effect: Creating Coherence in World Consciousness. Fairfield, IA, Maharishi International Universities Press, 1990

Buettner D: The Minnesota Miracle (the extraordinary story of how folks in this small town got motivated, got moving, made new friends, and added years to their lives). AARP Magazine, January/February, 2010, pp 32–36. Available at: http://www.aarp.org/health/longevity/info-01-2010/minnesota_miracle.html. Accessed February 2011.

Carroll RT: Transcendental meditation. The Skeptic's Dictionary, November 21, 2010. Available at: http://www.skepdic.com/tm.html. Accessed December 8, 2010.

Chao GT, Gardner PD: Young Adults at Work: What They Want, What They Get, and How to Keep Them. White paper prepared by Collegiate Employment Research Institute for the Study of Student Transitions for MonsterTRAK, 2008. Available at: http://ceri.msu.edu/publications/pdf/yadultswk3-26-09.pdf. Accessed December 8, 2010.

Erikson E: Childhood and Society. New York, WW Norton, 1963

Everett S, Price J: Students' perceptions of violence in public schools: the MetLife survey. J Adolesc Health 17:345–352, 1995

Futrell N: Violence in the classroom: a teacher's perspective, in Schools, Violence, and Society. Edited by Hoffman AM. Westport, CT, Praeger, 1996, pp 3–20

Guerra N: Preventing school violence by promoting wellness. Journal of Applied Psychoanalytic Studies 5:139–154, 2003

Hauser ST, Allen JP, Golden E: Out of the Woods: Tales of Resilient Teens. Cambridge, MA, Harvard University Press, 2006

Heath C, Heath D: Switch: How to Change Things When Change Is Hard. New York, Crown Business Publishing, 2010

Hodges E, Perry D: Victims of peer abuse: an overview. Reclaiming children and youth. Journal of Emotional and Behavioral Problems 5:23–28, 1996

Kelly EW, Greyson B, Kelly EF: Unusual experiences: near death and related phenomena, in Irreducible Mind: Toward a Psychology for the 21st Century. Edited by Kelly EF, Kelly EW, Crabtree A, et al. Lanham, MD, Rowman & Littlefield, 2007, pp 367–421

Kennedy R: 2 reasons for banning corporal punishment: an inappropriate disciplinary measure. About.com. 2010. Available at: http://privateschool.about.com/cs/forteachers/a/beating.htm. Accessed December 8, 2010.

Lasch C: The Culture of Narcissism: American Life in an Age of Diminishing Expectations. New York, WW Norton, 1978

Maddi SR, Khoshaba DM, Persico M, et al: The personality construct of hardiness. J Res Pers 36:72–85, 2002

Marans S: Listening to Fear: Helping Kids Cope, From Nightmares to the Nightly News. New York, Henry Holt, 2005

Menninger K: Man Against Himself. New York, Harcourt Brace, 1938

Olweus D: Bullying at School: What We Know and What We Can Do. Oxford, UK, Blackwell, 1993

Roland E, Bru E, Midthassel UV, et al: The Zero programme against bullying: effects of the programme in the context of the Norwegian manifesto against bullying. Social Psychology of Education: An International Journal 13:41–55, 2010

Safer M: The "Millennials" Are Coming: Morley Safer on The New Generation of American Workers. CBS News, May 23, 2008. Available at: http://www.cbsnews.com/stories/2007/11/08/60minutes/main3475200.shtml?tag=mncol;lst;2. Accessed December 8, 2010.

Sue DW, Sue D: Counseling the Culturally Different: Theory and Practice. New York, Wiley, 1999

Twemlow SW, Gabbard GO, Jones FC: Out-of-body experience: a phenomenological typology based on questionnaire responses. Am J Psychiatry 139:450–455, 1982

Vaillant GE: Adaptation to Life (1977; reprinted with new Preface). Cambridge, MA, Harvard University Press, 1995

Vernberg E, Gamm B: Resistance to violence interventions in schools: barriers and solutions. Journal of Applied Psychoanalytic Studies 5:125–138, 2003

Vernberg EM, Jacobs AK, Hershberger SL: Peer victimization and attitudes about violence in early adolescence. J Clin Child Psychol 28:386–395, 1999

Vernberg EM, Nelson TD, Fonagy P, et al: Victimization, aggression, and visits to the school nurse for somatic complaints, illnesses, and physical injuries. Pediatrics 127:842–848, 2011

Wilson EO: Biophilia. Cambridge, MA, Harvard University Press, 1984

World Health Organization: Preamble to the Constitution of the World Health Organization as adopted by the International Health Conference, New York, 19–22 June, 1946; signed on 22 July 1946 by the representatives of 61 States (Official Records of the World Health Organization, no. 2, p. 100) and entered into force on 7 April 1948

Index

*Page numbers printed in **boldface** type refer to tables or figures.*